Atlas of URETHROPLASTY

System requirement:

- Operating System—Windows XP or above.
- Web Browser—Internet Explorer 8 or above, Google Chrome, Mozilla Firefox.
- Essentia plugins—Java and Flash player.
  - Facing problems in viewing content—it may be your system does not have Java enabled.
  - If videos do not show up—it may be the system requires Flash player or need to manage Flash setting. To learn more about flash setting click on the link in the help section.
  - You can test Java and Flash by using the links from the help section of the CD/DVD.

Accompanying DVD-ROM is playable only in Computer and not in DVD player.

CD/DVD has autorun function—it may take few seconds to load on your computer. If it does not work for you, then follow the steps below to access the contents manually:

- Click on my computer.
- Select the CD/DVD drive and click open/explore—this will show list of files in the CD/DVD.
- Find and double click file—"launch.html".

For more information about troubleshoot of autorun click on:
http://support.microsoft.com/kb/330135

DVD Contents

S No	Video Name	Author Name
1	Anastomotic Urethroplasty	SB Kulkarni
1a	Inferior Pubectomy	SB Kulkarni
2	BMG Urethroplasty DOG and VOG by Muscle and Nerve Sparing Bulbar Technique	Guido Barbagli
3	Penile Fascio cutaneous Flap	Mc Aninch
4	Kulkarni Technique for Pan-urethral Structure	SB Kulkarni
5	Double BMG—Dorsal, Ventral	Enzo Palminteri
6	Perineal Urethrostomy	Guido Barbagli
7	Asopa's Urethroplasty	Guido Barbagli
8	Ist Stage Urethroplasty—BMG Graft	Jeremy Meyers
9	2nd Stage Urethroplasty	Guido Barbagli
10	Female Urethroplasty	Anne Cameron

Atlas of URETHROPLASTY

Editor

Rajesh Gulia

MBBS MS DNB (Urology-NBC) MNAMS (Genitourinary Surgery)
Senior Specialist
Chief (Urology) and Head
Reconstructive Urology, Unit II

Director
Kidney Center, Sector 34A
Chandigarh, India

Co-Editor

Richard Santucci MD FACS
Clinical Professor
Michigan State University College of Osteopathic Medicine

Specialist-in-Chief
Department of Urology
The Detroit Medical Center

Director, The Center for Urologic Reconstruction™

Detroit, MI, USA

Foreword

Sanjay B Kulkarni

JAYPEE BROTHERS MEDICAL PUBLISHERS (P) LTD

New Delhi • London • Philadelphia • Panama

Jaypee Brothers Medical Publishers (P) Ltd.

Headquarters
Jaypee Brothers Medical Publishers (P) Ltd.
4838/24, Ansari Road, Daryaganj
New Delhi 110 002, India
Phone: +91-11-43574357
Fax: +91-11-43574314
Email: jaypee@jaypeebrothers.com

Overseas Offices

J.P. Medical Ltd.
83, Victoria Street, London
SW1H 0HW (UK)
Phone: +44-2031708910
Fax: +02-03-0086180
Email: info@jpmedpub.com

Jaypee-Highlights Medical Publishers Inc.
City of Knowledge, Bld. 237, Clayton
Panama City, Panama
Phone: +1 507-301-0496
Fax: +1 507-301-0499
Email: cservice@jphmedical.com

Jaypee Medical Inc.
The Bourse
111, South Independence Mall East
Suite 835, Philadelphia, PA 19106, USA
Phone: +1 267-519-9789
Email: jpmed.us@gmail.com

Jaypee Brothers Medical Publishers (P) Ltd.
17/1-B, Babar Road, Block-B, Shaymali
Mohammadpur, Dhaka-1207
Bangladesh
Mobile: +08801912003485
Email: jaypeedhaka@gmail.com

Jaypee Brothers Medical Publishers (P) Ltd.
Bhotahity, Kathmandu, Nepal
Phone: +977-9741283608
Email: kathmandu@jaypeebrothers.com

Website: www.jaypeebrothers.com

Website: www.jaypeedigital.com

Inquiries for bulk sales may be solicited at: jaypee@jaypeebrothers.com

Atlas of Urethroplasty

First Edition: **2014**

ISBN: 978-93-5090-651-4

Printed at: Ajanta Offset & Packagings Ltd., New Delhi

Dedicated to

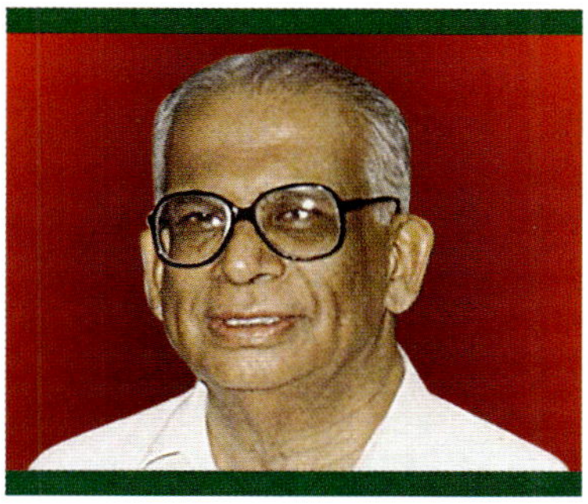

In the memory of

Professor Hattangadi Shashidhar Bhat

January 21st 1921–November 19th 2010

The one person who has shaped me into what I am today. He is none other than my "Guru"—Professor HS Bhat. It is from him, I learnt how to respect the human urethra. Apart from the many golden one liners, I would like to mention one. Regarding female urethra, he used to say "it is an outlet for many a problems in the ladies, so ensure that it is patent, lest you face the fallbacks of a blocked drain".

About urethral stricture, he would often say "traumatic strictures are curable but inflammatory strictures can only be palliated". On his response to the results of various urethroplasties, he would say "you can say a urethral stricture is cured only if it has a dilatation-free life of at least 10 years". In tune with his humane touch and the importance of SPC, he would say "after the age of 75 years, a patient of stricture urethra has no business to pass urine per urethra, he will be a burden on his family. Let him live happily on an SPC". He would always say place yourself in the patient's shoes and you can never go wrong!

Rajesh Gulia

Contributors

AL Vyas MS FRCS (England) FRCS (Glasgow)
Professor and Senior Consultant
Asopa Hospital and Research Center
Agra, Uttar Pradesh, India

Allen F Morey MD
Professor
Department of Urology
University of Texas Southwestern Medical Center
Dallas, Texas, USA

Allen McNeil Haraway MD
Fellow
University of Michigan
Ann Arbor, MI, USA

Anne Pelletier-Cameron MD
Assistant Professor
University of Michigan
Ann Arbor, MI, USA

Anthony Atala MD
WH Boyce Professor and Chair
Department of Urology
Director, Wake Forest Institute for Regenerative Medicine
Wake Forest University
Winston-Salem, NC, USA

BA Erickson MD
Assistant Professor
Department of Urology
University of Iowa Hospitals and Clinics
Iowa City, IA, USA

Chris M Gonzalez MD MBA
Professor
Department of Urology
Director, Genitourinary Reconstruction
Northwestern University
Chicago, IL, USA

Daniel D Dugi III MD
Assistant Professor
Department of Urology
Oregon Health and Science University
Portland, Oregon, USA

Geoffrey R Nuss MD
Fellow
Reconstructive Urology
Northwestern University
Chicago, IL, USA

Gerald H Jordan MD FACS FAAP (Hon) FRCS (Hon)
Professor
Department of Urology
Eastern Virginia Medical School (EVMS)
Genitourinary Reconstructive Surgery
Norfolk, Virginia, USA

GG Singhal MS FICS FAIS
Professor and Senior Consultant
Asopa Hospital and Research Center
Agra, Uttar Pradesh, India

Giuseppe Romano MD
Fellow Division of Urology Surgery
University of Vita-Salute San Raffaele
The Center for Reconstructive Urethral Surgery
Arezzo, Italy

Guido Barbagli MD
Professor, Division of Urology Surgery
University of Vita-Salute San Raffaele
Head, Center for Reconstructive Urethral Surgery
Arezzo, Italy

HS Asopa MS FRCS FRCS (Ed) FACS FICS (Hon) FAMS FNASc (India) DSc(Hc)
Professor
Department of Urology
Director and Chief Surgeon
Asopa Hospital and Research Center
Agra, Uttar Pradesh, India

Jeremy B Myers MD
Assistant Professor
The Center for Reconstructive Urology and Men's Health
The University of Utah
Department of Surgery
Salt Lake City, Utah, USA

JW McAninch MD FACS FRCS
Professor
Department of Urology
University of California, San Francisco
Chief
Department of Urology
San Francisco General Hospital
San Francisco
California, USA

Lucas R Wiegand MD
Fellow, Reconstructive Urology
Division of Urology Surgery
Washington University
School of Medicine
St. Louis, MO, USA

Mang L Chen MD
Assistant Professor
Reconstructive Urology
University of Pittsburgh Medical Center
Pittsburgh, PA, USA

Massimo Lazzeri MD PhD
Fellow, Division of Urology Surgery
Department of Urology
San Raffaele Hospital
Milan, Italy

Pankaj M Joshi MS DNB (Urology)
Consultant
Reconstructive Urology
Center for Urethral Reconstruction and Indian School of Urethral Surgery
Pune, Maharashtra, India

Rajesh Gulia MBBS MS DNB (Urology-NBC) MNAMS (Genitourinary Surgery)
Senior Specialist
Chief (Urology) and Head
Reconstructive Urology, Unit II
Director, Kidney Center, Sector 34A
Chandigarh, India

Ramón Virasoro MD
Urology Instructor
Eastern Virginia Medical School (EVMS)
Norfolk, Virginia, USA

Richard Santucci MD FACS
Clinical Professor
Michigan State College of Osteopathic Medicine
Specialist-in-Chief
Department of Urology
The Detroit Medical Center
Director, The Center for Urologic Reconstruction™
Detroit, MI, USA

Rodrigo A Campos MD
Research Fellow
University of Minnesota School of Medicine
Minneapolis, MN, USA

Ryan P Terlecki MD
Assistant Professor
Department of Urology
Wake Forest University
Winston-Salem, NC, USA

Salvatore Sansalone MD
Fellow, Division of Urology Surgery
University of Vita-Salute San Raffaele
The Center for Reconstructive Urethral Surgery
Arezzo, Italy

Sanjay B Kulkarni MS FRCS (Glasgow) Dip Urology (London)
Professor and Chief
Department of Urology
Center for Urethral Reconstruction and Indian School of Urethral Surgery
Pune, Maharashtra, India

Sean P Elliott MD MS
Associate Professor
Department of Urology
Director, Urologic Reconstruction
University of Minnesota School of Medicine
Minneapolis, MN, USA

Steven B Brandes MD FACS
Professor
Department of Urologic Surgery
Division of Urology Surgery
Washington University, School of Medicine
St. Louis, MO, USA

William O Brant MD
Assistant Professor
The Center for Reconstructive Urology and Men's Health
The University of Utah
Department of Surgery
Salt Lake City, Utah, USA

Foreword

I wish to congratulate my friends Dr Rajesh Gulia and Dr Richard Santucci for introducing *Atlas of Urethroplasty*.

Urethral stricture disease is known to mankind for more than 5000 years. In the past, patients were treated by dilation. The initial enthusiasm of direct visual internal urethrotomy (DVIU) slowly waned over a period of time. As the long-term success rates were not favorable. Now urethral stricture is considered an open surgical disease.

The book has been a hard work and contribution from renowned reconstructive urologists around the globe. The book has 15 chapters starting from the basics of anatomy to the complex procedures and tissue engineering. Each chapter is crafted by experts in their field. It narrates the detailed description of steps for performing a successful surgery. The book also provides a DVD on surgical techniques.

Urethral stricture disease is a challenging issue. Urethra is a nonforgiving organ and delicate care needs to be taken while performing urethroplasty. Failure of urethral surgery directly affects the quality of life of patient and family.

More urologists are diverting their attention to reconstructive urology.

Posterior urethroplasty after pelvic fracture urethral injury needs expert management. I suggest that all urologists should have adequate knowledge of standard steps of anastomotic urethroplasty in posterior urethra. I have detailed the steps in my chapter for reference. However, failures of surgery in pelvic fracture urethral distraction defect (PFUDD) are complex and hence it is advisable for urologists to personally train under experts for management of PFUDD surgery.

I believe that when there exists two options/surgeries for one problem, it means there is scope of improvement. It means no procedure is perfect. Today in reconstructive urology, we are moving towards standardization. For example, buccal grafts are widely recommended. Flaps are used rarely when there is problem of ischemia. Ventral onlay is performed for proximal bulbar strictures. Dorsal onlay buccal graft urethroplasty is widely practiced for bulbar strictures. Anastomotic urethroplasty is preferred mainly in traumatic strictures. Penile strictures can be approached by circumcision or by minimally invasive cosmetic perineal approach with invagination. One stage procedures are more successful than 2 or 3 stage procedures.

These clear concepts will assist urologists to perform majority of urethroplasty.

The basis of the book is to provide simple solution for complex urethral stricture disease. I am sure that it will help all urologists to have clear understanding of commonly performed urethroplasties.

Sanjay B Kulkarni
MS FRCS (Glasgow) Dip Urology (London)
Professor and Chief
Department of Urology
Center for Urethral Reconstruction and
Indian School of Urethral Surgery
Pune, Maharashtra, India

Preface

Need for Such a Book

Actually, there was no need of a separate book on stricture urethra. Not until then! When approached for writing a book in urology, I could not think of anything more close to my heart than urethroplasty; and while on this project, I realized–Not until now! Times have changed.

The level of specialization now talks of anterior urethral, bulbar urethral and posterior urethral surgeons. Can we be left behind? We have got to know more and more of less and less. We cannot restore the factory settings of any machine (human body being the most complex one manufactured by God) but we, can become the 2nd factory itself where such machines come for repair. Having been to one of the automobile factories, one wonders at the level of standardization. No wonder they are able to roll out such mean machines of perfection to the likes of Lamborghinis' and the Audis'. Our aim as urethral engineer is to standardize each procedure down to the finest detail much akin to the assembly line system. This will enable to significantly cut down the operating time and unnecessary tissue handling. All this translates into better results. In the beginning of my endeavor towards perfection, on seeing recordings of my own surgeries, I was surprised at the number of unnecessary steps and movements. Now, I have been able to engineer my own assembly line with reasonable time precision. And, in this small journey of mine, I must thank Professor Kulkarni, who never fails in stimulating your gray cells. Our aim should be to work at least at a 6 sigma level.

We must also realize that there are "n" number of procedures for treating "n" types of strictures and each has good results in the hand of their proponents. Our aim is not to confuse the young budding urethral engineer into the maze of the number of procedures available, but to present before him 10% of the procedures which if mastered can cure more than 90% of the strictures. The other 10% can be taken care of by the other 90% procedures available. Urethral stricture disease does not involve any hi-tech technology or implants. Hence, the absence of any company driven bias/ sponsorship. A urethral surgeon is a "poor" surgeon; the only satisfaction is the smile on the face of a patient when he keeps on voiding without any assistance—day after day, month after month, year after year. This puts a greater burden of moral responsibility on our shoulders in presenting this complex problem with utmost simplicity and clarity.

We must always constantly challenge our gray cells. I strongly believe that the best way to grow is to separately keep an hour or so daily when you can do the thinking cap. Read about your area of interest, see your own procedures, etc. We do come out with certain concepts, ideas which have proved to be logical and useful in certain cases (not necessary for it to have been subjected to the concept of evidence-based medicine). Some ideas may sound funny/bizarre/awkward at the moment, but could be the triggering point of another blast waiting to happen in some destined neurons.

The most exciting phrase to hear in science, the one that heralds new discoveries, is not "Eureka!" but "That's funny..."

— I Asimov

A word of advice for the young urethral surgeons–Press on. Nothing in the world can take the place of persistence. Talent will not; nothing is more common than unsuccessful men with talent. Genius will not; unrewarded genius is almost a proverb. Education alone will not; the world is full of educated derelicts. Persistence and determination alone are omnipotent—(C. Coolidge).

Rajesh Gulia

Acknowledgments

On a personal level, I would like to offer my sincere thanks to the support given to me by my colleague urologists—Dr Manoj Sharma and Dr Virendra Dhankhar. Had it not been for them, this project would not have seen the light of the day. My Co-editor Professor Richard Santucci has been the guiding force. His promptness in dealing with any deadline is remarkable. Dr Santucci would like to thank his family—Christine, Lauren, and Alison for their perseverance and support. "We all know it could not be done without you."

All the contributors were very helpful and prompt in their respective contributions, I have my greatest regards for them.

With love to Pinki, Kabir and Monchu, who always pushed me hard and gave me constant encouragement to excel. Not to speak of the family time lost which they sacrificed for the sake of this book.

Last but not least, I have no words for my publisher M/s Jaypee Brothers Medical Publishers (P) Ltd, New Delhi, India, who very patiently waited for the project to finish.

Rajesh Gulia

Contents

List of Abbreviations

ACSM	Acellular Corpus Spongiosum Matrix
BMG	Buccal Mucosal Graft
BXO	Balanitis Xerotica Obliterans
CIC	Clean Intermittent Catheterization
DED	De-epidermized Dermis
DVIU	Direct Vision Internal Urethrotomy
ECM	Extracellular Matrix
ED	Erectile Dysfunction
FDA	Food and Drug Authority
Fr	French
GAGs	Glycosaminoglycans
KUB	Kidney Ureter Bladder
LS	Lichen Sclerosis
LSA	Lichen Sclerosus et Atrophicus
LUTS	Lower Urinary Tract Symptoms
MCU	Micturating Cystourethrogram
MHz	Mega Hertz
MRI	Magnetic Resonance Imaging
OIU	Optical Internal Urethrotomy
OR	Operating Room
PAPA	Progressive Perineoabdominal Approach
PDS II	Polydioxanone
PFUDD	Pelvic Fracture Urethral Disruption Defect
PGA	Polyglycolic Acid
PHB	Polyhydroxybutyric Acid
PLA	Polylactic Acid
PLGA	Poly (lactic-co-glycolic acid)
RGU	Retrograde Urethrogram
RRP	Radical Retropubic Prostatectomy
SCC	Squamous Cell Carcinoma
SIS	Small Intestine Submucosa
STSG	Split Thickness Skin Graft
TURP	Transurethral Resection of the Prostate
USCs	Urine-derived Stem Cells
VCUG	Voiding Cystourethrography
XRT	External Radiation Therapy

Introduction

Urethroplasty is more art than science. Even in this modern day of molecular biology, routine space travel and ubiquitous computing, the field of urethroplasty is still a craft. It is performed full-time by a surprisingly small group of surgeons, perhaps 40(?), worldwide. However, we have calculated that at least in the United States, less than 2% of the urethroplasties that should be done are actually done. Most patients are treated with proven ineffective treatments: endlessly repeated courses of urethral dilation and urethrotomy. In the rest of the world, the number of urethroplasties performed is probably even lower. I need to upgrade the treatment of urethral stricture from "craft" to "science".

I have created the "Atlas of Urethroplasty" for just this reason. I desire to communicate the tools of urethroplasty to a wide audience, with the idea of revealing the secrets of expert craftspeople. I have chosen a world-class panel of authors to achieve this result. In this text you will learn the basic techniques (graft onlay, anastomotic, fasciocutaneous and Johanson urethroplasties) and how to apply them. Also, I have included intraoperative videos (more still are available on iclinics.org) and have strived to provide the tools that expert and novice surgeons alike can use to advance the field, and improve life for their patients.

Richard Santucci

CHAPTER 1

Back to the Basics: Penoscrotal Anatomy

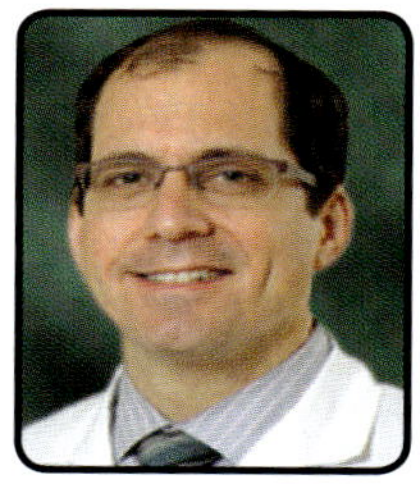

Steven B Brandes

Steven B Brandes, Lucas R Wiegand

Chapter Outline

- Genital Flap Selection
- Penoscrotal Fascial Anatomy
- Penile Vascular Anatomy
  - Arterial
  - Venous
- Scrotal Vascular Anatomy
  - Arterial
  - Venous
- Surgical Pearls
  - Arterial Anatomy and Implications for Urethral Stricture Repair
  - Venous Anatomy
  - Urethral Elasticity
  - Urethral Location within Corpus Spongiosum

Abstract

This basic anatomy knowledge and in-depth understanding is a must for anyone undertaking urethral reconstruction. This chapter helps one to master the concepts of the blood supply that allows flap to survive, grafts to take and the urethra to heal. As outlined in this chapter, the vascular anatomy is predictable and can be utilized to ensure a well-vascularized urethral repair. Also the author helps us to understand the clinical utility of these tissue planes which is evident when developing fasciocutaneous penile skin island flaps, as in an Orandi (vertical) or McAninch/Quartey (circular transverse) flap. Dissection in the correct plane will ensure well-vascularized flaps. It is debated which label is given to these correct planes (i.e. whether the anterior lamella of Buck's fascia or the tunica Dartos). Regardless, a plane can be developed between the skin and the Dartos-related fascial vascular structures and another can be developed between these and the deep penile structures which allows for creation of a well-vascularized penile skin flap. Of special importance is the subsection— "Surgical Pearls," in which the authors have diagrammatically highlighted the surgical applied anatomy in relation to various types of urethroplasties and their outcome.

Keywords

Dartos fascia, Buck's fascia, Tunica albuginea, Penile artery, Bulbar artery, Circumflex arteries, Dorsal median vein, Retrobalanic venous plexus, Posterior scrotal artery, Dual blood supply, Urethral elasticity.

INTRODUCTION

It is vital that anyone undertaking urethral reconstruction should have a thorough understanding of the blood supply that allows flap to survive, grafts to take and the urethra to heal. The male genitalia are well-vascularized with a redundant blood supply that has implications for reconstructive procedures, as detailed below.

GENITAL FLAP SELECTION

Genital skin and subcutaneous tissues are crucial for successful urethral reconstruction. A detailed understanding of the vascular supply can help to ensure long-term success of the repaired urethra. The ideal flap will have a vascular pedicle that is reliable and robust. As outlined below, the vascular anatomy is predictable and can be utilized to ensure a well-vascularized urethral repair.

PENOSCROTAL FASCIAL ANATOMY

The penile skin is elastic and has no adipose layer. Deep to the skin is the Dartos fascia, a loose areolar layer. The Dartos is also free of adipose tissue and freely moves over the underlying Buck's fascia or fascia penis. The

Dartos layer is continuous with the Scarpa's fascial layer of abdominal wall and continues into scrotum. In the perineum, it continues as Colles' fascia. Within this layer runs the superficial nerves and lymphovascular system. Buck's fascia covers the tunica albuginea of both corpora cavernosa as well as the corpus spongiosum. Buck's fascia is continuous with the external spermatic fascia in the scrotum **(Fig. 1.1)**.

The clinical utility of these tissue planes is evident when developing fasciocutaneous penile skin island flaps, as in an Orandi (vertical) or McAninch[1]/Quartey[2] (circular transverse) flap. Dissection in the correct plane will ensure well-vascularized flaps. It is debated which label is given to these correct planes (i.e. whether the anterior lamella of Buck's fascia or the tunica Dartos). Regardless, a plane can be developed between the skin and the Dartos-related fascial vascular structures, and another plane can be developed between these and the deep penile structures which allows for creation of a well-vascularized penile skin flap.

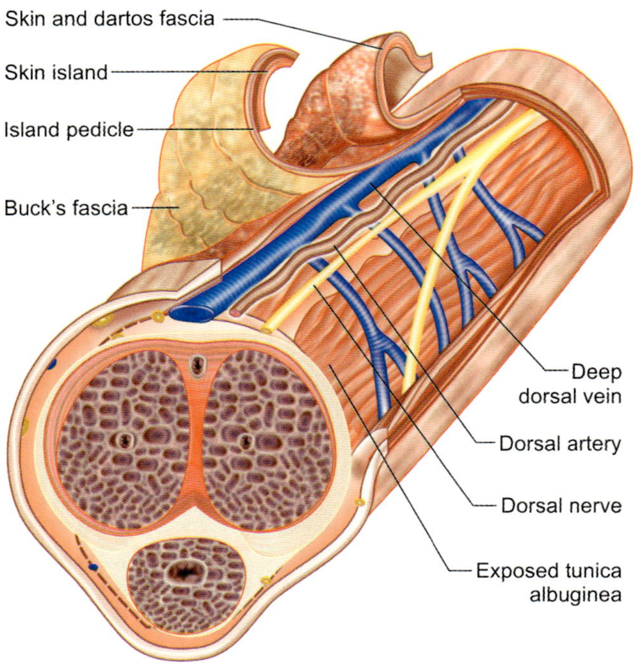

Fig. 1.1: Penoscrotal fascial anatomy
Source: McAninch JW, Morey AF. Penile circular fasciocutaneous skin flap in 1-stage reconstruction of complex anterior urethral strictures. J Urol. 1998;159(4):1209-13.

PENILE VASCULAR ANATOMY

Arterial

The blood supply to the penile skin derives from femoral arteries. There are two main blood supplies, the superficial and deep external pudendal arteries. Superficial to Scarpa's fascia, these arteries run from lateral to medial, and enter base of the penis. There, they give off scrotal branches and then divide into dorsolateral and ventrolateral axial penile arteries that run superficial to the anterior lamella of Buck's fascia and within the tunica Dartos fascia **(Fig. 1.2)**.[3] These axial penile arteries then give off superficial branches to form the subdermal plexus, which supplies the penile skin **(Figs 1.3A and B)**. The perforators that connect the subcutaneous and subdermal arterial plexuses are so small that an avascular plane can be developed between the skin and Dartos. The axial penile arteries continue to the foreskin as preputial arteries and also send perforating branches through Buck's fascia to provide collateral circulation with the dorsal arteries **(Fig. 1.4)**. It is important to keep in mind that the circulation comes from lateral part and base of the penis when developing axial penile skin flaps so that they can be mobilized and transposed appropriately.

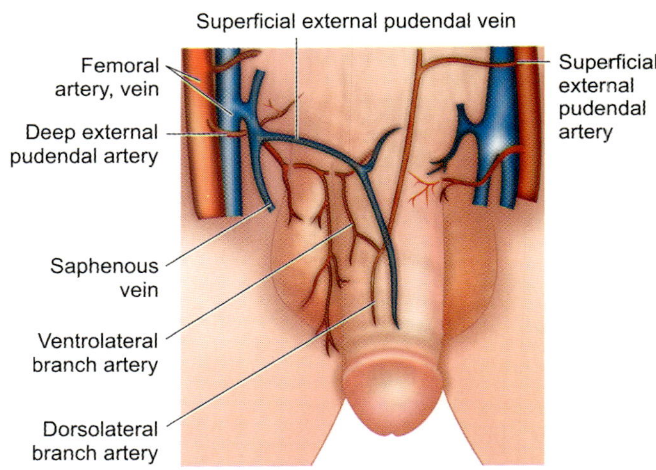

Fig. 1.2: Penile vascular anatomy
Source: Jordan GH, Stack RS. General concepts concerning the use of genital skin islands for anterior urethral reconstruction. Atlas Urol Clin North Am. 1997;5:23-44.

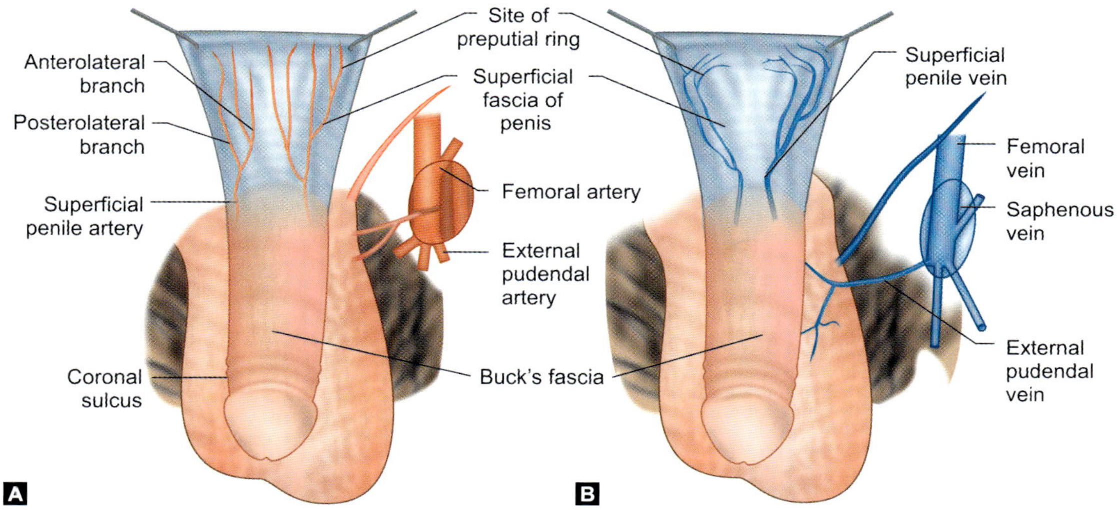

Figs 1.3A and B: Dartos vascular anatomy. (A) Arterial; (B) Venous
Source: Quartey JK. Microcirculation of the penile and scrotal skin. Atlas Urol Clin North Am. 1997;5:23.

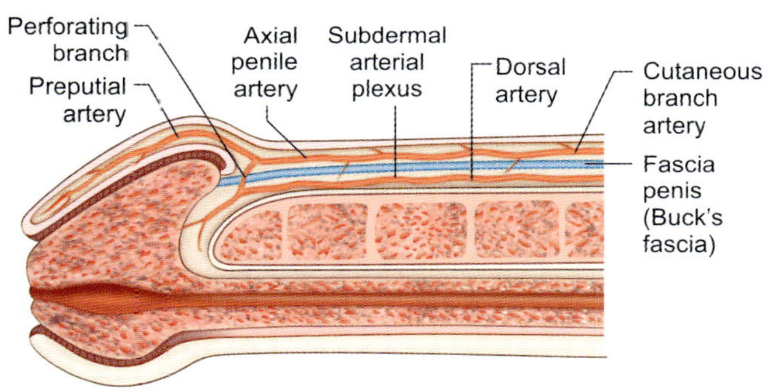

Fig. 1.4: Penile arterial microcirculation
Source: Quartey JK. Microcirculation of the penile and scrotal skin. Atlas Urol Clin North Am. 1997;5:23.

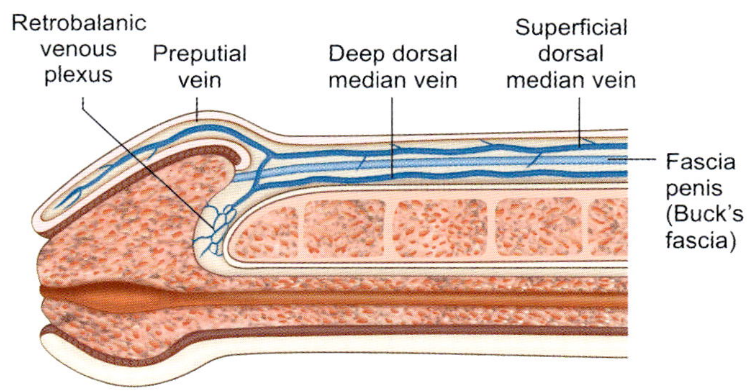

Fig. 1.5: Penile venous microcirculation
Source: Quartey JK. Microcirculation of the penile and scrotal skin. Atlas Urol Clin North Am. 1997;5:23.

Venous

The glans and corpus spongiosum drain into the retrobalanic venous plexus, which lies in the space between proximal part of the glans and the distal corpora cavernosa. From there it divides into the superficial and deep dorsal median veins. The deep dorsal median vein runs proximally down the penis deep to the anterior lamella of Buck's fascia, eventually travels through the suspensory ligament of the penis and finally empties into dorsal vein complex plexus beneath the pubic symphysis **(Figs 1.5 and 1.6)**.

The superficial dorsal median vein receives blood from the retrobalanic plexus or can take off directly from the deep dorsal median vein. Regardless, it pierces Buck's fascia to travel superficially within the tunica Dartos to base of the penis. There may be multiple superficial veins in a variable pattern that drain ultimately through base of the penis and into the external pudendal veins. The preputial veins may drain directly through base of the penis or may combine with the other superficial veins **(Figs 1.2 and 1.3)**.

Other venous drainage includes the subdermal venous plexus which drains through many large veins at base of the penis and venae comitantes which run with the axial penile arteries **(Fig. 1.7)**. There are not generally connections between the subdermal plexus and the Dartos-based venous drainage, although there is an occasional large communication.

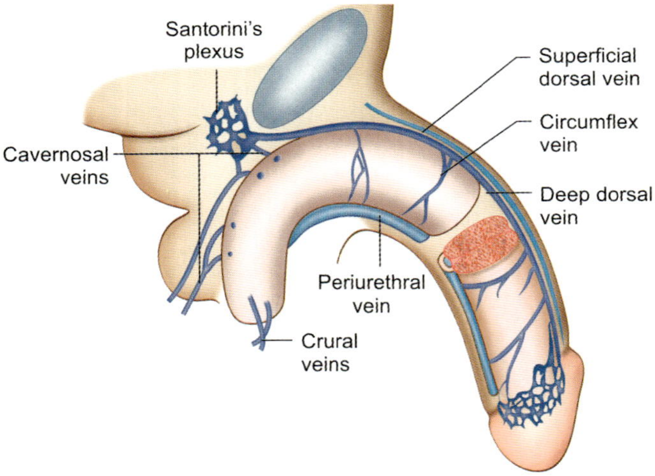

Fig. 1.6: Penile venous anatomy
Source: Quartey JK. Microcirculation of the penile and scrotal skin. Atlas Urol Clin North Am. 1997;5:23.

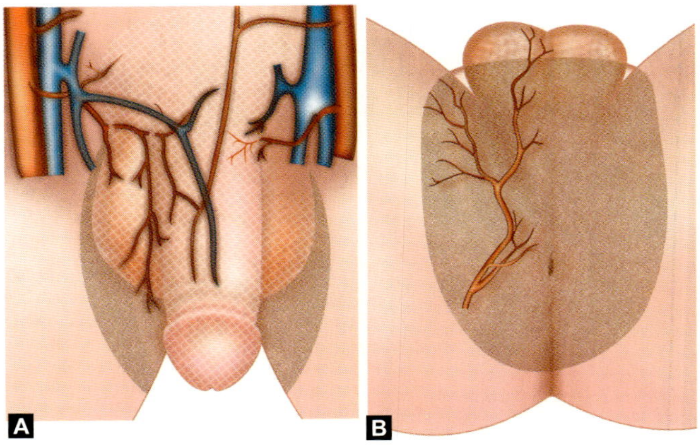

Figs 1.8A and B: (A) Anterior; (B) Posterior scrotal circulation—crosshatched area is anterior and dotted area is posterior circulation
Source: Jordan GH, Stack RS. General concepts concerning the use of genital skin islands for anterior urethral reconstruction. Atlas Urol Clin North Am. 1997;5:23-44.

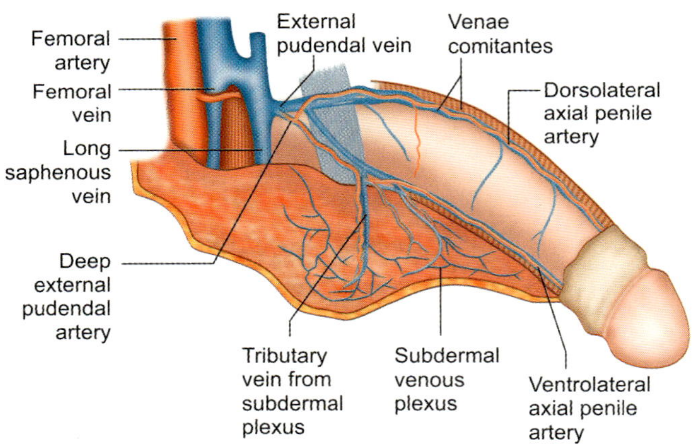

Fig. 1.7: Superficial venous penile drainage
Source: Quartey JK. Microcirculation of the penile and scrotal skin. Atlas Urol Clin North Am. 1997;5:23.

SCROTAL VASCULAR ANATOMY

Arterial

The scrotum's arterial blood supply is from two main sources, the femoral artery via the external pudendal arteries and the internal iliac artery via the internal pudendal artery.

The anterior scrotum is nourished by the anterior scrotal arteries, branches of the superficial and deep external pudendal arteries. These arteries are variable in course. Within the scrotum, near the penoscrotal junction, superficial branches supply a subdermal plexus that travel toward apex of the scrotum to anastomose with the posterior circulation **(Fig. 1.8A)**.[4]

In the perineum, the internal iliac artery continues as the internal pudendal artery. After emerging from Alcock's canal, it travels through the perineal membrane to continue as the perineal artery **(Fig. 1.8B)**. The course of this artery is between ischiocavernosus and bulbospongiosus muscles, in the membranous layer of the superficial perineal fascia. From there, posterior scrotal arteries are given off in a variable pattern and travel toward apex of the scrotum. Interconnections are made with the anterior circulation, as well as across the central septum combining left and right-sided circulations. In addition, it has been shown **(Figs 1.9A and B)** that the scrotal raphe receives branches through a separate branch of the perineal artery.[5]

Scrotal skin island flaps that are based on the Dartos fascia can bring a well-vascularized flap to the bulbar urethra, but is often not long enough to reach the anterior urethra. A Blandy flap for perineal urethrostomy can also be fashioned from the posterior circulation by making an inverted "U"-shaped incision.

Venous

The anterior scrotum is drained by veins in the subdermal plexus and then come together at the base of scrotum. From there they travel to the external pudendal veins and

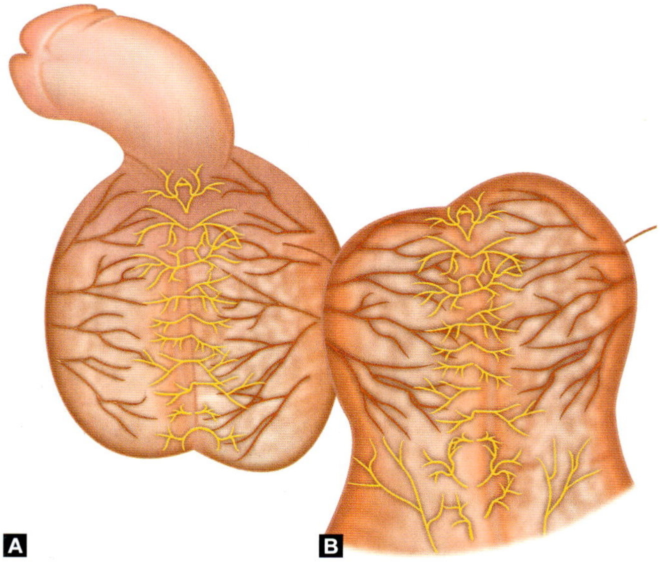

Figs 1.9A and B: Scrotal raphe branches of posterior scrotal artery. (A) Anterior scrotum; (B) Posterior scrotum (Red—anterior or posterior scrotal branches, Yellow—median raphe branches)
Source: Carrera A, Gil-Vernet A, Forcada P, et al. Arteries of the scrotum: a microvascular study and its application to urethral reconstruction with scrotal flaps. BJU Int. 2008:103;820-4.

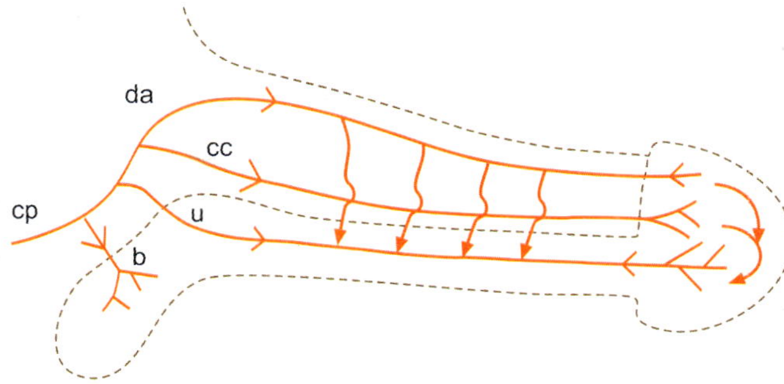

Fig. 1.10: Bidirectional arterial flow to the urethra (cp: Common penile; da: Dorsal artery of the penis; cc: Central cavernosal; **u:** Urethral artery and b: Bulbar artery)
Source: Brandes SB. Urethral Reconstructive Surgery. Totowa, NJ: Humana Press; 2008.

ultimately to the femoral veins. The posterior scrotum is emptied by coalescence of subdermal plexus veins into the perineal vein and finally the internal pudendal vein, mirroring course of the arterial system **(Figs 1.8A and B)**.

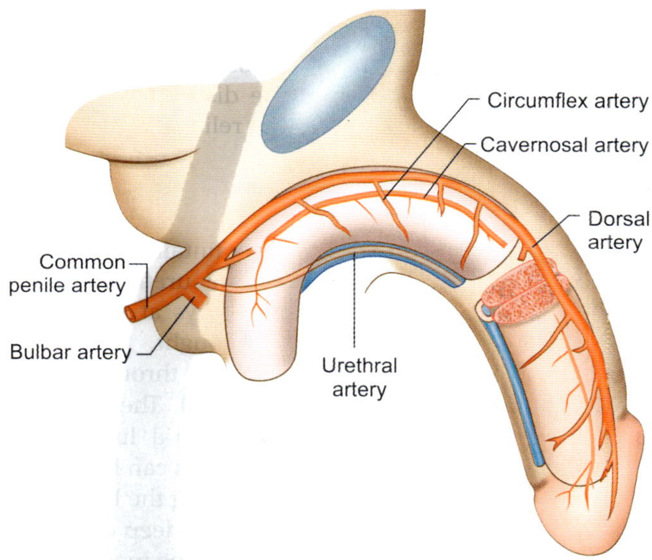

Fig. 1.11: Arterial anatomy of the urethra
Source: Jordan GH, Stack RS. General concepts concerning the use of genital skin islands for anterior urethral reconstruction. Atlas Urol Clin North Am. 1997;5:23-44.

SURGICAL PEARLS

Arterial Anatomy and Implications for Urethral Stricture Repair

One of the unique properties of the urethra that is crucial to reconstruction is its dual blood supply. This allows extensive mobilization and division of the urethra without compromising distal vascular flow. The distal and proximal urethra are maintained by two related blood supplies, but with the proximal being nourished in an antegrade fashion and the distal, retrograde fashion **(Fig. 1.10)**.[6]

The arterial supply is from the internal iliac to the internal pudendal artery. After giving off perineal, posterior scrotal and central scrotal arteries, the internal pudendal continues as the common penile artery. The common penile artery **(Fig. 1.11)** first gives off bulbar and urethral artery and then continues to split into the central cavernosal artery and the dorsal artery of penis. The bulbar and urethral arteries supply the proximal corpus spongiosum. The urethral artery continues within the spongy tissue in a variable location **(Figs 1.12A and B)**.[7]

The paired dorsal arteries travel down shaft of the penis beneath the anterior lamella of Buck's fascia and ultimately form multiple small branches that supply the glans penis. Blood then flows in a retrograde fashion proximally down the corpus spongiosum. Along the way, the dorsal artery also gives off a variable number of

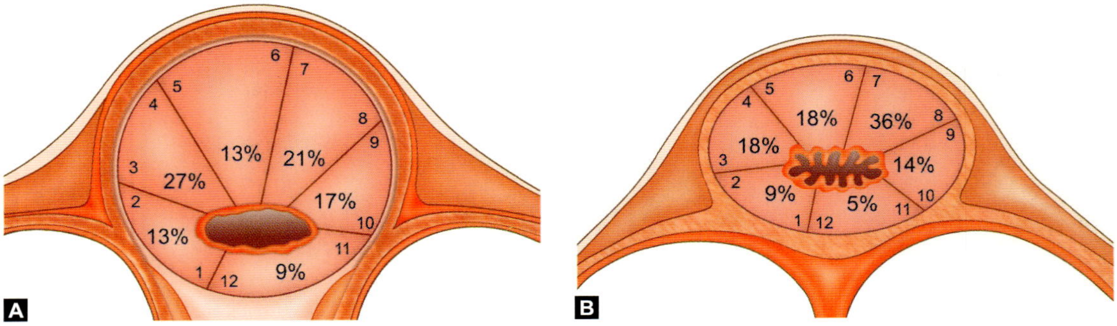

Figs 1.12A and B: Urethral arterial location. (A) Bulbar urethra; (B) Pendulous urethra
Source: Redrawn from Chiou RK, Donovan JM, Anderson JC, et al. Color Doppler ultrasound assessment of urethral artery location: potential implication for technique of visual internal urethrotomy. J Urol. 1998;159(3):796-9.

circumflex arteries that travel ventrolaterally and help to supply the corpus spongiosum. Another source of blood supply to the spongy tissue is via perforators between the corpora cavernosa (central cavernosal arteries) and the corpus spongiosum. However, the distribution of these small vessels is neither constant nor reliable.

Urethrotomy

During anastomotic urethroplasty, maintaining adequate blood flow is crucial. As stated, the urethral arteries travel in a variable location, not always at the 3- and 9 o'clock position as previously thought. Rather, the arteries are distributed almost equally throughout the corpus spongiosum **(Figs 1.12A and B)**. These arteries can be superficial and near the urethral lumen. The location and depth of the urethral arteries can be seen by ultrasound. While this can help in guiding the location of urethrotomy, it is more important to cut deep enough to allow the urothelium to open without being too deep into the spongiosum (which can bleed aggressively).

Anterior Urethroplasty/Excision and Primary Anastomosis

Mobilization of the urethra in conditions with poor distal retrograde blood flow in patients with severe hypospadias and deficient distal spongiosum can lead to bulbar urethral ischemia **(Figs 1.13A to D)**.[8] In cases like this, anastomotic urethroplasty can lead to complications such as necrosis or restricture.[9] These patients may be better served with substitution urethroplasty, flap onlay or even a staged approach. In patients with poor bipedal blood supply, it is important to maintain blood supply through the bulbar arteries and perforating vessels **(Fig. 1.14)**.

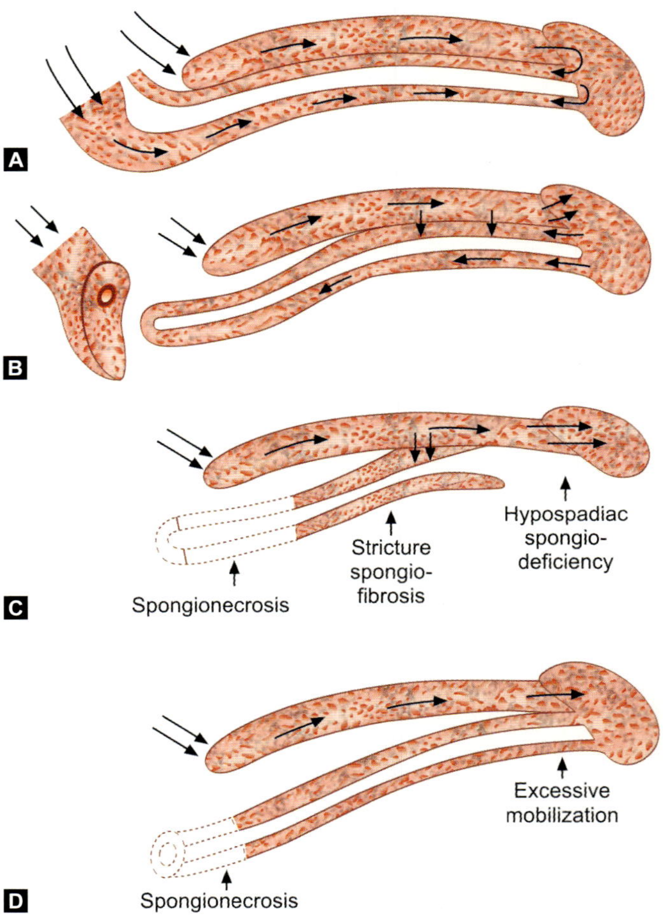

Figs 1.13A to D: Bipedal blood flow in anastomotic urethroplasty. (A and B) With loss of bulbar artery inflow, the proximal bulbar urethra relies on retrograde flow; (C and D) If the retrograde supply is deficient by hypospadias, spongiofibrosis or mobilization, ischemia can develop
Source: Yu G, Miller HC. Critical Operative Maneuvers in Urologic Surgery. St Louis: Mosby; 1996.

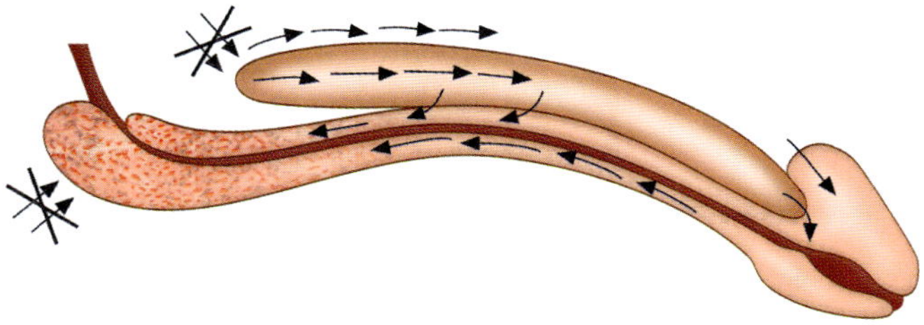

Fig. 1.14: With bilateral internal pudendal inflow loss (X marks), there can be ischemia of the proximal urethra after excision/primary anastomosis (hatch marks)
Source: Brandes SB. Urethral Reconstructive Surgery. Totowa, NJ: Humana Press; 2008.

Posterior Urethroplasty

Posterior urethroplasty is usually required after posterior urethral distraction defects from pelvic trauma. The pelvic trauma can cause concomitant vascular injury, of which bilateral internal pudendal arterial injury or iatrogenic thrombosis is of particular importance to the reconstructive urologist. To ensure that patients scheduled for posterior urethroplasty have a good outcome without excessive risk of ischemia-related restricture, selected patients require a vascular work-up. Jordan et al. noted that children, the elderly, patients with bilateral internal pudendal injury, failed prior urethroplasty, decreased erections, or a cold or insensate glans, were at increased risk for posterior urethral ischemia and stenosis. Patients with risk factors are studied as per **Flow chart 1.1**, and revascularized 3–6 months prior to urethroplasty, if necessary.

Postprostatectomy Stricture

Patients that are postprostatectomy and have both a urethral stricture and sphincter-deficiency incontinence can also be a challenge regarding the maintenance of adequate urethral blood flow. When stress incontinence is treated with artificial urinary sphincter after anastomotic urethroplasty, the arterial inflow can be compromised by the circumferential compression from the cuff, leading to cuff erosion. It is recommended that the bulbar arteries should be maintained here for anastomotic urethroplasty in order to help the blood supply proximal to the cuff, which might otherwise be dependent on the retrograde blood flow from the distal urethra.

Venous Anatomy

Flow chart 1.1: Evaluation of arterial inflow prior to posterior urethroplasty

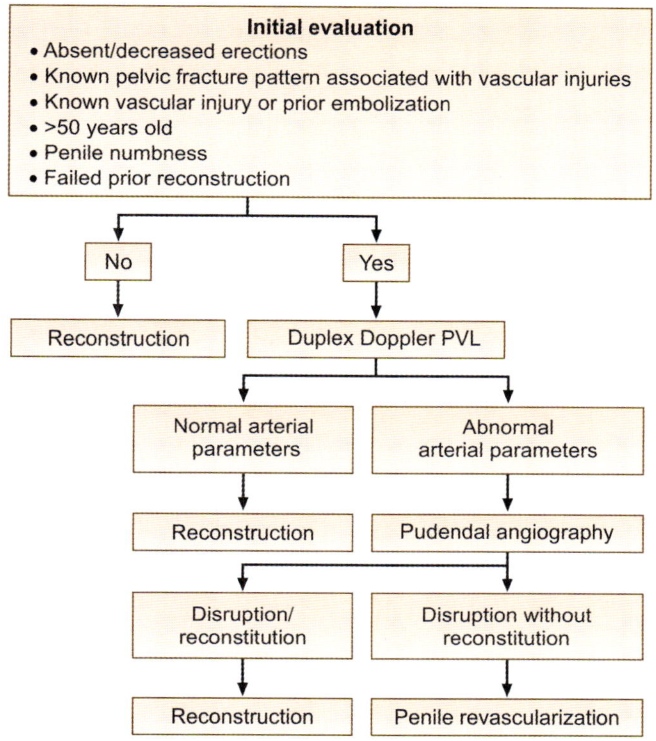

Source: Jordan GH. Reconstruction for urethral stricture. Atlas Urol Clin North Am. 1997;5(1).

The corpus spongiosum has a venous drainage pattern that is essentially the same as that of the glans penis and other deep structures. This is usually through the periurethral veins, circumflex veins emptying into the paired para-arterial veins that run with the dorsal arteries, and the deep and superficial dorsal veins. The corpora cavernosa are drained by emissary veins which feed cavernosal veins and travel to base of the penis to drain independently into the dorsal vein complex. There are free communications between all of the veins, which eventually end in the superficial and deep dorsal median veins. The deep dorsal median vein is deep to Buck's fascia and ultimately drains through the dorsal vein complex. There may be multiple superficial dorsal median veins, and they are superficial to Buck's fascia and drain to the right or left superficial external pudendal vein **(Figs 1.6 and 1.15)**.[10]

Urethral Elasticity

Excision and primary anastomosis (EPA) relies upon the natural elasticity of the corpus spongiosum and urethra to allow bridging of the area excised with a tension-free anastomosis of normal urethra. Sampaio et al.

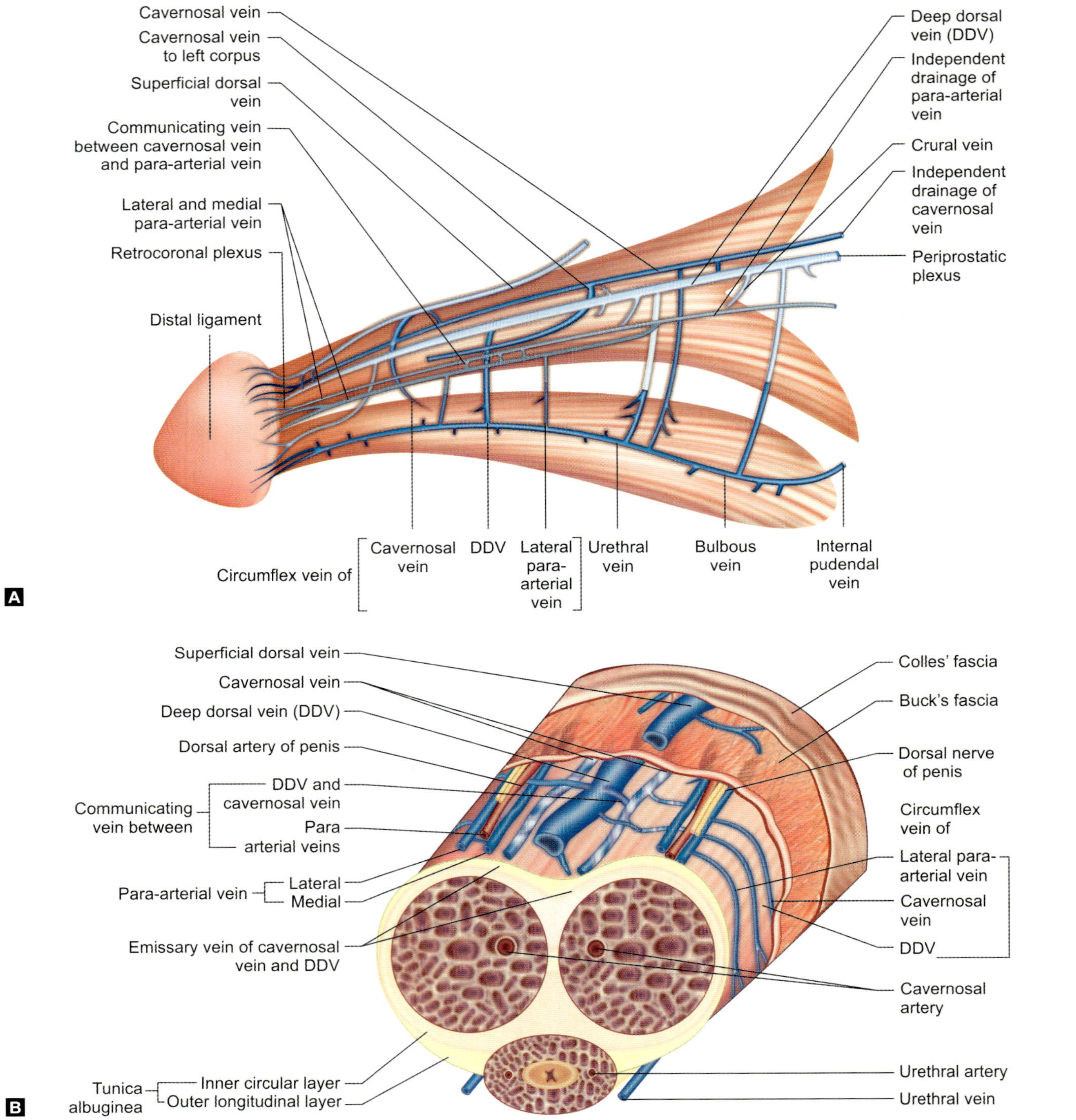

Figs 1.15A and B: Deep venous anatomy of the penis

Source: Hsu GL, Hsieh CH, Wen HS, et al. Penile venous anatomy: An additional description and its clinical implication. J Androl. 2003;24(6):921-7.

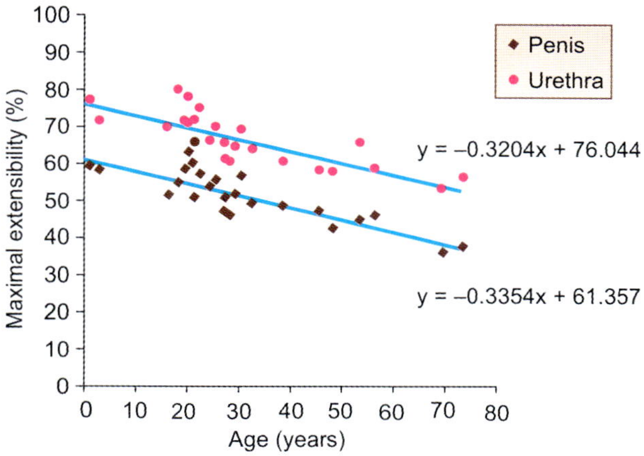

Fig. 1.16: Extensibility by age. Top line is urethral extensibility and bottom line is penile extensibility. Age is on the x-axis and shows decreased extensibility with increasing age

Source: Da Silva EA, Sampaio FJ. Urethral extensibility applied to reconstructive surgery. J Urol. 2002;167(5):2042-5.

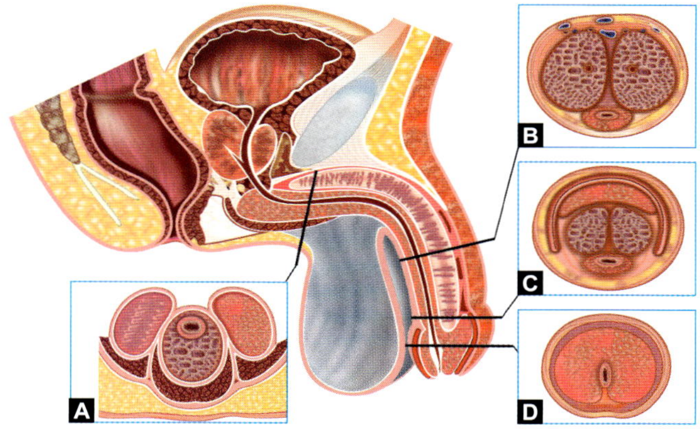

Figs 1.17A to D: Anatomic location of urethra within the corpus spongiosum by cross-section. (A) The bulbous urethra; (B) Penile shaft; (C) Coronal margin; (D) Glans

Source: Jordan GH, Virasoro R, Eltahawy EA. Reconstruction and management of posterior urethral and straddle injuries of the urethra. Urol Clin North Am. 2006;33:97-109.

Table 1.1: Estimated amount of urethral mobilization required to bridge a 1 cm urethral gap

Age (Year)	*Estimated linear regression ratio*
1	1:3.2
10	1:3.4
20	1:3.7
30	1:4.0
40	1:4.5
50	1:5.0
60	1:5.7
70	1:6.6

Source: Da Silva EA, Sampaio FJ. Urethral extensibility applied to reconstructive surgery. J Urol. 2002;167(5):2042-5.

demonstrated the expected extensibility of the urethra and penis in fresh cadavers. There were two main findings:

1. The urethral extensibility of the urethra exceeds that of the penis **(Fig. 1.16)**.
2. The urethral and penile extensibility decrease with age **(Table 1.1)**. Based upon these findings, the estimated amount of urethral mobilization, needed for EPA, can be determined (on average about 1:4, but varies with age as per **Figure 1.16.**[11] Knowledge of these principles can lead to decreased complications such as chordee, ischemia-related restenosis, dehiscence and meatal retraction.

Urethral Location within Corpus Spongiosum

In the penis, the urethra is very central, so there is generally insufficient spongiosum ventrally to perform an adequate spongioplasty for a ventral graft (buccal or skin). For this reason, penile grafts are placed within the split urethral plate (as in the Asopa technique) or placed dorsally, quilted to the corpora cavernosa. Moving proximally, the spongy tissue is thicker and the urethra is located more eccentric and dorsal **(Figs 1.17A to D)**.[12] Thus, the bulb makes an excellent location for a ventral onlay graft with spongioplasty, while the penis does not. The disadvantage of making a ventral urethrotomy for graft placement is that the spongiosum is very thick here and can bleed profusely. For this reason, we prefer a dorsal urethrotomy and dorsal graft placement, in order to avoid brisk bleeding.

REFERENCES

1. McAninch JW, Morey AF. Penile circular fasciocutaneous skin flap in 1-stage reconstruction of complex anterior urethral strictures. J Urol. 1998;159(4):1209-13.
2. Quartey JK. Microcirculation of the penile and scrotal skin. Atlas Urol Clin North Am. 1997;5:23.
3. Jordan GH, Stack RS. General concepts concerning the use of genital skin islands for anterior urethral reconstruction. Atlas Urol Clin North Am. 1997;5:23-44.
4. Jordan GH. Reconstruction for urethral stricture. Atlas Urol Clin North Am. 1997;5(1).

5. Carrera A, Gil-Vernet A, Forcada P, et al. Arteries of the scrotum: a microvascular study and its application to urethral reconstruction with scrotal flaps. BJU Int. 2008;103: 820-4.
6. Brandes SB. Urethral Reconstructive Surgery. Totowa, NJ: Humana Press; 2008.
7. Chiou RK, Donovan JM, Anderson JC, et al. Color Doppler ultrasound assessment of urethral artery location: potential implication for technique of visual internal urethrotomy. J Urol. 1998;159(3):796-9.
8. Yu G, Miller HC. Critical operative maneuvers in urologic surgery. St Louis: Mosby; 1996.
9. Complications of interventional techniques for urethral stricture. In: Carson CC (Ed). Complications of Interventional Techniques. New York: Igaku-Shoim; 1996.p.89.
10. Hsu GL, Hsieh CH, Wen HS, et al. Penile venous anatomy: an additional description and its clinical implication. J Androl. 2003;24(6):921-7.
11. Da Silva EA, Sampaio FJ. Urethral extensibility applied to reconstructive surgery. J Urol. 2002;167(5):2042-5.
12. Jordan GH, Virasoro R, Eltahawy EA. Reconstruction and management of posterior urethral and straddle injuries of the urethra. Urol Clin North Am. 2006;33:97-109.

Infection is rarely the cause of urethral strictures in the modern developed world. Historically, and in some countries to this day, gonococcal urethritis was a significant cause. Gonoccocal urethral strictures are located in the region of paraurethral glands (Littre glands) as these are inflamed during the infection. There is no evidence of a relationship between nongonococcal urethritis (due to *Chlamydia*, ureaplasma and mycoplasma) and stricture development. Similarly, tuberculosis is an uncommon cause of urethral stricture in the modern era.

Lichen sclerosus et atrophicus (LSA) is a frequent cause of strictures in Western countries. It affects the glans and the meatus, but can also produce a panurethral stricture. The more proximal strictures may occur as a result of chronic obstruction and inflammation of the Littre glands. Primary urethral cancer is a rare cause of urethral stricture.

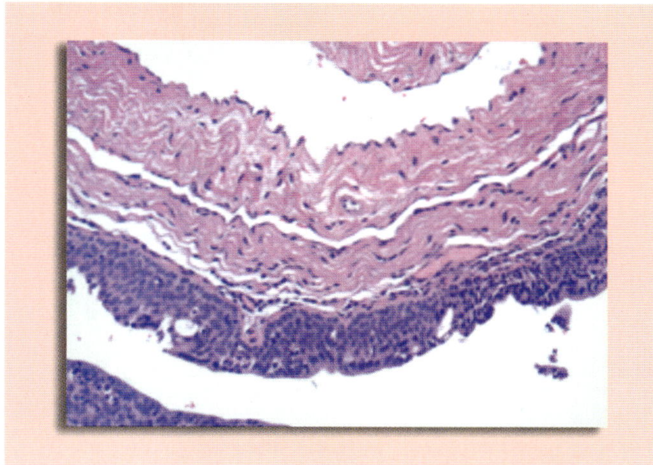

Fig. 2.2: Photomicrograph of normal urethra—pseudostratified columnar epithelium

Acknowledgment: J Carlos Manivel, MD, Department of Pathology, University of Minnesota.

Posterior Urethral Stricture

Posterior urethral strictures are secondary to pelvic fracture or iatrogenic causes. Approximately 4–14% of pelvic fractures are associated with posterior urethral injury.[12] The urethra is torn when the pelvic fracture causes the anterior and posterior urethra to move in different directions. There is debate about whether all of these injuries occur above the genitourinary diaphragm or whether some may occur below the voluntary sphincter.[13] When they occur above the diaphragm, they can be associated with a pelvic hematoma that displaces the prostate cephalad. This hematoma then matures into a dense scar. Therefore, these are best termed as urethral disruption defects rather than urethral strictures. Iatrogenic posterior urethral strictures are most commonly due to prostate cancer treatment and less commonly due to surgical treatment of benign prostatic hyperplasia. Radical prostatectomy results in bladder neck contracture in 8.4%.[14] With short-term follow-up, radiation appears to result in stricture in 1.7–12% depending on the type of treatment but rates continue to rise over long term in the few studies with data beyond 10 years.[14,15]

HISTOLOGY

Urethral stricture is a complex process involving several histologic changes that result in a fibrotic process of the corpus spongiosum and narrowing of the urethral lumen caliber.

The normal urethral tissue from inside to outside is formed by a pseudostratified columnar epithelium, a basal membrane and the spongiosum which is a complex connective tissue layer rich in vascular sinusoids and smooth muscle **(Fig. 2.2)**. The connective tissue is composed of fibroblasts and an extracellular matrix that contains collagen, proteoglycans, elastic fibers and glycoproteins. The concentration of elastic fibers is particularly high in the spongiosum, explaining in part its high degree of extensibility.[16]

After a noxious event, the epithelium changes from the pseudostratified columnar type to stratified squamous epithelium.[17] This is a more fragile epithelium which tends to ulcerate, permitting focal extravasation of urine during voiding which produces a subepithelial fibrosis. The fibrosis is a result of increased collagen production and a shift from a predominance of elastic collagen type III to inelastic collagen type I, both replacing the normal smooth muscle.[18,19] All of these changes are more evident in traumatic strictures than in those due to other etiology[20] **(Fig. 2.3)**.

PATHOPHYSIOLOGY OF STRICTURE URETHRA

Mundy[21] proposed a model of stricture formation in which the microscopic foci of fibrosis grow and coalesce over a period of years, forming macroscopic plaques, which may then constrict the urethra, if they form a complete ring around circumference of the urethra **(Flow chart 2.1)**. Pathogenic models include overexpression of connective tissue growth factor,[22] and changes in nitric oxide synthase metabolism, which stimulate abnormal collagen synthesis.[23]

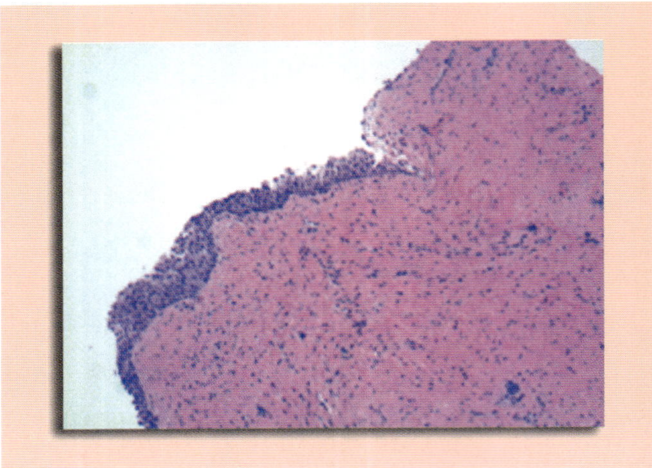

Fig. 2.3: Photomicrograph of urethral spongiofibrosis

Acknowledgment: J Carlos Manivel MD, Department of Pathology, University of Minnesota.

Flow chart 2.1: Pathophysiology of stricture development

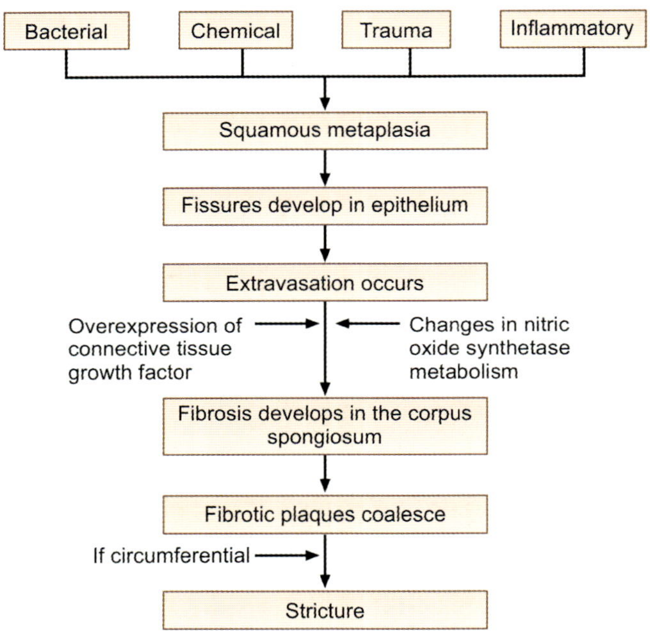

Source: Mundy AR, Andrich DE. Urethral strictures. BJU Int. 2010;107:6-26.

Of note, the location of paraurethral glands (Littre glands) coincides with site of stricture when the cause is infection, implicating these as a possible cause. These glands are concentrated in the bulbar urethra, extending deeply into the corpus spongiosum and are distributed circumferentially around the urethra. In gonococcal urethritis, these glands form abscesses and resulting spongiofibrosis.

Classification

The ideal grading system would classify urethral strictures based on preoperative clinical and radiologic findings. It would be a tool to aid in selection of the appropriate reconstruction technique and might even help to predict success rates with various surgeries; higher grade strictures would correlate with more a challenging reconstruction. To date, no such tool exists. Instead, we have classification systems based on intraoperative findings or pathologic findings, which cannot aid in preoperative planning. There are classification systems based on ultrasound findings; however, ultrasounds are usually done intraoperatively and although they may guide intraoperative decisions they cannot shape preoperative patient counseling. Of note, the number and variety of classifications systems speaks to the failure of any single system to successfully meet the stated goals.

One important classification is the distinction between disease of the anterior and posterior urethra. Urethral stricture generally refers to anterior urethral disease, which involves fibrosis of the corpus spongiosum. In contrast, posterior urethral stricture results generally from (1) a urethral disruption defect after pelvic fracture, (2) radiation stenosis or (3) a postoperative bladder neck contracture. Thus, these more specific terms which speak to the unique etiologies in the posterior urethra are usually preferred over the generic term urethral stricture.

In 1983, Devine et al.[24] proposed a classification of urethral strictures based on the extent of spongiofibrosis and the anatomy of stricture. A few years later, Jordan et al.[25] added a treatment algorithm based on this classification **(Figs 2.4A to F)**. The major limitation, as discussed above, is that this is largely based on intraoperative or pathologic findings.

For this reason some authors proposed a classification according to the sonographic degree of stenosis,[26] stenosis length and involvement of the spongiosum.[27] Adoption has been slow because the examination is operator-dependent; the results are very subjective and thus are not reproducible.

Barbagli has developed a classification system for inflammatory stenosis produced by LSA.[28] Although unique to a single etiology, this classification system can prove to be helpful in staging and thus selecting appropriate management in these particularly challenging strictures. Similarly, Pasandoro has recognized that prostatic urethral strictures are especially challenging to

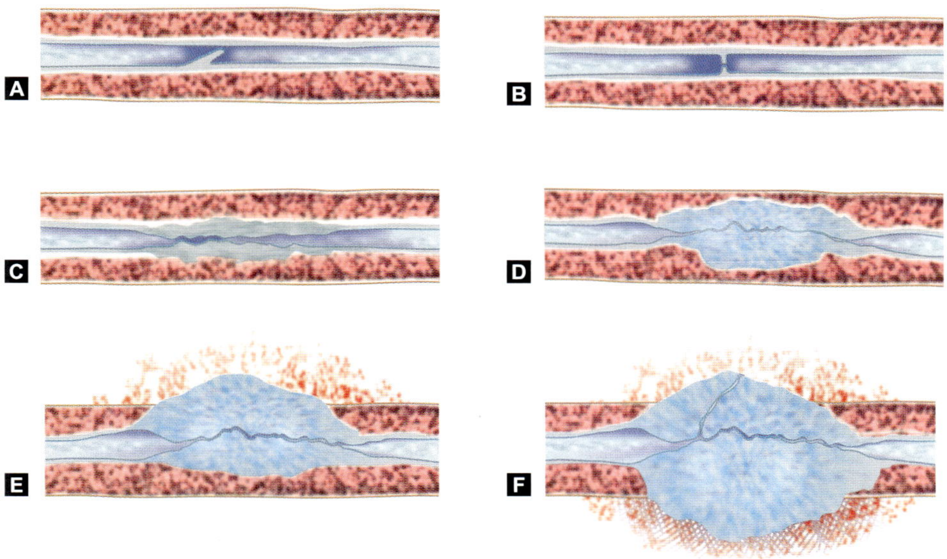

Figs 2.4A to F: Classification of anterior urethral stricture disease according to the anatomical. (A) Epithelial fold; (B) Epithelial scar; (C) Initial spongiofibrosis; (D) Full-thickness spongiofibrosis; (E) Progressive spongiofibrosis involving tissues outside the corpus spongiosum; (F) Spongiofibrosis occupies the entire corpus spongiosum forming a complex stricture with potential fistula formation

Source: From Schlossberg SM, Jordan GH. Urethral stricture. In: Rakel RE, Bope ET (Eds). Conn's Current Therapy. Amsterdam: Elsevier; 2005.

manage and has proposed a unique classification system for these.[29]

ECONOMIC IMPACT

The cost related to the treatment of urethral stricture disease in the US was estimated to be close to $200 million in 2002, principally due to ambulatory surgery, with a yearly individual cost of disease of about $6,000. The cost of this pathology is considerably lower than for other more common urological diseases like nephrolithiasis, but is quite significant for an often-overlooked disease.[30]

If we generally categorize urethral stricture management as endoscopic [dilation or direct vision internal urethrotomy (DVIU)] and urethral reconstruction, then we find that the majority of board-certified urologists in the US choose to perform repeated endoscopic procedures rather than reconstruction.[31] This may in part be due to an understanding that dilation/DVIU are minimally invasive, easy to perform, repeatable, have good results and are a low cost procedures. Urethroplasty is more complex, requires surgical expertise, and may be believed to have more complications and be more expensive. However, careful study reveals several misconceptions. Steenkamp et al.[32] reported a 60% success rate at 12 months for short (1–2 cm) strictures of the bulbar urethra treated with DVIU, with the success rate declining over longer-term follow-up. Likewise, Pasandoro et al.[33] report lower success rates with long-term follow-up, specifically 32% at 98 months. Recently Santucci et al.[34] report only an 8% success rate at 7 months of follow-up after a first urethrotomy. Thus, the average success rate after a single DVIU is likely to be close to 35%[35] depending on the location, length, etiology and grade of spongiofibrosis. Subsequent DVIUs have a higher failure rate than initial DVIU;[34] after a third DVIU the success rate is close to 0%.[33,34,36]

Urethroplasty is a more complex surgery than DVIU, requires a specially-trained urologist, and has potentially more complications, but the results are superior. Urethroplasty has reported lifetime success rates ranging from 75% to close to 100%. Several authors report over 95% success rates at 4–5 years follow-up using buccal mucosal free grafts in the Barbagli procedure[37] or with excision and primary anastomosis (EPA).[38]

How do Costs Compare for these Two Procedures?

In the United States the cost of performing one DVIU has been calculated as $5,421, and the cost of urethroplasty with its longer operative time and hospital stay as $16,093. Using a decision analysis approach in a theoretical patient with a less than 2 cm bulbar urethral stricture, Rourke and Jordan assumed the success rate of initial DVIU to be 27 versus

96% with EPA and calculated the least costly approach over the long-term. Under these assumptions and factoring in complication rates from the literature, the cost of a strategy of immediate urethroplasty was $16,444, whereas the cost of a strategy of initial DVIU was $17,747, reflecting increased costs with repeat procedures. In this study, the authors concluded that initial urethroplasty was preferred for short segment bulbar strictures. Initial DVIU was preferred only when the long-term success of DVIU exceeded 40%.[39]

Wright et al.[40] in a slightly different model estimated costs from a societal perspective, including the costs of procedures and office visits, as well as lost wages from convalescence. In this model, the success rate of initial urethroplasty was again assumed to be excellent (95%), but the success rate of initial DVIU was set higher than in Rourke and Jordan's study, at 50%. Here they conclude that the most cost-effective approach was one DVIU before urethroplasty. They noted that the incremental cost of performing a second DVIU before attempting urethroplasty was $141,962 for each additional successfully voiding patient. Urethroplasty as primary therapy was cost-effective only when the expected success rate of the first DVIU was less than 35%, very close to the 40% threshold set by Rourke and Jordan.

It must be pointed out that these models analyze the best-case scenario for DVIU—a less than 2 cm bulbar stricture. Initial urethroplasty is likely to be favored in longer segment strictures or in penile urethral strictures where even though the success of urethroplasty is not 95%, the success of DVIU is dismal. In summary, the most cost-effective approach to managing urethral strictures as a society would include earlier referral for urethroplasty.

EDITORIAL COMMENTS

Dr Rajesh Gulia

The histological characteristics of the urethral mucosa helps us in understanding the various phases of stricture. Also it explains why certain area of the urethra are more prone to urethral stricture disease. Columnar and cylindrical epithelium is an unusually good breeding ground for gonococci. It lines the urethra from the external meatus to the membranous portion. The innumerable glands and crypts interspersed among the columnar cells offer favorable habitat for inflammatory foci, notably in the bulbous urethra. In the membranous urethra because of the absence of glandular structures, this area is resistant to infection and stricture in this location is less frequent.

The pathology of urethral stricture is that of chronic urethritis plus scar formation. Now, not all patients who have chronic urethritis ultimately develop a urethral stricture and we do see stricture developing in a period of weeks in the presence of unusually acute urethral infections. This can be clearly understood if we understand the sequence of the pathological process involved as very beautifully worked out by Oberlander.

If the glandular exudate can drain into the canal, intraglandular or intracryptic inflammation continues as a chronic catarrh (glandular urethritis of Oberlander), if the gland orifices are plugged by firm exudate, a glandular abscess or colloidal cyst is formed (dry urethritis of Oberlander). Further, the gland may be obliterated by scar or may return to normal.

Oberlander designated as soft infiltration that lesion which urethroscopically appears as a reddened mucosa dotted by still more red suppurating duct orifices and with slight sclerosis of the walls indicated by diminution of the normal folds and urethral striae.

The next stage or hard infiltration of Oberlander is characterized urethroscopically by loss of striae or folds, a rigid urethral wall against the striking pallor of which the reddened orifices of inflamed glands stand out in sharp contrast. There may be erosions, ulcerations, granulations or papillomata. Increased scar formation with resulting anemia explains the mucosal pallor. Infection accounts for ulceration and erosion while various stages of the repair process produce granulations and, if exaggerated, papillomata. Intensification of this latter process, the hard infiltration of Oberlander, results in the condition we observe clinically as stricture.

In the transition from chronic urethritis to clinical stricture the Finger-Gujon theory assumes the urethritis to be always a sclerotic process, the degree of stricture being proportional to the duration of the inflammation. Since sclerotic repair is proportional to the severity of the inflammation and we do see stricture developing in a period of weeks in the presence of unusually acute urethral infections whereas chronic urethritis may persist for years without stricture formation, Guiard's theory—that stricture is dependent upon the severity of the localized infection—may be universally applied.

In the clinical scenario, when a patient presents with symptoms of dysuria to his family physician he is prescribed a course of antibiotics (which is inadequate for this pathological process of urethritis), he gets symptomatically better, but the underlying intraglandular and intracryptic inflammation continues subclinically. Each time the symptoms of urethritis recur he is again prescribed an inadequate course of antibiotics. Thus the process continues and predisposes him to a prolonged underlying sclerotic process leading on to stricture formation. Thus we must not underestimate the rational

CHAPTER 3

Imaging in Stricture Urethra

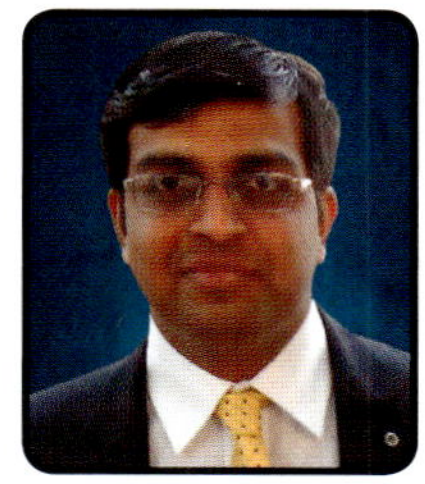

Pankaj M Joshi

Sanjay B Kulkarni, Pankaj M Joshi

Chapter Outline

Abstract

Imaging in stricture urethra is of utmost importance. Retrograde urethrogram is the basic and most important investigation. It is essential that a urologist does the retrograde urethrogram under fluoroscopy, rather than leave it to radiologists, judgment. It should be done in aseptic precautions. Sonourethrography is helpful in assessing stones, diverticulum, severity of spongiofibrosis and length of stricture. A well done combined antegrade and retrograde urethrogram in pelvic fracture urethral disruption defect (PFUDD) gives a fair idea about the length of gap. MRI should be performed in complex and redo PFUDD related posterior urethral strictures. Penile Doppler in PFUDD is essential for understanding vasculogenic impotence. It should be performed in all patients with PFUDD.

Keywords

Retrograde urethrogram (RGU), Antegrade urethrogram, Micturating cystourethrogram (MCU), Up and downogram, Pericatheter urethrogram, Color Doppler of penis, Urethrosonography, Spongiofibrosis, MR urethrography, Neurogenic impotence.

INTRODUCTION

Stricture of the urethra causes obstruction to the flow of urine. Stricture is a local disease of the urethra but can become systemic in cases where it leads to urinary retention and back pressure changes. Imaging in stricture depends upon the site and suspected causes of stricture. In this review, we will take you through the various modalities of radiological importance which help us in diagnosis and management of stricture. We would start from simple to more complex investigations.

X-RAY KIDNEY, URETER, BLADDER

A patient of stricture disease, which is long standing may have development of urinary calculi. They may be present in the bladder or the kidneys. While the bladder calculi are due to obstruction, stricture can cause recurrent urinary tract infections and possibility of kidney stone formation.

RETROGRADE URETHROGRAM

This is the basic and most important investigation in evaluation of the stricture disease. It simply means opacification of the urethra by means of a radiocontrast agent with subsequent photography. Urethrogram can be classified into various categories:

- Elective versus emergency
- Antegrade versus retrograde
- Combined up and downogram.

While elective urethrogram is carried in cases of suspected stricture, emergency urethrograms are done in the casualty trauma departments in cases of suspected urethral injuries after pelvic trauma or perineal trauma.

Technique

Urethrogram is an invasive procedure which needs to be done by taking utmost care and precautions. It is essential to have the patient well informed about the procedure and the complications. Usually urethrogram is best avoided in presence of infections as it may cause intravasation of bacteria and bacteremia. However, routine examination of urine is not required, and good clinical judgment is fair enough for the procedure.

It is always recommended that the urethrogram should be performed by the treating urologist or a urology trainee rather than leaving it upon the radiologist's judgment. Performing retrograde urethrogram (RGU) under fluoroscopy guidance gives accurate information about the distensibility of urethra which may not be seen in static images.

Utmost care must be taken to use all aseptic technique while performing the urethrogram. The patient should be placed supine and the genitals should be painted with antiseptic solution, povidone-iodine being authors' choice.

Position

Urethra is a tubular structure which lies in the midline. However, it has its natural curvature along the bulbar region with two dilated parts, the bulb and the fossa navicularis. Obtaining the urethrogram in supine position will cause overlapping of the bulbar and penile urethra and will not give the correct diagnosis. In order to straighten the urethra, two steps are crucial:

1. *Positioning the patient in oblique position at approximately 20°*: The question is right oblique or left oblique. In the radiology suites where the fluoroscopy machine is organized, usually the screening arm is placed on left of the patient or on the opposite side of table. It is clumsy to stand on the side of machine and do the urethrogram. Right-handed surgeons would always prefer the right oblique position, while left-handed surgeons may prefer to use the left oblique position.
2. *Straighten the penis*: In order to get a good representation of the urethra, the penis needs to be straightened. This can be done by using hand; however, it may cause the hand shadow on the urethrogram and there is a risk of radiation exposure. Hence various techniques can be used as using a gauze piece around the glans and stretching the penis, using Foley's catheter with balloon inflated with 2 cc of saline placed in navicularis fossa with a pull applied to the Foley's or by using the Brodney's clamp.

Materials

We can use a simple Foley's catheter adaptor to cannulate the meatus, some authors recommend Foley's catheter to be inflated in the fossa navicularis. Problem comes in patients of severe lichen sclerosus where there is meatal stenosis and difficulty in cannulating the meatus. Here we can use the inner sheath of intravenous catheter routinely used for gaining access to a vein or a small 6 French infant feeding tube which is cut at approximately 2.5 cm distance from the hub.

Contrast: Diluted diatrizoate meglumine is widely used. It has been proved beyond doubts that nonionic contrast had less complication when given intravenously as compared to the ionic contrasts. Same may be applied in case of urethrograms.

Films

Scout film: Before doing a urethrogram, it is essential to take a plain X-ray of the desired region to rule out presence of calculi and calcifications as they may cause confusion in interpreting the urethrogram.

Patient is placed in oblique position and contrast is injected into the urethra with continuous fluoroscopic monitoring. Excessive pressure is avoided while injecting, so as to prevent intravasation and extravasation. The stricture is visualized, the site identified and the contrast would be seen passing beyond the stricture into the proximal urethra and bladder. If the patient has a suprapubic catheter, then antegrade urethrogram could be done so as to get a clear picture of full length of the stricture. In a classical case of panurethral stricture due to lichen sclerosis, a well done RGU will show irregular urethral mucosa with contrast entering the glands of Littre **(Figs 3.1A and B)**.

MICTURATING CYSTOURETHROGRAM

Having diagnosed a stricture in the urethra, efforts should not be made to insert a feeding tube in the bladder to get a micturating film as it may cause false passage and damage

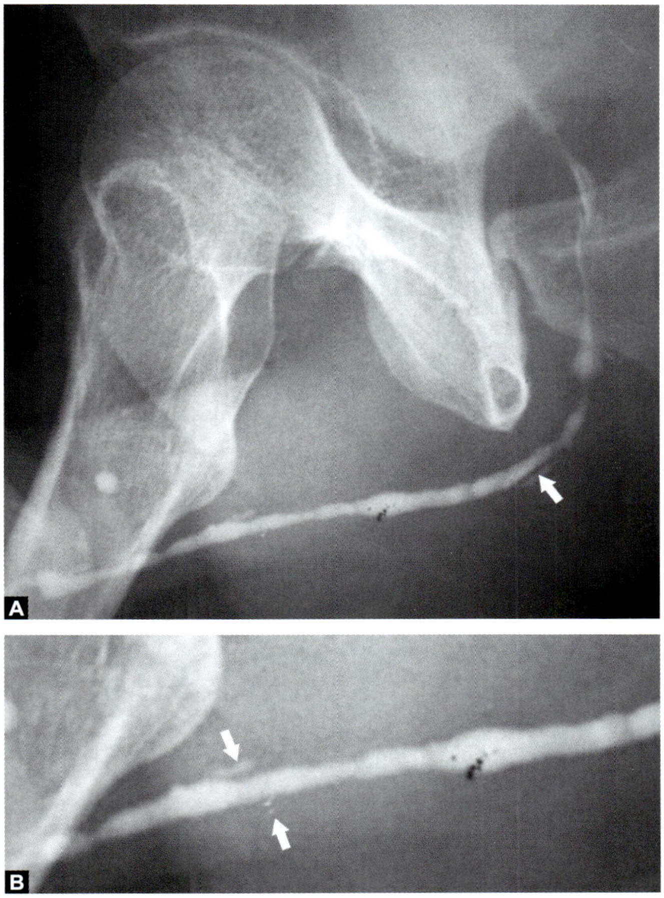

Figs 3.1A and B: Panurethral stricture involving whole of the anterior urethra, usually seen in lichen sclerosus. Note the irregular urethral mucosa and contrast entering the glands of Littre all along the urethra (arrow heads)

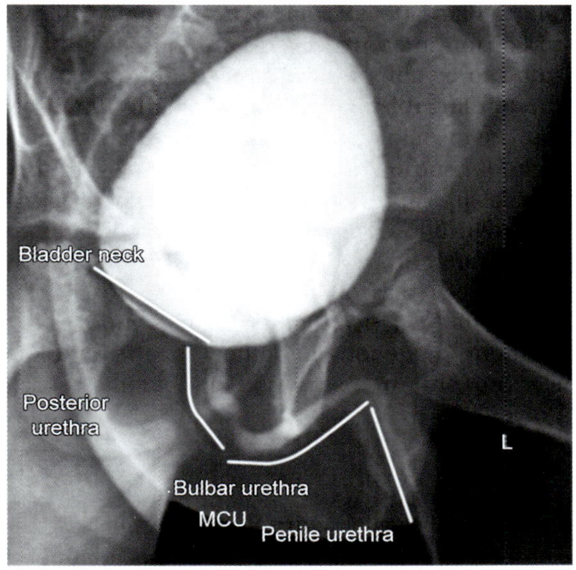

Fig. 3.2: Micturating cystourethrogram (MCU) showing the parts of urethra and bladder neck

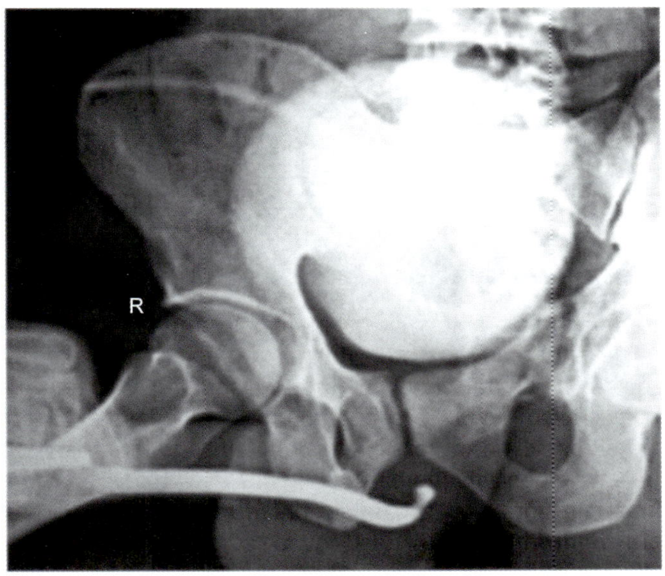

Fig. 3.3: Ascending and descending urethrogram in pelvic fracture urethral distraction defect

to the urethra. In case the patient has a suprapubic catheter or if the bladder can be filled easily from below just by injecting contrast, micturating film can be obtained **(Fig. 3.2)**. It helps in highlighting proximal extent of the stricture, nature of bladder as to presence of reflux or diverticulum. It helps if the patient is given an alpha-blocker 30 minutes prior, as it helps the bladder neck to open. Also sometimes a suprapubic puncture is resorted to, to fill the bladder in case of failure of access from below and in the absence of a suprapubic catheter.

UP AND DOWNOGRAM

In cases of pelvic fracture with urethral distraction defects (PFUDDs), patients who are referred ones usually have a suprapubic catheter. A plain X-ray reveals healing fracture of the pelvis.

Steps

Urethrogram in such scenario is often labeled as up and downogram **(Fig. 3.3)**. Patient is placed in supine position. Parts are painted with povidone-iodine. It is important to fill the bladder slowly. Hence, 500 ml of sterilized normal saline connected to an intravenous infusion set is connected to the suprapubic catheter with contrast added to the normal saline. It is allowed to flow slowly and bladder examined periodically under fluoroscopy.

Once the bladder is full, bladder neck is assessed. Contrast is seen flowing in the posterior urethra. Patient is then given an oblique position and contrast injected through the urethra. Fluoroscopic image then shows gap between the proximal and distal ends of urethra.

Issue arises when bladder neck does not open. In such cases we could resort to the use of alpha blockers and repeat the urethrogram or rather as a routine give an alpha blocker before a micturating cystourethrogram (MCU).

Features to be Seen in a Urethrogram

- To assess the continuity of urethra
- The length of gap between the proximal and distal ends
- State of bladder, presence of diverticulum, stones, bladder capacity
- Bladder neck—open or closed.

PERICATHETER URETHROGRAM

This is a procedure which is done in follow-up period of patients who undergo complex urethral reconstruction or after redo surgeries. All aseptic precautions are taken. There are two ways of doing this procedure:

1. Use an infant feeding tube or cannula of an intravenous access sheath and inject contrast around the catheter from the meatus.
2. If the patient has suprapubic catheter, then we could fill the bladder with contrast and ask the patient to void. The contrast usually highlights the urethra around per urethral catheter.

The purpose of this procedure is to look for any leaks from the urethra.

NORMAL ANATOMY OF THE URETHRA ON URETHROGRAM

Urethra in an adult male is approximately 17–20 cm in length. Urethra is divided into two parts: anterior urethra and posterior urethra **(Fig. 3.4)**.

Anterior urethra is divided into.

- *Penile urethra*: It extends from fossa navicularis to penoscrotal junction **(Fig. 3.5)**
- *Bulbar urethra*: It is from penoscrotal junction to membranous urethra **(Fig. 3.6)**

Posterior urethra is divided into:

- *Membranous urethra*: It is approximately 1 cm in length, sphincteric area.
- *Prostatic urethra*: It is part of the urethra within the prostate.

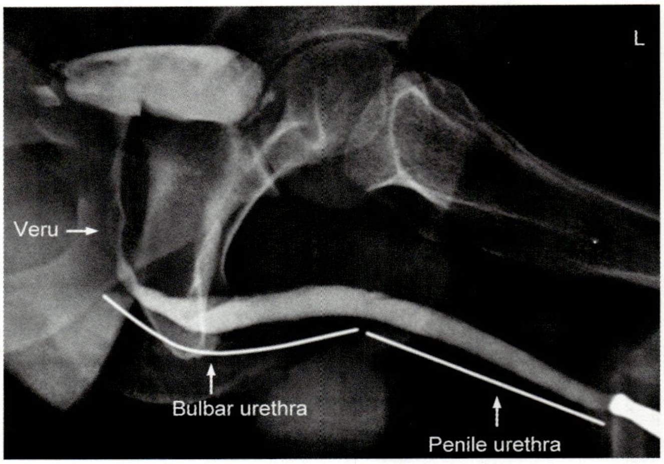

Fig. 3.4: A normal retrograde urethrogram showing parts of urethra and verumontanum. Starting at this landmark extending distally for about 1–1.5 cm, shows position of the external urethral sphincter, the membranous urethra

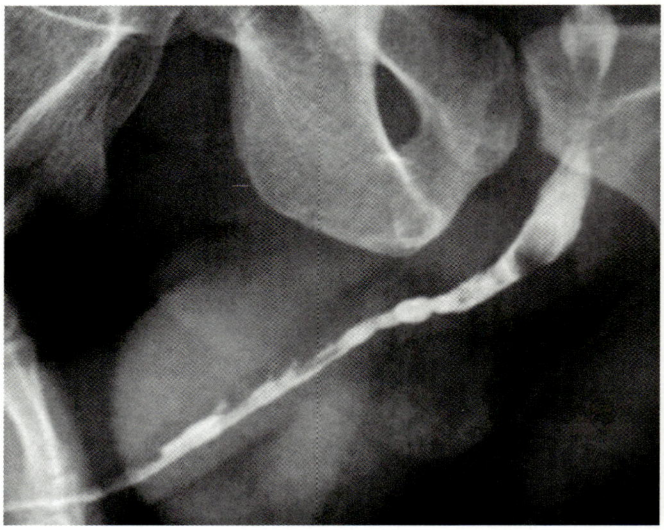

Fig. 3.5: Stricture involving the penile and distal bulbar urethra

Complications of Urethrogram

- Excessive use of force may cause urethral bleeding
- Extravasation
- Venous intravasation
- Vasovagal reaction due to pain.

Pitfalls in Urethrogram

- In case of lichen sclerosus where there is a stricture from fossa navicularis itself, by using an infant feeding tube, the initial stricture may be missed.

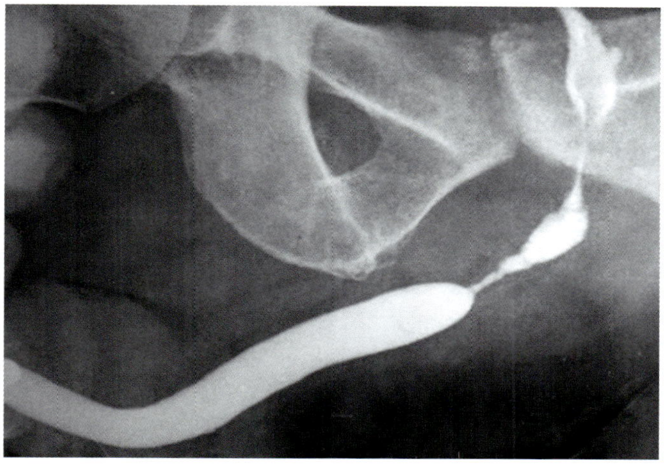

Fig. 3.6: Proximal bulbar urethral stricture

- Extravasation may blur the image and may make interpretation difficult.
- Failure to take a plain X-ray prior may make subsequent interpretation difficult in case of calcification or calculi.
- Failure to straighten the penis may cause overlapping of the curvature and false interpretation.

ULTRASONOGRAPHY

There are three ways in which ultrasound is useful in stricture disease:

1. Ultrasound of the kidney, ureter and bladder (KUB).
2. Color Doppler of penis.
3. Sonourethrography in anterior strictures.

Abdominal Ultrasound

Sonography of the abdomen and pelvis is necessary to check the back pressure changes in the upper tracts like bilateral hydroureteronephrosis.

Significant postvoid residual urine volume indicates significant obstruction and/or decompensated detrusor. Bladder wall thickness is also an important measurement.

Color Doppler of the Penis

Color Doppler of penis is performed in all patients of pelvic fracture urethral injury. Color Doppler is done to measure flow and velocities in cavernosal arteries pre- and postpapaverine injections. Patients with pelvic fracture may have arteriogenic insufficiency leading to impotence. Patients with bilateral affection need revascularization procedure prior to urethroplasty. Otherwise, they may land with bulbar urethral necrosis following mobilization and proximal transection of the bulbar urethra as this part gets its blood supply in a retrograde fashion through corpora cavernosa into glans and penile urethra. As this retrograde blood supply is inadequate, the bulbar urethra undergoes necrosis or stenosis.

Normally the systolic velocity in the cavernosal artery should be 30–35 cm/sec. A difference of more than 10 cm/sec indicates presence of arterial stenosis.

Penile Doppler in cases of pelvic fracture injury also has medicolegal implications. Impotence in cases of pelvic fracture is due to the initial injury itself. Hence, documenting the arteriogenic impotence is necessary preoperatively. It also helps in patient counseling.

Thus, penile Doppler is useful to identify patients at risk of bulbar urethral necrosis and impotence. It is an essential tool in patient counseling. Thus, a patient of arteriogenic impotence is informed that he will have to first undergo urethral reconstruction, and may subsequently require penile prosthesis after successful urethral surgery. He needs to be informed that as per literature, impotence is related to the initial injury and not as a result of surgery.

Urethrosonography

The use of ultrasonography to evaluate anterior urethral strictures was first reported by McAninch et al. in 1988. He suggested that sonourethrography was consistently more accurate in estimating stricture length than urethrography **(Figs 3.7A and B)**. It is a dynamic three-dimensional study and can be repeated without risk of radiation exposure. Sonourethrography is preferable to radiographic RGU to evaluate patients with suspected anterior urethral strictures. Initially using a 5 MHz linear-array transducer applied over dorsum of the penis, the contemporary technique involves use of a 7.5 MHz linear-array transducer applied directly to ventrum of the penis, scrotum and perineum. Initial studies suggested injecting saline in urethra. Recent literature suggests use of lignocaine jelly in the urethra.

Morey AF and McAninch JW et al.[1,2] in their prospective study in 1997 and review article in 2000 concluded that sonographic staging of anterior urethral strictures offers clinically important information that may be useful in guiding reconstructive therapy, and also suggested excisional therapy for strictures appearing sonographically to be 25 mm or less, and substitution urethroplasty for longer strictures.

Advantages of Sonourethrography

- Accurate length of stricture
- Length of spongiofibrosis

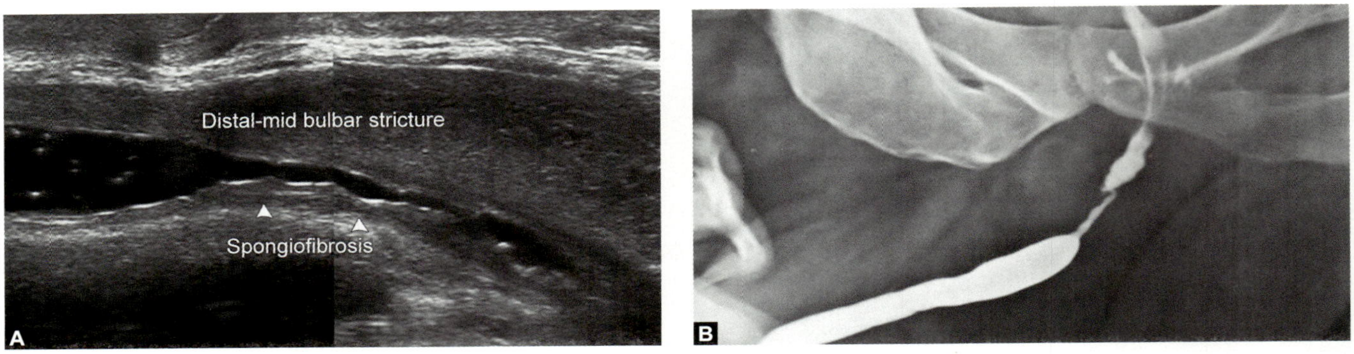

Figs 3.7A and B: Bulbar urethral stricture—sonourethrogram and retrograde urethrogram (RGU). Point to note is the spongiofibrosis extends well beyond the measured length of stricture on RGU

- Depth of spongiofibrosis
- Associated abnormalities like diverticulum, stones
- No radiation exposure.

Disadvantages of Sonourethrography

- Operator dependent
- As of now it had limited role in evaluation of posterior strictures.

MAGNETIC RESONANCE IMAGING

Magnetic resonance imaging (MRI) can be used in two ways as far as stricture disease is concerned. There are papers regarding magnetic resonance urethrography. The current use of MRI is in cases of posterior strictures after pelvic trauma and complex redo surgeries of PFUDDs **(Fig. 3.8)**. Preoperative MRI can provide useful information that might help to determine the appropriate surgical repair. It has the following advantages:[3]

- It correctly estimates length of the urethral defect
- Type and degree of prostatic displacement
- Precisely delineates the site and density of scar tissue
- Reveals the presence of paraurethral false tracks
- MRI can identify cause of post-traumatic impotence such as avulsion of the corpus.

To authors' understanding of stricture disease, routinely MRI is required in few selected cases. A good reconstructive urethral surgeon has all the tools in his armamentarium by which he can perform from simple to advanced procedures such as transpubic urethroplasty. This is a part of progressive perineal approach. Truly authors use MRI only in complex redo cases or in patients who are operated outside their set-up and they suspect that the posterior urethra was directly anastomosed to bladder bypassing the prostatic urethra.

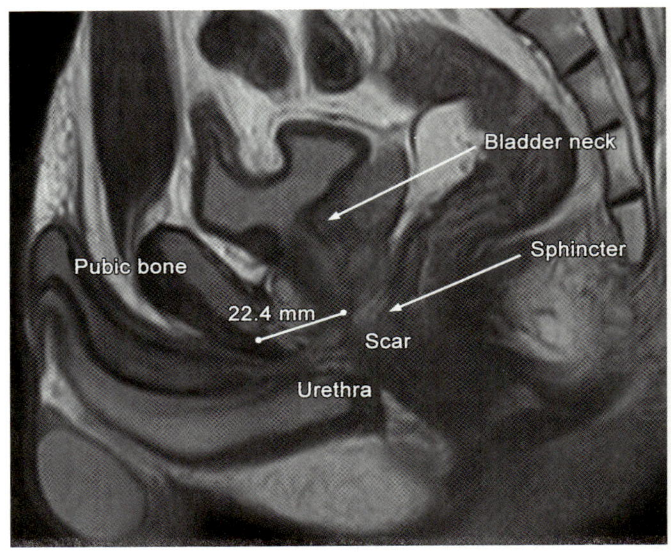

Fig. 3.8: An MRI done in a complex redo case

CONCLUSION

So to conclude, imaging forms an important part in evaluation and decision making in stricture urethra. Ascending urethrogram remains an indispensable, simple, affordable and reproducible investigation that forms the cornerstone of stricture disease evaluation.

EDITORIAL COMMENTS

Dr Rajesh Gulia

Decoding Erectile Dysfunction in PFUDD

As a urethral reconstructive surgeon, one should have the basic knowledge of how to interpret a well done penile

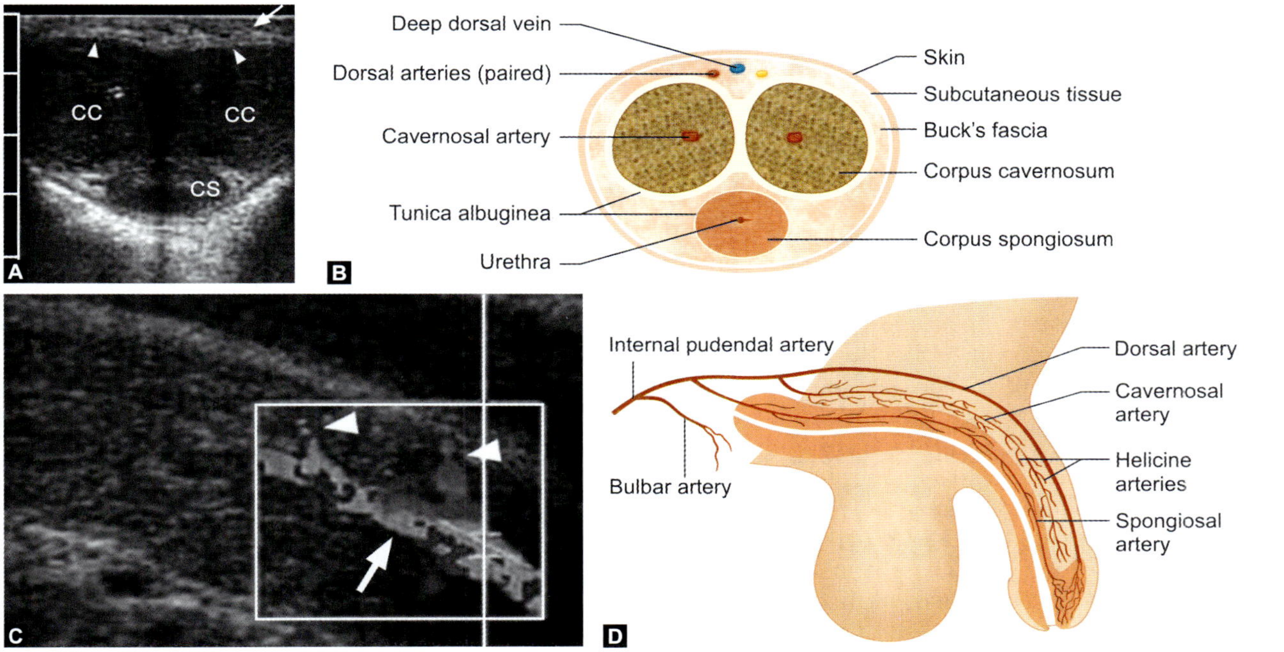

Figs 3.9A to D: Normal sonogram of penis. (A) Transverse gray-scale ultrasound of the penis demonstrates the two corpora cavernosa (CC) surrounded by the tunica albuginea (arrowhead). The corpus spongiosum (CS) is seen inferior to the corpora cavernosa. All three corpora are surrounded by the Buck's fascia (arrow); (B) The corresponding line diagram; (C) Longitudinal color flow Doppler ultrasound of normal cavernosal bodies and flow through cavernosal artery (arrow) and the helicine branches (arrowheads); (D) The corresponding line diagram of blood supply to the penis

Doppler study and to extract the required information. One cannot underestimate its importance in prognosticating the outcomes in PFUDD cases, especially so in patients with decreased erections, (or a cold or insensate glans), failed prior urethroplasty and the elderly.

Normal Sonogram of the Penis

Below is shown how a *normal sonogram of the penis* looks like **(Figs 3.9A to D)**.

Doppler Findings in Various Phases of Erection

Also important is to understand the *Doppler findings in various phases of erection,* as illustrated in **Figures 3.10A to D**.

Certain Points in Interpretation of Penile Doppler

Peak flow rates less than 25 cm/sec are abnormally low, and peak flow rates greater than 35 cm/sec are normal, but the range of 25–35 cm/sec is equivocal. The parameters that indicate the presence of arterial disease are:

- A subnormal clinical response to vasoactive agents
- A less than 60% increase in diameter of the cavernosal artery
- A peak systolic velocity of the cavernosal arteries less than 25 cm/sec
- Recently, Speel et al.[4] reported that acceleration time was the most valid parameter to detect cavernous atherosclerotic pathology. Blood flow velocity in the cavernous artery following pharmacostimulation was determined with duplex ultrasonography in 106 patients with erectile dysfunction (ED). The cutoff point for acceleration time to discriminate between atherosclerotic and nonatherosclerotic ED was determined at acceleration time 100 milliseconds or greater. Sensitivity was 66% and specificity was 71%.

In the presence of normal arterial function, Doppler findings suggestive of an abnormal venous leak are:

- Persistent end diastolic velocity of the cavernosal artery greater than 5 cm/sec
- Demonstration of flow in the deep dorsal vein
- The development of diastolic flow reversal after an injection has been found to be a reliable indicator of venous competence.

Although the accurate diagnostic procedure for venous leak diagnosis is infusion cavernosometry after maximal vasodilatation, this is rarely employed owing to poor surgical results of venous leak repair.

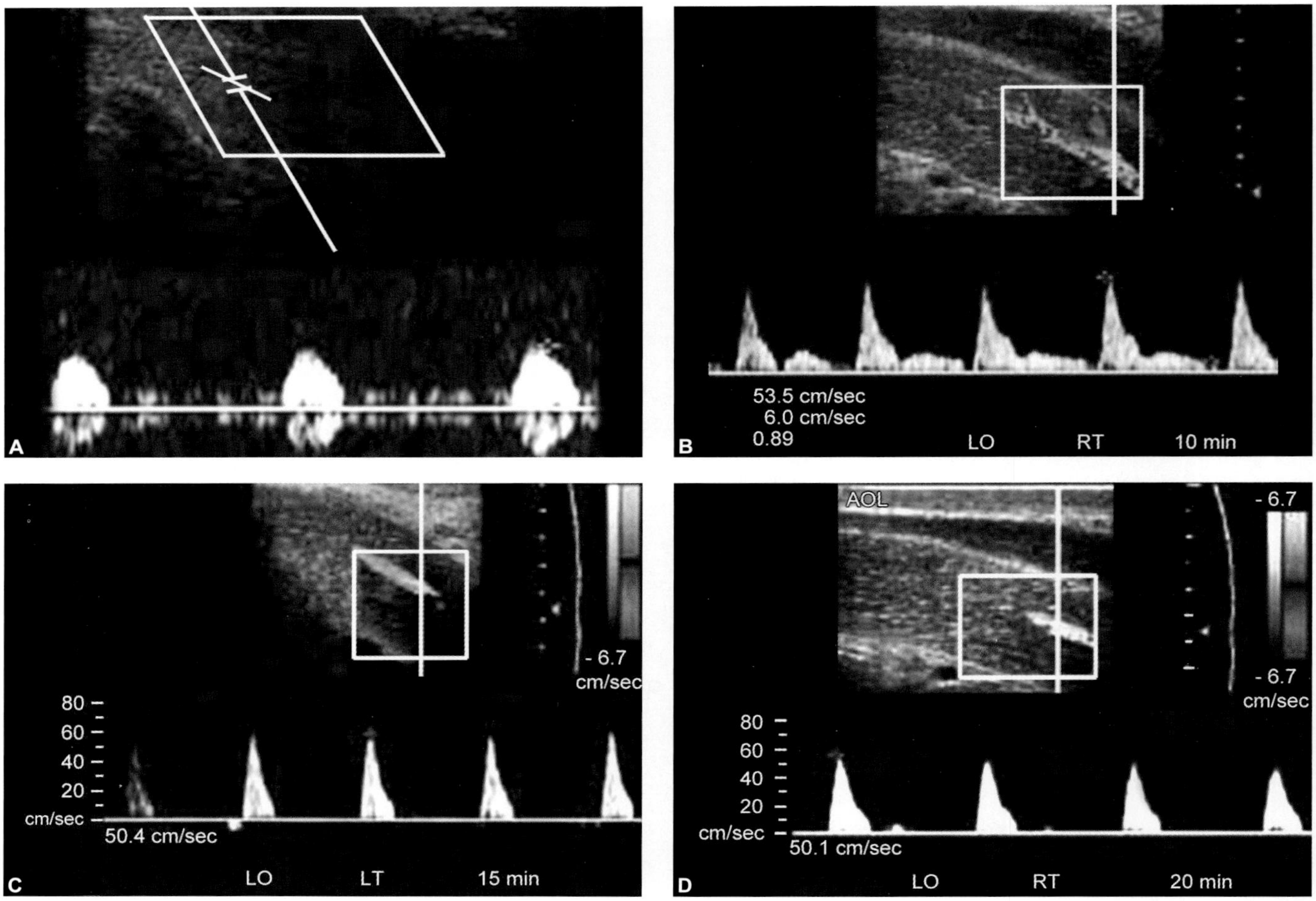

Figs 3.10A to D: Phases of erection. (A) Flaccid phase—spectral Doppler waveform demonstrates high resistance waveform. Velocities are in the range of 5–15 cm/sec; (B) Filling phase—spectral Doppler waveform demonstrates increased systolic velocity and increased diastolic flow; (C) Tumescent phase—the systolic velocities stabilize, diastolic flow decreases or becomes reversed; (D) Rigid phase—spectral Doppler waveform demonstrates very high resistance waveform with no diastolic flow and minimal systolic flow. The peak systolic velocities decrease

Procedure of Penile Doppler (Steps)

High-frequency (7.5–14 MHz) linear-array transducers are used to obtain high-resolution images of the penis. The cavernosal artery is visualized on the medial portion of the corpora cavernosa. Owing to the variation in peak systolic velocity (PSV) of the cavernosal artery at different locations across shaft of the penis (PSV is higher proximally), PSV should be consistently measured at junction of the proximal one-third and distal two-thirds of the penile shaft. Cavernosal artery velocities in healthy volunteers measure 10–15 cm/sec in the nonerect condition. Cavernous arteries should be identified and their action potential dimension is measured. When pharmacological testing is required, papaverine injection 30–60 μg (1–2 ml) is injected to one of the corpora cavernosa laterally in distal part of the penis with a 30-gauge needle. Injection should always be made in the distal two-thirds part of the penis on one side only because of the presence of a septum in between the two corpora cavernosa in proximal part of the penis, which is deficient distally, thus allowing bilateral perfusion of the injected vasoactive substance. Besides papaverine, other vasoactive agents used are prostaglandin E1, 10–20 mg and trimix (combination of papaverine, phentolamine and prostaglandin E1). Trimix is reserved for those patients who do not respond to prostaglandin.

Neurogenic Impotence

Having stressed the importance of vascular work-up in PFUDD, the majority of patients after the primary injury have neurogenic impotence (in some series up to 90%). These are the patients more likely to respond to sildenafil/ self-injection therapy with vasoactive agents, than those with arterial damage. A favorable response to these may predict spontaneous resumption of normal erectile function over time. Though it is stressed that first surgery does not contribute to any potent person becoming impotent, in a redo urethroplasty, the chances of fresh ED are higher. Bilateral pubic rami fracture was also associated with a high incidence of impotence.

Disruption of the cavernosal nerves lateral to the prostatomembranous urethra behind the symphysis pubis is the most likely cause of impotence in this injury. The cavernosal nerves are a part of the autonomic nervous system and incorporate both sympathetic and parasympathetic fibers. They regulate blood flow during erection and detumescence. The dorsal somatic nerves are branches of the pudendal nerves. They are primarily responsible for penile sensation.

Acknowledgments

To all the patients with stricture urethra.
Yogesh Sovani for images of sonourethrography.

REFERENCES

1. Morey AF, McAninch JW. Role of preoperative sonourethrography in bulbar urethral reconstruction. J Urol. 1997;158(4):1376-9.
2. Morey AF, McAninch JW. Sonographic staging of anterior urethral strictures. Review article. J Urol. 2000; 163(4):1070-5.
3. Mamdouh M, Koraitim, Ihab SR. Role of magnetic resonance imaging in assessment of posterior urethral distraction defects. Urology. 2007;70(3):403-6.
4. Speel TG, van Langen H, Wijkstra H, et al. Penile duplex pharmacoultrasonography revisited: revalidation of the parameters of the cavernous arterial response. J Urol 2003;169(1):216-20.

4

CHAPTER

The Role of Urethrotomy and Other Minimally Invasive Interventions

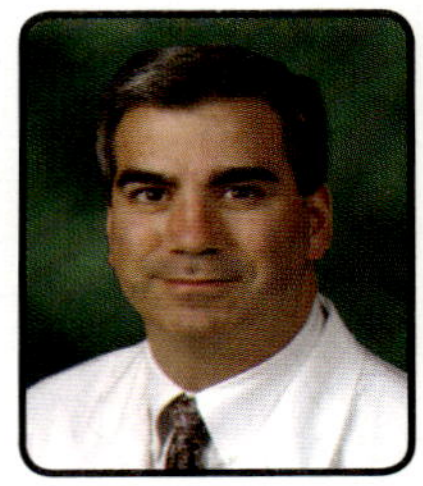

Richard Santucci

Richard Santucci, Mang L Chen

Chapter Outline

Abstract

Though urethroplasty offers cure, this chapter very vividly highlights the role of direct visual internal urethrotomy (DVIU). The correct technique of doing it, and the end point of the cut which is very vital in giving successful outcomes. Also highlighted are the other minimally invasive procedures like urethral stenting. Their role and place in the armamentarium of a urethral surgeon. Endoscopic realignment in cases of pelvic floor urethral distraction defect (PFUDD) is being talked about in workshops and is the hot topic wherever stricture urethra is discussed. Another promising procedure seems to be endoscopic urethroplasty. It has been explained in detail by the author. Every urethral surgeon must be aware of these procedures.

Keywords

Urethral dilatation, DVIU, Urethral stent, Endoscopic realignment, Endoscopic urethroplasty.

INTRODUCTION

Male urethral stricture disease causes significant obstructive and irritating voiding symptoms that are physically, mentally and financially exhausting. It has a prevalence as high as 0.6% (in US males treated at Veteran's hospitals) and accounts for about 5,000 inpatient and 150,000 outpatient US visits yearly, with an estimated annual cost of US $ 6,000 per patient[1] per year (year 2000). The prevalence, incidence and economic impact of this disease are expected to rise with an ever-aging population. Minimally-invasive therapies including urethral dilations, urethrotomy, urethral stents and other endoscopic treatment modalities are popular methods of management, although it is important to note that their success rates are low—no higher than 50% at best, and as low as 0% at worst.

In this chapter, we will discuss endoscopic treatment options for patients with "inflammatory" or idiopathic anterior urethral strictures. We submit that these are best used for: (1) short strictures, (2) strictures recurrent after urethroplasty and (3) patients who are unfit for open urethroplasty.

URETHRAL DILATION AND DIRECT VISUAL INTERNAL URETHROTOMY

Introduction

Urethral dilation arguably arose from urethral catheter development.[2] In their infancy, urethral catheters routinely dislodged. This led to the development of the first retention balloon catheter by JE Rebard in 1853. Comfortable latex catheters with intravesical balloons were later developed and popularized by Dr Frederic Foley in 1935. However, prior to this, balloon-attached catheters were used for urethral dilation. English military surgeon James Guthrie described balloon urethral dilation in 1825. Urethral dilation has since evolved into a wire-guided procedure with controlled balloon expansion and gradually enlarging catheter-shaped followers made up of plastic and metal.

Blind urethrotomy was practiced for over a century prior to the development of appropriate visual and cutting tools.[3] Sachse in 1973 performed the first direct visual internal urethrotomy (DVIU) with a specially designed scalpel. DVIUs are now performed with either an endoscopic scalpel or laser fiber.

Results of Dilation and Urethrotomy

The long-term outcomes between dilations and urethrotomies are very similar and have a high recurrence or failure rate. Steenkamp et al. prospectively evaluated 210 men with strictures who were randomized to receive either urethral dilations or internal urethrotomies and followed them every 3 months for the 1st year and annually thereafter for several years.[4] They concluded that the failure rate at 12 months was 40% for short strictures and 80% for longer strictures. The failure rate was also time-dependent since most strictures recurred within 6 months, and those who did not fail after 12 months were stricture free for longer periods of time. The same investigative group reported on the efficacy of repeat dilations and urethrotomies.[5] In the subpopulation who remained stricture-free 3 months after initial dilation or urethrotomy, 55–60% were disease-free at 2 years and 50–60% were disease-free at 4 years. After a second procedure, the subpopulation of patients who were stricture-free 3 months later remained stricture-free 30–50% of the time at 2 years and 0–40% at 4 years. After a third procedure, the stricture-free rate at 2 years was 0%. Santucci and Eisenberg confirmed the low success rate of urethrotomy by performing a retrospective chart review of 76 stricture patients who underwent urethrotomy.[6] They found that the stricture-free rate after the initial urethrotomy was 8% with a median time to recurrence of 7 months. The stricture-free rate after the second urethrotomy was even lower at 6% with a median time to recurrence of 9 months. Third urethrotomies had a stricture-free rate of 9% with a median time to recurrence of 3 months. Patients undergoing their fourth and fifth urethrotomies had stricture recurrence. In general, after an unsuccessful initial urethrotomy or dilation, open repair should be sought. In the subset of very long strictures, perhaps greater than or equal to 4 cm, the urologist should strongly consider initial open repair since the chance of urethrotomy failure is so high in this population.

Procedure/Technique of Dilation/Urethrotomy

Dilation can be done by cystoscopically placing a wire past the stricture and into the bladder followed by serial dilations with increasingly larger dilators, or balloon dilating catheters. A urethral catheter with an opening at the tip (Council catheter) is then advanced over the wire and into the bladder. We prefer to use a commercial catheter tip punch device to convert any catheter we like into a "Council catheter" (Cook Medical; Bloomington, IN). This procedure is done with local anesthesia in the supine position.

Visual urethrotomy oftentimes requires sedation or general anesthesia with patient in the dorsal lithotomy position. A 22 F cystoscope is then used to cannulate the urethra and identify the stricture. We then place a wire into the bladder, and the endoscopic scalpel or laser fiber is advanced into view. We next incise the stricture at the 10, 12 and/or 2 o'clock position depending on the size and density of the stricture. Care is taken to make an adequate incision—enough to cut through the stricture but not to overly violate the corpus spongiosum or enter the corpus cavernosa.

All patients get preoperative antibiotics within 1 hour prior to the procedure. Those with urinary tract infections get a therapeutic course of culture specific antibiotics prior to urethral manipulation.

Postoperative Care after Dilation/Urethrotomy

Dilation is an outpatient procedure. In general, patients go home with a urethral catheter for 3–4 days. They are given postoperative pain medication and an oral antimicrobial like nitrofurantoin for as long as the catheter remains, although we acknowledge that no trials exist to support the utility of postprocedure antimicrobials in this population. We then follow the patients every 3 months with uroflow, postvoid residual, and symptom check to assess for disease recurrence, which for most will inevitably occur. We find value in the uroflow pattern since recurrence shows as a flattened prolonged curve.

Alternatives to Dilation/Urethrotomy

Urethral stricture management very much depends on location and length of stricture. Since dilation and urethrotomy are often used to treat short strictures of the bulbar urethra or bladder neck (prostate surgery), alternatives include the following: (1) chronic urethral catheterization; (2) periodic clean intermittent catheterization (CIC) to maintain patency; (3) urethral stenting; (4) endoscopic urethroplasty; (5) suprapubic cystostomy tube; and (6) open urethroplasty with buccal mucosa onlay, skin graft onlay, fasciocutaneous flap, or scar excision and primary anastomosis.

STENTS

Introduction

Urethral stenting was first described in 1980 by Fabian for treatment of prostatic urethral strictures.[7] About a decade later, reports arose about the benefit of stenting in urethral stricture disease[8] and detrusor sphincter dyssynergia.[9] These initial reports were favorable, but with longer follow-up; complications such as pain, infection, stent migration, restenosis, and encrustation or stone formation became much more prevalent. The FDA therefore recommended that stents should not be used in stricture patients under 30 years of age, strictures longer than 3 cm, or strictures located in the penile urethra. Urolume [American Medical Systems (AMS); Minnetonka, MN] is a permanent implantable urethral stent most often used for urethral strictures. Authors never or almost never use the Urolume system for urethral strictures, favoring definitive surgical repair instead.

Results of Urethral Stents

The North American Study Group long-term data on urethral stents revealed that the overall complication rate was more than 70% over 11 years.[10] A subsequent study from the Netherlands found that only 2 of the 15 (13%) patients implanted had subjectively satisfactory results at 10 years.[11] Due to their ease of use, stents are often overutilized and misused for various urethral strictures that could have been more appropriately managed with other techniques. In general, experts in urethral reconstruction do not use urethral stents for bulbar urethral strictures. Furthermore, urethral stents should never be used for penile urethral strictures or urethral scarring after pelvic floor urethral distraction defects (PFUDDs).

Urethral stents may have some utility in patients with anastomotic stricture after radical prostatectomy since other treatments in this patient population can have an unacceptably high morbidity rate. Eisenberg et al. supported posterior urethral stent placement in patients with prior prostate cancer therapy as long as the surgeons expect, and the patients accept a high complication and failure rate.[12]

Procedure/Technique for Urethral Stent Placement

Stent placement is an outpatient procedure that is often done with local/spinal anesthesia, sedation or general anesthesia. Patients are placed in dorsal lithotomy and the stricture is identified cystoscopically. We then place a wire into the bladder and dilate the urethra to 30 F with urethral dilators or optical urethrotomy. Stricture length is then approximated with the AMS measuring catheter or a ureteral measuring catheter. We then select a stent that is 1 cm longer than the estimated stricture length. Urolume comes with a 24 F delivery system that includes its own telescope and outer sheath. This system is then inserted into the urethra and the stent is deployed starting 5 mm proximal to and ending 5 mm distal to the stricture. For longer strictures, overlapping stents are used and they must overlap by 5 mm. Avoid incorporating the membranous urethra, since incontinence can result.

Postoperative Care after Urethral Stents

All patients receive perioperative antibiotics and are told to avoid straddling activities like bicycling or horseback riding. We try not to perform any urethral intubation (i.e. catheter or cystoscopy) for 4–6 weeks to allow urothelial incorporation of the stent. Patients are then followed every 3–6 months to assess for symptom recurrence and complications.

Alternatives to Urethral Stent Procedure

Alternatives are similar to those listed for dilation and DVIU. However, given that more appropriate stenting is now done for posterior urethral strictures associated with prostate cancer therapy, alternatives include: (1) suprapubic cystostomy; (2) endoscopic management, urethral catheterization, CIC, urethral dilation, or DVIU; or the standard (3) open repair with scar/stricture excision with or without prostatectomy and primary anastomosis.

ENDOSCOPIC REALIGNMENT OF PFUDD

Introduction

In discussing urethral stricture disease, we must always be clear about the differences between inflammatory strictures (true strictures) and distraction injuries (not true strictures) that occur after pelvic fracture. Pelvic fracture urethral distraction defects occur in approximately 10% of patients with pelvic fractures **(Fig. 4.1)**. Immediate management includes retrograde urethrogram **(Fig. 4.2)** with either early primary realignment or suprapubic cystostomy. Definitive management, which is undertaken 2–6 months after the inciting event, involves scar excision and primary anastomosis. Many citations espouse the efficacy of endoscopic incision ("cut to the light" procedures) and laser ablation of PFUDDs, but most experts avoid them except in rare recurrent strictures or extremely flimsy strictures.

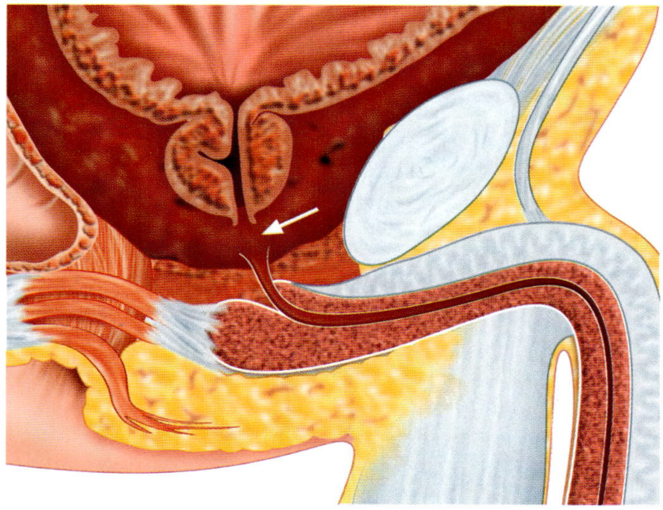

Fig. 4.1: Pelvic floor urethral distraction defect. Anatomic illustration reveals complete separation between membranous urethra and prostatic urethra (arrow), although most defects occur at the bulbomembranous urethral junction

Results of Endoscopic Realignment of PFUDD

Early primary realignment was examined by Elliott et al. who retrospectively reviewed 53 patients with PFUDDs who underwent primary realignment within 6 hours after injury.[13] Mean follow-up was 10.5 years and strictures were seen in 36 of the 53 patients (66%). Of these 36 patients, 23 (64%) required either no procedure or outpatient dilation; 13 (36%) required operative intervention. Of these 13 patients, 9 (69%) were managed endoscopically and 4 (31%) underwent open repair. A smaller study from Israel looked at early endoscopic realignment in 11 patients suffering from PFUDDs and found similar stricture results with 5 patients (45%) developing strictures.[14] Generally speaking, if early primary realignment can be easily achieved, we would do it since it may obviate the need for surgery (40–60% of cases) and facilitate open surgery by positioning the disrupted urethral ends closer together.

A study from Egypt by Shawky reviewed endoscopic management of post-traumatic urethral obliteration.[15] Overall, there were 396 patients, 79 (20%) of whom failed initial DVIU and subsequently required endoscopic resection of scar. After a mean follow-up of 2 years, 46 of these 79 patients (58%) were subjectively voiding satisfactorily. The remaining 33 patients (42%) required open urethroplasty. A similar study from the Mayo Clinic looked at pediatric post-traumatic urethral obliteration and found that laser or cold knife resection for re-establishing urethral continuity failed in all 22 patients.[16] Only 2 out of 22 patients (9%) were able to maintain urethral patency, and this was only possible with periodic self-catheterization. The remaining patients underwent open repair. We must emphasize that scar excision and primary anastomosis is the gold standard treatment for PFUDDs with a stricture-free rate of about 85%.

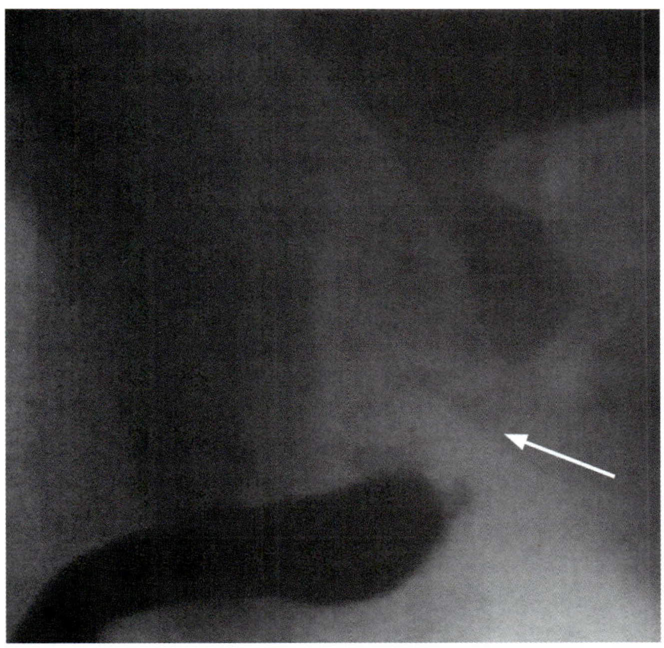

Fig. 4.2: Retrograde urethrogram (RUG) showing complete disruption of urethral continuity (arrow). Bladder opacification is not from RUG contrast but from prior IV contrast that has been renally cleared

Procedure/Technique for Endoscopic Realignment of PFUDD

In suspected urethral injuries, we perform a retrograde urethrogram in the trauma bay. If contrast makes it into the bladder, a single careful attempt at retrograde urethral catheter insertion is made. If this fails, we attempt a bedside placement of a Council catheter using flexible cystoscopy. If this fails, we either place a suprapubic cystostomy tube, or if possible, take the patient immediately to the operating room (OR) for another attempt at cystoscopy using rigid instruments. If this fails, we place a suprapubic tube in the OR.

In those patients who are going to the OR urgently for an exploratory laparotomy, we still attempt primary endoscopic realignment **(Fig. 4.3)** as long as the patient is stable from a general surgery standpoint. Techniques to place the catheter can be assisted by several maneuvers. First we attempt a flexible cystoscope at the bedside. Then we attempt a rigid cystoscopy in the OR (this may not be possible if the patient cannot be put in lithotomy). Next, we attempt a flexible cystoscopy through the suprapubic tract, which may require dilation of the tract over a wire. Next we attempt a two-cystoscope technique where the flexible cystoscope is passed from above and the rigid cystoscope from below **(Fig. 4.4)**. We can turn off the light of suprapubic flexible scope, aiming toward the light of rigid scope.

However, describing the procedure is much easier than doing the procedure since navigating through hematoma and soft tissue injury is frequently unproductive, frustrating and even dangerous. We seldom work for longer than 30 minutes at a time, favoring placement of a suprapubic tube and trying again in 2–3 days if the initial attempts fail. While we have not seen evidence of infection or other harm from absorption of cystoscopic fluid into the hematoma, we are concerned that overly prolonged attempts may harm the patient.

Procedure/Technique for Endoscopic Incision of PFUDD

We must be again clear that we favor the treatment of PFUDD with urethroplasty. In some rare or unusual cases, incision of the defect is preferred, including patients who cannot tolerate lithotomy position, who refuse surgery, or who suffer failure after definitive urethroplasty. Under spinal or general anesthesia, patient is placed in the dorsal lithotomy position. We perform cystoscopy to identify the obliterated urethral lumen, which often will have a tiny fistula through the scar, especially if his urine is not diverted with a suprapubic tube **(Fig. 4.5)**. If a guidewire cannot be placed from below, then we perform flexible cystoscopy from above and attempt to pass the wire from above. We favor a slightly stiffer "hydrophilic" guidewire (Boston Scientific; Natick, MA) over the less stiff hydrophilic gulidewire (Terumo Medical; Somerset, NJ). If this fails, two methods may be used. Often there is a residual tiny lumen. If so, we will make small, judicious, careful and superiorly-oriented cuts with the urethrotome in hopes of breaking into a wider lumen that will allow wire passage. Caution is advised with this maneuver. If this fails then a "cut to the light" or "cut to the sound" technique may be used. We then cannulate the suprapubic cystostomy

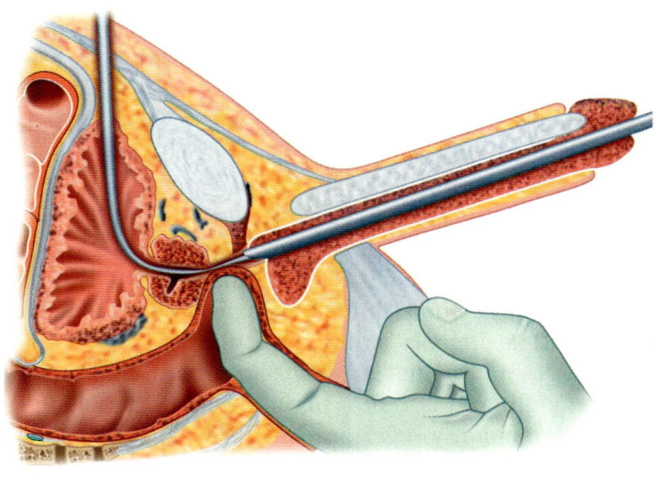

Fig. 4.3: Primary endoscopic realignment with use of a curved sound and cystoscope. Concomitant digital rectal examination may assist in re-establishing urethral continuity

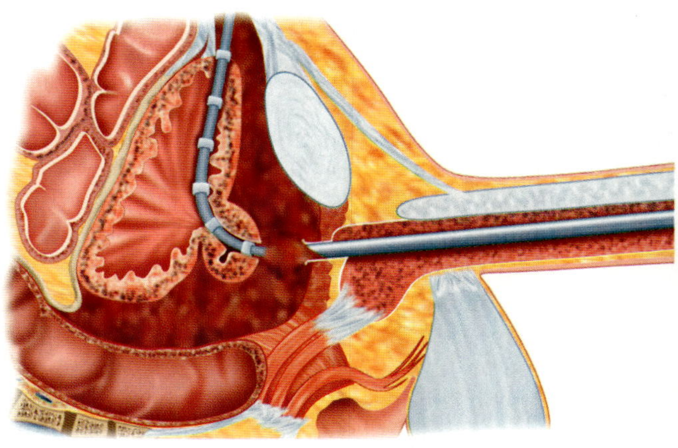

Fig. 4.4: Cut to the light procedure with a suprapubic flexible cystoscopy and urethral rigid cystoscopy

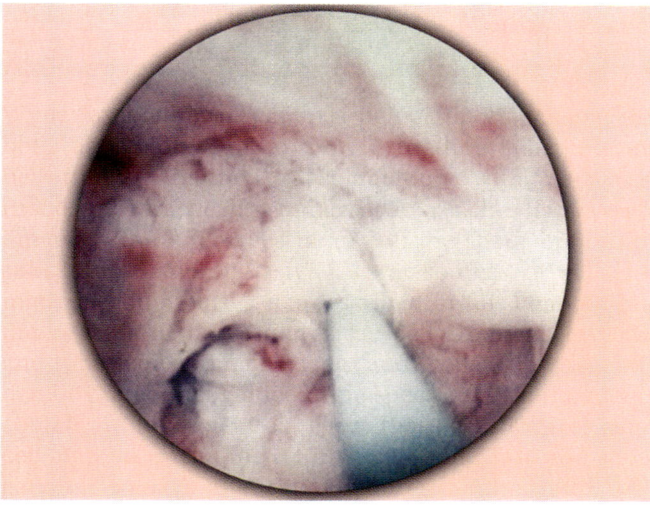

Fig. 4.5: Wall of scar seen with pelvic fracture urethral disruption defect (PFUDD). The wire is placed through a pinhole fistula into the bladder, if possible, to facilitate endoscopic scar excision or direct visual internal urethrotomy (DVIU)

tract with a curved metal sound (Bard; Covington, GA) and direct it toward the bladder neck. Concomitant digital rectal examination allows palpation of the metal sound and blind but judicious urethrotomy toward the sound tip is carried out until urethral continuity can be established **(Fig. 4.3)**. We sometimes use fluoroscopy for visualization, if the obliterated segment is long. If the obliterated segment is short, suprapubic cystoscopy will illuminate proximal end of the scar tissue and we will essentially cut to the light. Once urethral continuity is established, we place a Council catheter over the wire. We also replace the suprapubic tube.

Postoperative Care

All patients are given perioperative antibiotics and prophylactic nitrofurantoin for as long as the catheter is in place. We leave the catheter for a short period of time—72 hours. We then remove the urethral catheter and clamp the suprapubic tube. If the patient voids satisfactorily, the suprapubic tube is removed a few weeks later. Close follow-up is initiated and if the stricture recurs, either repeat incision (not preferred) or urethroplasty (preferred) are performed.

Alternatives to Endoscopic Realignment of PFUDD

Alternatives to endoscopic realignment and endoscopic urethroplasty for PFUDDs include lifelong suprapubic cystostomy urinary diversion, DVIU/dilation with self-catheterization, or the gold standard delayed posterior urethroplasty. If the initial attempt at bedside retrograde catheter insertion fails, we favor managing the PFUDD with a suprapubic cystostomy tube with planned scar excision and primary anastomosis in 6–12 weeks. Such timing allows most of the urgent medical issues to resolve so that the patient can tolerate a 2–4 hour operation in the extended dorsal lithotomy position. Delayed open reconstruction is the better option because elective operative intervention shortly after the inciting trauma can add unnecessary stress to an already stressed body. Authors have been unimpressed with the data supporting self-instrumentation with urethral catheters to "stabilize the scar". Patients despise the technique as they find it painful and inconvenient, and authors have not seen good results in their many hundreds of patients.

ENDOSCOPIC URETHROPLASTY

Introduction

Endoscopic urethroplasty is defined as performing graft placement after DVIU using minimally invasive techniques. Its advantages over open urethroplasty include a smaller learning curve, shorter operative time and faster postoperative recovery. Peterson and Lunstam in 1977 performed the first endourethral urethroplasty by securing split-thickness skin grafts (STSGs) to urethral catheters inserted after performing DVIU.[17] Similarly, Gaur reported using STSG on modified urethral catheters that have two balloons: one to keep the catheter in the bladder and the other to keep the STSG apposed to the graft bed.[18] Though the idea was novel at the time, the results were unacceptable with poor graft take due to the frequent movement and resultant shear forces between graft and recipient bed. Naude described a more involved procedure with better graft fixation using a specifically designed graft delivery device that allowed endoscopic suture placement to secure the skin graft to the raw DVIU site.[19] In attempts to minimize morbidity, Le Roux in 2005 described endoscopic urethroplasty using small intestinal submucosa (SIS) grafts[20] instead of skin grafts.

Results of Endoscopic Urethroplasty

The largest study was performed by Naude who reported on his first 53 patients who underwent endoscopic skin-graft urethroplasty. At 2-year follow-up, the overall graft take was 95%, though this was broken down into types of urethral strictures treated. Patients with inflammatory or iatrogenic strictures all (100%) maintained their urethral patency. Of those with PFUDDs, approximately 50% maintained their patency.

Using the Naude technique, Le Roux's 2005 study on nine inflammatory stricture patients having SIS grafts endoscopically placed showed overall poor results; stricture recurrence was found in six patients (67%) within 3 months of surgery, two (22%) were disease free at 1 year, and one was lost to follow-up. Of the six patients, three (50%) had undergone open urethroplasty and two were awaiting urethroplasty. The remaining patient elected periodic self-dilation. Despite advances in endoscopic urethroplasty, we must emphasize that we strongly favor open urethral reconstruction due to its well-established high success rates, low morbidity and overall patient satisfaction.

Procedure/Technique of Endoscopic Urethroplasty

As with all endoscopic procedures, patients are sedated or generally anesthetized and placed in the dorsal lithotomy position. Optical urethrotomy is performed with an urethrotome at site of the stricture. However, the cut is made at the ventral aspect at the 6 o'clock position as opposed to the traditional 12 o'clock incision. A specially designed needle and suture is then placed in the perineum and directed toward the proximal end of the stricture; this is guided by feel and by cystourethroscopy. The surgeon now secures the suture with a transcystoscopic grasper and pulls it through the urethra. This "proximal" suture is inserted through the "proximal" graft and graft carrying device. The surgeon then places the graft carrying device and adhered graft alongside the cystoscope and pushes a transcystoscopic needle with suture through distal end of the stricture and through the perineum. The final result is a suture at the distal and proximal aspect of the graft with "tails" at the two perineal needle sites which are tied together, fixing the graft in place. Finally, a suprapubic catheter is inserted.

Postoperative Care after Endoscopic Urethroplasty

The suprapubic tube and specific graft carrying device are removed after 2 weeks. Patients are thereafter followed with urethroscopy at 6 weeks and 3 months postoperatively. Flow rates and postvoid residuals are recorded every 6 months for several years.

Alternatives to Endoscopic Urethroplasty

Endoscopic urethroplasty has been used to treat inflammatory strictures and PFUDDs. Treatment options for inflammatory strictures include those listed for dilation and DVIU. Treatment options for PFUDDs include primary realignment, primary suprapubic cystostomy, dilation/DVIU, and suprapubic cystostomy with delayed anastomotic urethroplasty. Given our long-term success with open urethral reconstruction and its associated mild and well-tolerated morbidity (pain, 1–2 weeks of urethral catheterization, infection, difficulty in eating if buccal mucosa is harvested), we do not perform endoscopic urethroplasty.

CONCLUSION

Dilation and urethrotomy will provide lasting cure in a minority of patients. Failure is generally only a matter of time. Solutions for decreasing re-stricture rates have been sought and include prolonged postdilation urethral catheterization, periodic but regular CIC, and intraurethral steroid injections with unimpressive results.[21] The fact remains though that urethral stricture is an open surgical disease. However, these endoscopic procedures will likely have a role in the initial or palliative management of primary or recurrent urethral strictures in patients unwilling or unfit to undergo definitive surgical repair.

REFERENCES

1. Santucci RA, Joyce GF, Wise M. Male urethral stricture disease. J Urol. 2007;177:1667-74.
2. Patel SR, Caldamone AA. The history of urethral catheterization. Med Health RI. 2004;87:240-2.
3. Smith PJ, Kaisary AV, Ball AJ. Late results of optical urethrotomy. J R Soc Med. 1984;77:105-7.
4. Steenkamp JW, Heyns CF, DeKock ML. Internal urethrotomy versus dilation as treatment for male urethral strictures: a prospective randomized comparison. J Urol. 1997;157:98-101.
5. Heyns CF, Steenkamp JW, DeCock ML. Treatment of male urethral strictures: is repeated dilation or internal urethrotomy useful? J Urol. 1998;160:356-8.
6. Santucci RA, Eisenberg L. Urethrotomy has a much lower success rate than previously reported. J Urol. 2010;183:1859-62.
7. Fabian KM. The intraprostatic "partial catheter" (urological spiral). Urologe A. 1980;19:236-8.
8. Milroy EJ, Chapple CR, Cooper JE. A new treatment for urethral strictures. Lancet. 1988;1:1424-7.
9. Shaw PJ, Milroy EJ, Timoney AG. Permanent external striated sphincter stents in patients with spinal injuries. Br J Urol. 1990;66:297-302.
10. Shah DK, Paul EM, Badlani GH. North American Study Group: 11-year outcome analysis of endourethral prosthesis for the treatment of recurrent bulbar urethral stricture. J Urol. 2003;170:1255-8.

11. De Vocht TF, van Venrooij GE, Boon TA. Self-expanding stent insertion for urethral strictures: a 10-year follow-up. BJU Int. 2003;91:627-30.
12. Eisenberg ML, Elliott SP, McAninch JW. Preservation of lower urinary tract function in posterior urethral stenosis: selection of appropriate patients for urethral stenosis. J Urol. 2007;178:2456-61.
13. Elliott DS, Barrett DM. Long-term follow-up and evaluation of primary realignment of posterior urethral disruptions. J Urol. 1997;157:814-6.
14. Sofer M, Mabjeesh NJ, Ben-Chaim J. Long-term results of early endoscopic realignment of complete posterior urethral disruption. J Endourol. 2010;24:1117-21.
15. Shawky AE. Endoscopic treatment of post-traumatic urethral obliteration: experience in 396 patients. J Urol. 1995;153:67-71.
16. Tollefson MK, Ashley RA, Routh JC. Traumatic obliterative urethral strictures in pediatric patients: failure of the cut to light technique in long-term follow-up. J Urol. 2007;178:1656-8.
17. Peterson S, Lunstam S. Endourethral urethroplasty: a simple method for treating urethral retraction. J Urol Nephrol. 1977;83:659-62.
18. Gaur DD. Endourethral urethroplasty—use of a new catheter. J Urol. 1983;130:905-8.
19. Naude JH. Endoscopic skin-graft urethroplasty. World J Urol. 1998;16:171-4.
20. Le Roux PJ. Endoscopic urethroplasty with unseeded small intestinal submucosa collagen matrix grafts. J Urol. 2005;173:140-3.
21. Hradec E, Jarolim L, Petrik R. Optical internal urethrotomy for strictures of the male urethra. Effect of local steroid injection. Eur Urol. 1981;7:165-8.

5

CHAPTER

Fossa Navicularis and Meatal Strictures

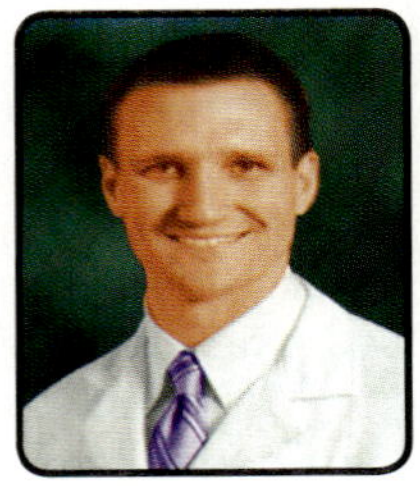

Geoffrey R Nuss

Geoffrey R Nuss, Chris M Gonzalez

Chapter Outline

Abstract

This chapter addresses the isolated strictures of the meatus and fossa navicularis, which are a unique challenge for the reconstructive urologist. Because of the distal location, reconstructive efforts require attention to establish not only urethral integrity, but also the cosmesis of the urethral meatus, glans, and penile shaft. Ideally, the meatus should be widely patent and located anatomically distal to the coronal sulcus in an attempt to recreate normal glans anatomy and facilitate a normal urinary stream. Described herein are few procedures in detail which come very handy in these type of strictures. Armenakas modified the Jordan technique, which resulted in glans preservation and better cosmesis. Other procedures described are—extended meatotomy, ventral transverse island penile skin flap, single and multistage buccal mucosal graft ventral onlay urethroplasty. A must read for any urethral surgeon.

Keywords

Meatal stricture, Fossa navicularis stricture, Lichen sclerosus (LS), Meatotomy, Extended meatotomy, Genital skin flap urethroplasty, Staged graft inlay urethroplasty, Armenakas urethroplasty, Ventral transverse island penile skin flap, Glans preserving urethroplasty.

INTRODUCTION

Isolated strictures of the meatus and fossa navicularis (FN) are a unique challenge for the reconstructive urologist. Because of the distal location, reconstructive efforts require attention to establish not only urethral integrity, but also cosmesis of the urethral meatus, glans and penile shaft. Ideally, the meatus should be widely patent and located anatomically distal to the coronal sulcus in an attempt to recreate normal glans anatomy and facilitate a normal urinary stream.

It has been estimated that isolated strictures of the meatus and FN can comprise up to 18% of anterior urethral strictures.[1] The etiology of distal urethral stricture disease varies and includes lichen sclerosus (LS), previous urethral instrumentation (iatrogenic), complications from previous hypospadias repair and rare conditions such as prior condyloma treatment and isolated urethral trauma.[2] Of these etiologies, LS appears to be the most common cause identified, responsible for 12–42% of isolated strictures of the FN or meatus.[1,2] Strictures due to LS are particularly difficult to treat due to the tissue destruction and high probability for disease recurrence.[3]

Urethroplasty techniques for strictures of the meatus and FN vary widely and include meatotomy, extended meatotomy, and various substitution techniques including genital skin flap urethroplasty, extragenital and genital patch graft urethroplasty, and staged graft inlay urethroplasty. This chapter reviews the available urethroplasty techniques for isolated strictures of the meatus and FN.

HISTORY

There have been multiple different reconstructive techniques described to address isolated strictures of the

FN and meatus over the past half-century. Early efforts focused on making a ventral urethrotomy and rotating or advancing a penile skin flap into the defect.[4-7] In 1967, Cohney described "urethroplasty" as a surgical procedure which involved a penile skin flap, derived from the preputial skin, folded upon itself to create both the ventral surface of the reconstructed urethra as well as its overlying penile skin coverage.[4] Critics of this procedure noted that it resulted in glans torsion and had a high rate of flap necrosis, presumably from compression of the vascular supply as it was folded upon itself.[5] Blandy and Tresidder described a procedure in which a ventral U-shaped penile skin flap was created and advanced into the ventral urethrotomy. They noted that this was simple to perform; however, the neomeatus opened in a subcoronal position creating a cosmetically undesirable hypospadiac meatus.[5] Brannen, observing that the subcoronal meatus was not an optimal cosmetic outcome, modified the technique described by Blandy and Tresidder. The U-shaped preputial flap was advanced into the ventral urethrotomy in a similar fashion; however, two additional epithelial incisions were made on either side of the ventral midline on the preputial shaft skin, creating an epithelial strip. This strip was then advanced into the meatal defect, thus recreating an orthotopic meatus.[6] In 1984, De Sy described a modification to the technique given by Brannen, utilizing a ventral U-shaped flap and a ventral epithelial strip. However, the epithelial layer on ventral portion of the flap was removed prior to closing lateral edges of the glans over repair. This was done in an effort to create a more anatomic appearing ventral glans.[7] Ultimately, all of these techniques were criticized for their complexity as well as suboptimal functional and cosmetic outcomes, and were subsequently modified or abandoned.[8]

More recently, the modified substitution techniques have gained wider favor among reconstructive urologists. In 1987, abandoning the rotational and advancement flap techniques, Jordan described a repair using a ventral transverse island penile skin flap. This technique eliminated glans torsion by mobilizing and closing the glans over the stricture repair and minimized flap ischemia by creating a wide vascular pedicle.[8] Armenakas subsequently reported a modified approach to Jordan's description; instead of dividing the glans prior to stricturotomy, glans is dissected off of underlying urethra intact and placed over ventral onlay of the fasciocutaneous flap.[9]

Current reconstructive techniques to address strictures of the FN employ modifications of these earlier techniques with the use of a fasciocutaneous skin flap or graft as an onlay. Furthermore, meatotomy and extended meatotomy represent options for limited meatal or distal FN repairs, respectively. As with any anterior urethral stricture, the etiology, length, location and surgeon preference should dictate the surgical approach.

TECHNIQUE

Extended Meatotomy

The most basic approach to the very distal FN stricture is extended meatotomy. If the stricture only affects the urethral meatus, simple meatotomy successfully corrects the stenotic segment. However, as the stricture extends proximally into the FN, extended meatotomy may be needed. In this procedure, the urethra is incised ventrally from the meatus and ultimately into the glans until the urethra and glans tissue are both found to be supple and patent. All scar tissue is sharply excised. The cut edges of the urethral mucosa are then reapproximated to the surrounding healthy glans tissue with interrupted, 4-0 absorbable suture **(Figs 5.1 and 5.2)**. We have found that dorsal incision of the urethral plate or glans is not useful with this procedure. A urethral catheter may be left for 1–2 days, but it is not usually necessary, especially for these relatively short strictures. Extended meatotomy may be a useful approach in patients with limited distal FN strictures, those who may not be candidates for a more complex urethroplasty or patients who have had multiple failed prior attempts at distal urethral reconstruction.[10] The success rate of extended meatotomy has been reported to

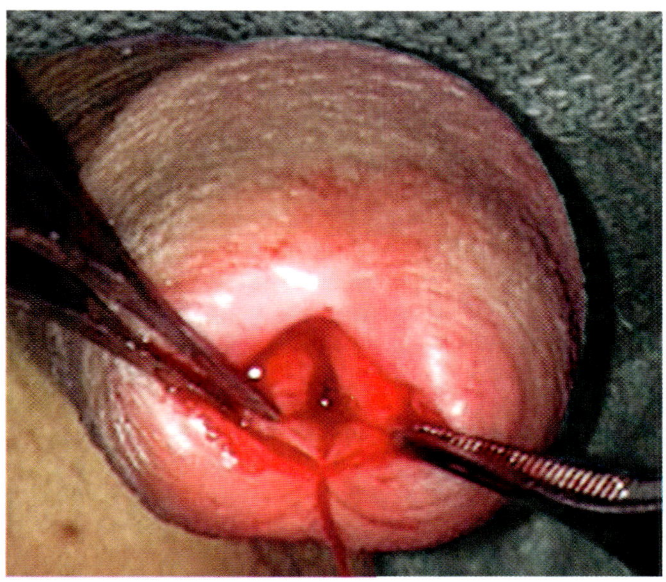

Fig. 5.1: Extended meatotomy. The healthy urethral mucosa is approximated to cut edge of the glans

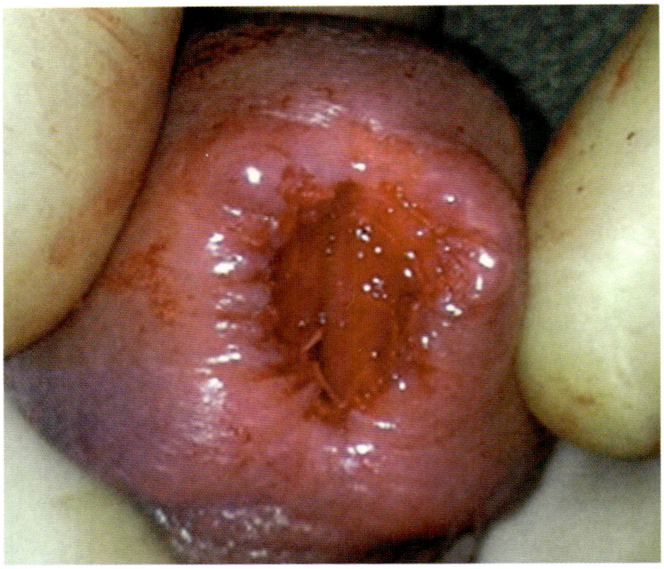

Fig. 5.2: Extended meatotomy. Note that the healthy urethral mucosa is reapproximated to the surrounding glans tissue with interrupted absorbable sutures

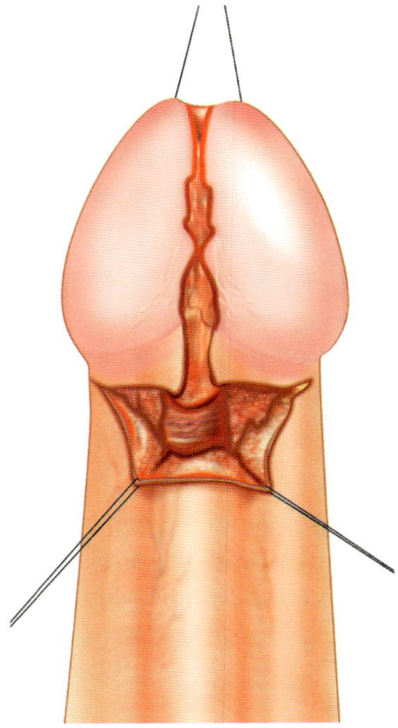

Fig. 5.3: Transverse island skin flap urethroplasty. A ventral subcoronal incision is made in the penile skin to expose the urethra, and a ventral urethrotomy is made through the strictured segment

be as high as 88%.[10] Potential drawbacks to this procedure are urinary spraying due to the proximal location of the neomeatus as well as a potentially unfavorable cosmetic appearance. These outcomes should be discussed with the patient prior to reconstruction.

Ventral Transverse Island Penile Skin Flap

This procedure is best suited for the FN strictures. First described by Jordan and modified by Armenakas, this technique utilizes an axial fasciocutaneous skin flap with the tunica dartos as the vascular pedicle.[8] First, a ventral subcoronal transverse incision is made to expose the urethra and the strictured segment. Next, the glans is divided and a longitudinal ventral urethrotomy is made through the strictured segment and extended into approximately 1–1.5 cm of healthy urethra proximally **(Fig. 5.3)**. A fasciocutaneous skin flap arising from the penile shaft bordering the proximal edge of the skin incision is fashioned and rotated on its dartos pedicle into the ventral urethral defect **(Fig. 5.4)**. The divided glans edges are then mobilized and reapproximated to cover the flap in a tension-free closure **(Fig. 5.5)**. Complications from this repair are largely related to flap ischemia and include stricture recurrence and fistula formation. Success rates have been reported to be as high as 96% and 83% at a mean follow-up of 30.2 months and 10.2 years, respectively.[11,12] This technique should be avoided if the presence of LS is evident or if the penile skin appears to be deficient.

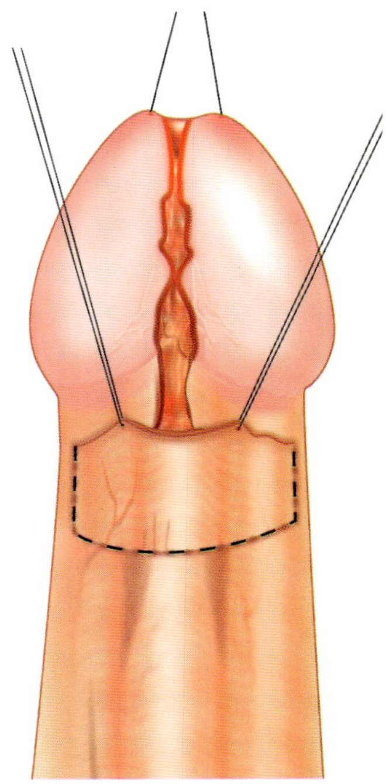

Fig. 5.4: Transverse island skin flap urethroplasty. The flap is outlined and its vascular pedicle is based on the tunica dartos

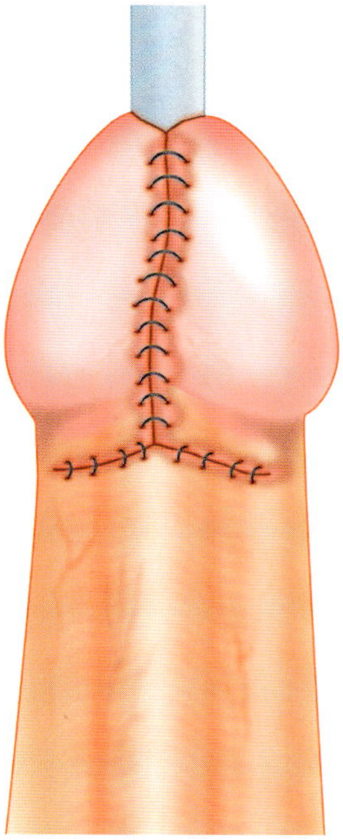

Fig. 5.5: Transverse island skin flap urethroplasty. The mobilized glans is closed over the ventral flap onlay

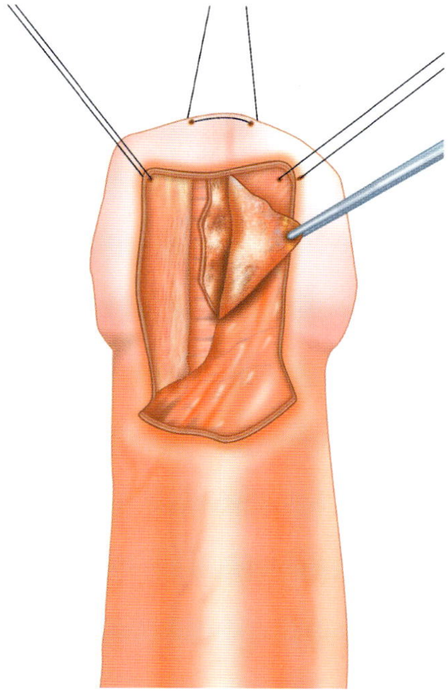

Fig. 5.6: Modified transverse island skin flap urethroplasty. The intact glans has been dissected off the urethra. The flap is then tunneled under the glans and sewn to the ventral urethrostomy

Modified Transverse Island Skin Flap Procedure

It is designed to preserve integrity of the overlying ventral glans, which has also proven useful for FN strictures.[9] In this procedure, the distal urethra is exposed through a transverse subcoronal penile skin incision. Next, the intact glans is dissected off the urethra creating a "glans cap". A ventral urethrotomy is made, and a fasciocutaneous flap is created from the ventral penile skin in a similar fashion to the previously described transverse island flap.[8] The fasciocutaneous skin flap is tunneled under the intact glans, and sutured to healthy epithelium of the ventral urethrotomy with 5-0 absorbable suture. Care should be taken to excise all strictured urethra and nonviable spongiosum **(Fig. 5.6)**. If stricture involves the meatus, flap is brought under the glans cap to meatus and sutured to surrounding healthy glans epithelium to create ventral portion of the neomeatus. The reported success rate of this approach is 94.7% at a mean follow-up of 42.7 months. Complications specific to this repair include transient spraying of the urinary stream, fistula formation and potential glans torsion due to the postoperative edema.[9] As with all techniques involving genital fasciocutaneous flaps, patients with LS and deficient penile skin should be offered an alternative technique utilizing extragenital tissue.

Buccal Mucosal Graft Urethroplasty

The concern for the relatively high rate of long-term failure of distal urethroplasty secondary to lichen sclerosis, previous urethroplasty, or deficient genital skin,[13,14] has led to the increasing use of buccal mucosal graft (BMG) for both single and multistaged substitution urethroplasty over the past several years. A multistaged approach is reserved for obliterative strictures, strictures due to extensive LS, and strictures as a result of failed hypospadias repair.

Single Stage Buccal Mucosal Graft Ventral Onlay

For the single-stage technique, the native dorsal urethral plate is left *in situ* and a ventral onlay graft is performed. To begin, a circumcising incision is made on the penile shaft. The skin and dartos fascia are sharply dissected away from the underlying urethra. To expose distal portion of the FN, the ventral glans is divided or dissected intact off the urethra. We prefer to keep the glans penis intact during this dissection as it provides for a better vascular bed over the graft and better overall cosmetic appearance. Once entirety of the strictured segment is exposed, a longitudinal ventral urethrotomy is made extending through the stricture into healthy urethral mucosa and corpus spongiosum. The scarred corpus spongiosum and urethral mucosa are then judiciously excised, taking care to preserve as much urethral plate as possible **(Fig. 5.7)**. The proximal and distal portion of the urethrotomy should calibrate to 24 F, using bougienage. To estimate dimensions of the buccal graft required for repair, length of the stricture and width of the urethral plate are measured. Generally, a 2–2.5 cm wide area of buccal mucosa is adequate depending on width of the remaining urethral plate. Once the graft is harvested and prepared, it is sewn into the ventral urethral defect using 5-0 polyglactin **(Fig. 5.8)**. The glans is then replaced over the repair and a 16 F catheter is used to stent the urethra. The penile skin is then reapproximated using a running absorbable stitch. Typically, there is no need for tissue interposition to provide vascular support or prevent fistula formation due to robust coverage of the intact ventral glans over repair. However, if the procedure is a redo urethroplasty or extensive tapering of the urethral plate is involved, the penile skin can be degloved, and a tunica vaginalis flap harvested from one of the testis and placed over the repair. A compressive dressing is used to cover the wound for 2 days and the catheter is left in the urethra for 2 weeks.

Complications: These include stricture recurrence, wound dehiscence, catheter induced erosion of the neomeatus and urethrocutaneous fistula. Although, there are few reports in the literature that have specifically addressed distal urethroplasty, one recent multi-institutional study have found an overall success rate of 66% for single-staged buccal graft reconstruction of the FN.[2]

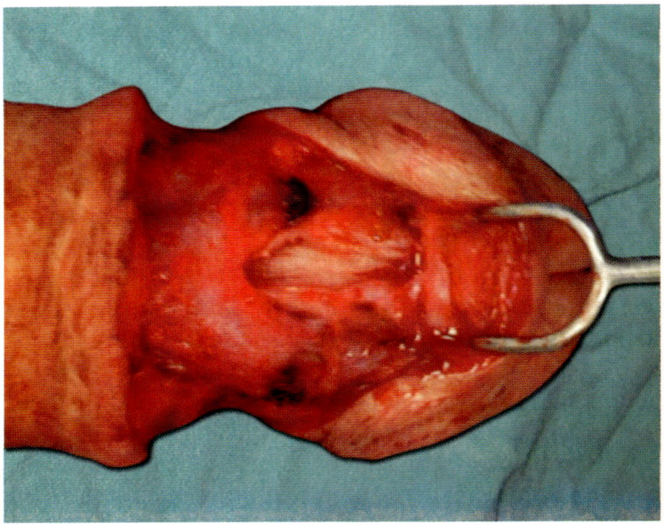

Fig. 5.7: Single stage buccal graft onlay urethroplasty. The glans has been mobilized off the urethra to expose the strictured segment. A ventral stricturotomy is made and the scarred tissue is excised, leaving the urethral plate

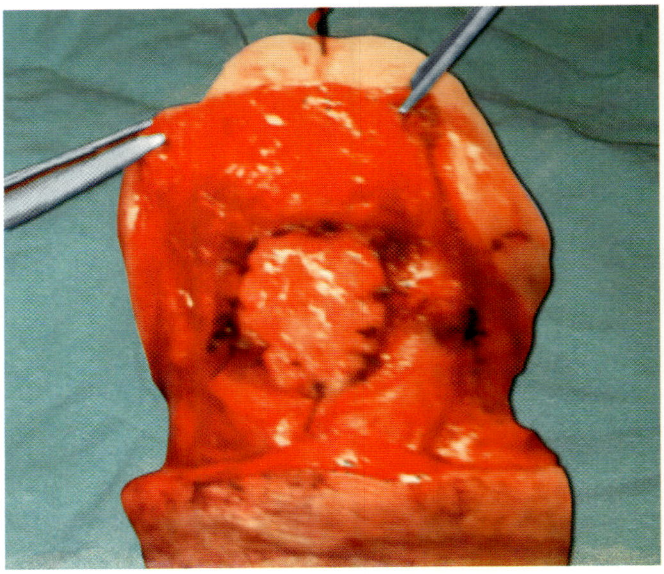

Fig. 5.8: Single stage buccal graft onlay urethroplasty. The buccal graft has been approximated to the ventral stricturotomy

Multistaged Distal Urethral Reconstruction

In our experience, obliterative strictures due to failed previous hypospadias repair or LS require a staged approach, as the native urethral plate and surrounding blood supply and tissue coverage is not suitable for incorporation into the reconstructed urethra in one operation. For strictures due to LS, it is important to excise as much, if not all, of the diseased tissue, as recurrence is common if diseased tissue is left *in situ*. Similarly, strictures due to failed hypospadias repair typically have extensive scarring and nonviable tissue, and if not excised, may contribute to stricture recurrence. A full thickness graft of skin or oral mucosa should be utilized in these procedures with care being taken to avoid genital skin, if LS is present. Split thickness skin grafts tend to contract too much and in the authors' experience should not be used for staged repair of the distal urethral stricture.

Technique: To begin, a urethrotomy is made through the ventral penile shaft extending into the strictured urethral segment. Next, 0-chromic stay sutures are placed through the incised penile skin edges on either side of the

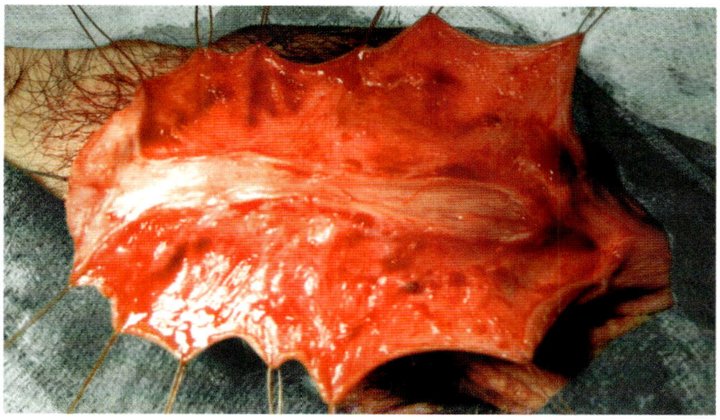

Fig. 5.9: Staged urethral reconstruction. The majority of diseased urethra has been excised, leaving just the urethral plate. The paired chromic stay sutures are placed through lateral edges of penile skin and aid in retraction during the operation as well as securing dressing following the procedure

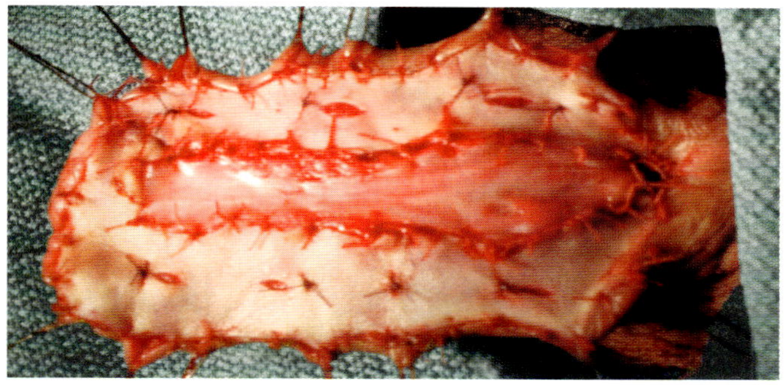

Fig. 5.10: Staged urethral reconstruction. The graft has been fixed to the edges of healthy penile skin and urethral plate with interrupted absorbable suture. Pie-crusting incisions and quilting stitches help in affixing graft to the host bed

exposed urethra for retraction and later to serve as bolster sutures. The nonviable urethral tissue and penile skin are then dissected off the ventral glans and corpora. If the existing urethral plate appears viable, it is left in place. The dimensions of the urethral defect are then measured and an appropriately sized full thickness graft is harvested. Full thickness graft width should be approximately 3 cm if the urethral plate was excised, as some contraction may occur. This will provide an eventual urethral plate that, once tubularized, will be approximately 22–24 F in caliber. The graft is then sutured to the penile skin edges laterally, using a combination of interrupted and running 5-0 polyglactin. If the urethral plate is left intact the graft can be divided and placed alongside the plate **(Fig. 5.9)**. A urethrostomy is created with healthy genital skin and urethral mucosa at the proximal most portion of the stricturotomy. Several small perforations, or pie-crusting incisions, are made in the graft to help in preventing seroma or hematoma formation which would inhibit inosculation of the graft. Quilting sutures are placed every square centimeter in order to optimize apposition of the graft to its host bed **(Fig. 5.10)**.

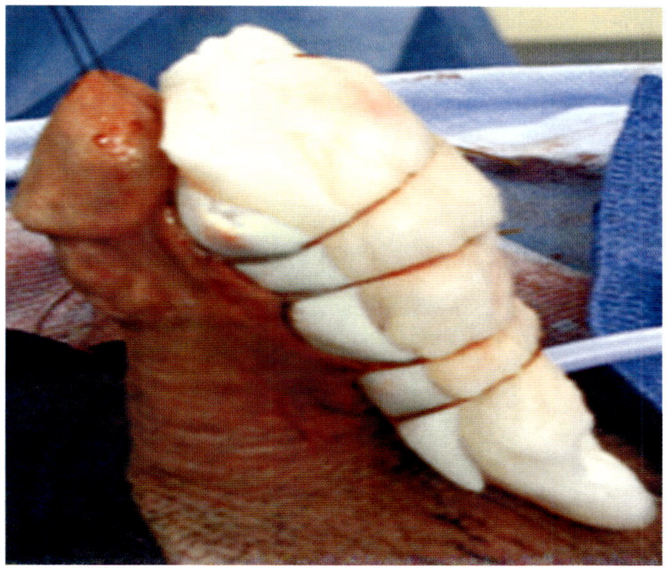

Fig. 5.11: Staged urethral reconstruction. Wound dressing consists of Xeroform® gauze and sterile cotton soaked in mineral oil and saline. The chromic bolster sutures are then tied around the dressing. The catheter arises from the urethrostomy below the dressing. The wound and catheter are then wrapped in the sterile Coban®

A 16 F catheter is placed in the urethrostomy, and the graft is covered with Xeroform® gauze followed by cotton soaked in saline and mineral oil. The bolster sutures are then tied around to dressing followed by Coban® dressing **(Fig. 5.11)**. This dressing provides compression and moisture for optimal graft healing. The dressing and catheter both are removed 4 days following the procedure. Patients are advised to refrain from sexual activity for 4 weeks following the first stage urethroplasty. If the graft appears to be healing well and the urethrostomy is patent, the second stage reconstruction can be considered 4–6 months following the first operation. Occasionally, additional revisions may be necessary, in order to replace nonviable graft tissue or to revise the urethrostomy site. Generally this is most applicable in poorly controlled diabetic patients and active smokers that is why we require a normal hemoglobin A_{1c} level and smoking cessation prior to surgery. In the case of failed hypospadias repair where the host tissues are often scarred and blood flow compromised, some graft slough or excessive contraction may occur, leaving an inadequate urethral plate and the need for multiple procedures to provide adequate tissue coverage. In the case of strictures due to LS, disease recurrence, typically seen within 6 months, may require additional excision and grafting leading to a multistaged approach. In either case, excision of scarred or diseased tissue and further grafting may be necessary and should be actively monitored between reconstructive stages **(Fig. 5.12)**.

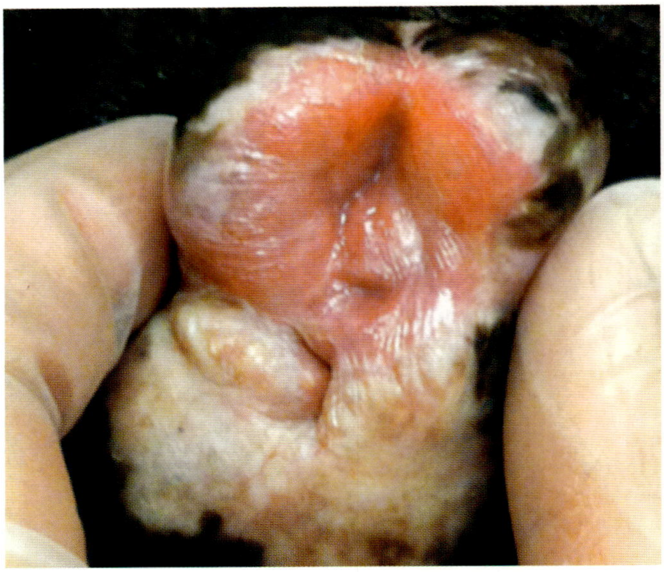

Fig. 5.12: Lichen sclerosus recurrence after first stage urethroplasty. Note the healthy buccal mucosa graft on the ventral fossa navicularis. The LS has progressed to involve the tissue surrounding the urethrostomy

The second stage: The final stage of urethral reconstruction involves mobilizing the existing graft tissue into a tube and covering the neourethral repair with as many layers of healthy tissue as possible. Prior to incision, the proximal urethrostomy is calibrated with a 24 F bougie à boule to ensure patency. A U-shaped incision is made along interface of the graft and penile skin from just distal to coronal sulcus to the urethrostomy site **(Fig. 5.13)**. The graft is then mobilized from the incised penile skin edges laterally down to Buck's fascia. Care must be taken to preserve blood supply laterally to the penile skin and medially to the graft. Around the urethrostomy site, penile skin and subcutaneous tissue are incised to free the mucosal border. One layer subepithelial closure with a running 5-0 polyglactin suture followed by harvest and placement of a tunica vaginalis flap over the neourethral suture line best prevents fistula formation in authors' experience. Multiple layers of closure over the initial suture line should be avoided as this causes excessive narrowing of the neourethral lumen. The dartos is then subsequently closed in at least two layers followed by penile skin closure.

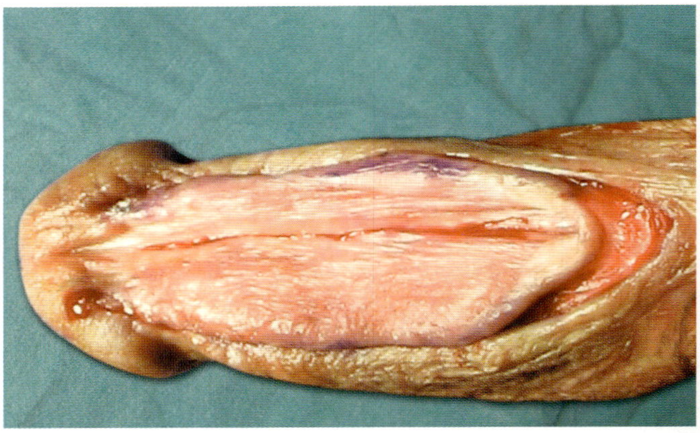

Fig. 5.13: Staged urethral reconstruction. The incision is made along the interface of the graft, penile skin and around the urethrostomy. The graft will then be mobilized and tubularized

In order to develop an orthotopic meatus, glans wings are mobilized laterally on either side of the urethral plate. The degree to which this can be accomplished depends on the size of the glans as well as the quality of the graft. Many times, a hypoplastic glans, as is often seen in men with previous pediatric penoscrotal hypospadias disease, presents a challenge to properly mobilize this tissue in order to create an orthotopic meatus. Likewise, graft contracture or scar may limit width of the distal most portion of the graft, and thus cannot be mobilized and rolled further to prevent meatal stenosis. In these situations, further staged procedures can be considered. The glans is then reapproximated in a tension-free fashion over the reconstructed neourethra using 4-0 polyglactin suture. The neourethral meatus is imbricated to the surrounding glans epithelium with interrupted 5-0 polyglactin suture.

A 16 F catheter is then placed through the urethra. Owens® gauze soaked in benzoin is placed around the wound, and the penile shaft is wrapped with sterile Coban.® The dressing is left in place for 2 days and the catheter for 2 weeks. Patients should refrain from heavy physical or sexual activity for 4 weeks. We do not obtain routine postoperative imaging; however, if patients complain of lower urinary tract symptoms or have recurrent urinary tract infections, office cystoscopy is performed to evaluate for stricture recurrence.

Complications: Complications following closure of the staged urethroplasty include stricture recurrence, wound dehiscence, urethrocutaneous fistula formation and rarely curved penile erections. In our experience, similar to others, the best success rates have been achieved with staged buccal graft reconstruction of the FN as compared to genital or extragenital skin.[15,16]

EDITORIAL COMMENTS

Dr Rajesh Gulia

Etiology of stricture is shifting from infective to inflammatory and iatrogenic causes. Stricture of FN is most often caused by lichen sclerosus et atrophicus and instrumentation.[17]

These, the distal most urethral strictures have proven a waterloo for many a urethral surgeons. Here it is not only important to maintain urethral continuity, but to preserve cosmesis of the glans. One should make an attempt to try to find the proximal extent of the stricture. Clinically if the ventral surface of the glans feels indurated then he is not a candidate for extended meatotomy.

Where possible the glans preserving methods should be used as cosmesis ultimately depends on the integrity of the glans. Once it is cut and resutured, invariably the distal most suture is always at a higher risk of giving way. Hence, in such cases I prefer using a monofilament absorbable suture (Polydioxanone, PDS). Being monofilament the chances of infection in this area (more prone to bacterial colonization) are less with this suture. Secondly, glanular area requires extended support, which is provided by this suture.

Having stressed on the importance of glans preserving methods, one must not underestimate the place of extended meatotomy. This is especially so in complex or reoperative cases, when the patient has gone under the knife a couple of times and want one definitive solution. This is a wee bit akin to offering perineal urethroplasty. However, the patient must be counseled about the urinary spraying (due to proximal location of the neomeatus) and cosmetic appearance.

REFERENCES

1. Fenton AS, Morey AF, Aviles R, et al. Anterior urethral strictures: etiology and characteristics. Urology, 2005;65:1055.
2. Meeks JJ, Barbagli G, Mehdiratta N, et al. Distal urethroplasty for isolated fossa navicularis and meatal strictures. BJU Int. 2011.
3. Venn SN, Mundy AR. Urethroplasty for balanitis xerotica obliterans. Br J Urol. 1998;8:735.
4. Cohney BC. A penile flap procedure for the relief of meatal stricture. Br J Urol. 1963;35:182.
5. Blandy JP, Tresidder GC. Meatoplasty. Br J Urol. 1967;39:633.
6. Brannen GE. Meatal reconstruction. J Urol. 1976;116:319.
7. De Sy WA. Aesthetic repair of meatal stricture. J Urol. 1984;132:678.
8. Jordan GH. Reconstruction of the fossa navicularis. J Urol. 1987;138:102.
9. Armenakas NA, Morey AF, McAninch JW. Reconstruction of resistant strictures of the fossa navicularis and meatus. J Urol. 1998;160:359.
10. Morey AF, Lin HC, DeRosa CA, et al. Fossa navicularis reconstruction: impact of stricture length on outcomes and assessment of extended meatotomy (first stage Johanson) maneuver. J Urol. 2007;177:184.
11. Onol SY, Onol FF, Onur S, et al. Reconstruction of strictures of the fossa navicularis and meatus with transverse island fasciocutaneous penile flap. J Urol. 2008;179:1437.
12. Virasoro R, Eltahawy EA, Jordan GH. Long-term follow-up for reconstruction of strictures of the fossa navicularis with a single technique. BJU Int. 2007;100:1143.
13. Andrich DE, Dunglison N, Greenwell TJ, et al. The long-term results of urethroplasty. J Urol. 2003;170:90.
14. Dubey D, Vijjan V, Kapoor R, et al. Dorsal onlay buccal mucosa versus penile skin flap urethroplasty for anterior urethral strictures: results from a randomized prospective trial. J Urol. 2007;178:2466.
15. Mangera A, Patterson JM, Chapple CR. A systematic review of graft augmentation urethroplasty techniques for the treatment of anterior urethral strictures. Eur Urol. 2011;59:797.
16. Barbagli G, De Angelis M, Palminteri E, et al. Failed hypospadias repair presenting in adults. Eur Urol. 2006;49: 887.
17. Singh SK, Agrawal SK, Mavuduru RS. Management of the stricture of fossa navicularis and pendulous urethral strictures. Indian J Urol. 2011;27 (3):371-7.

6

CHAPTER

Anastomotic Urethroplasty

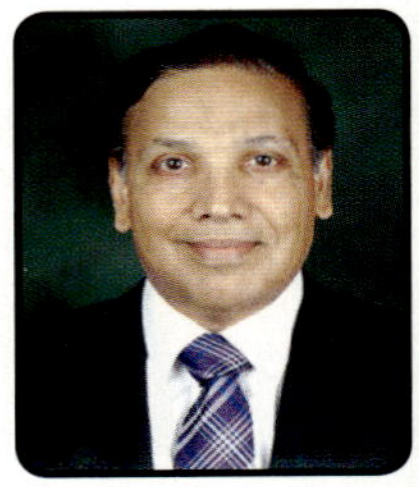

Sanjay B Kulkarni

Sanjay B Kulkarni

Chapter Outline

Abstract

Anastomotic urethroplasty should be only done for traumatic strictures. In pelvic floor urethral distraction defect (PFUDD), progressive perineoabdominal approach should be performed. Important successive steps include bulbar urethral mobilization, crural separation, inferior pubectomy, corporal rerouting, transpubic urethroplasty and omental wrapping. Results of anastomotic urethroplasty depend on the type, length and site of urethral stricture, surgical technique, previous surgery and urethral vascularity. An adequate urethral mobilization without tension, an excision of scar tissue, and a precise mucosa approximation are the pillars of a successful anastomotic urethroplasty. Failures after the anastomotic urethroplasty and other associated complications still pose considerable challenges to the reconstructive urologist. This chapter addresses the steps, recent concepts and techniques of anastomotic urethroplasty. Practical surgical tips are illustrated by the master himself.

Keywords

Anastomotic urethroplasty, Perineoabdominal progressive approach (PAPA), Scar excision, Bulbar urethral mobilization, Crural separation, Inferior pubectomy, Supracrural rerouting, Transpubic urethroplasty, Traumatic strictures, Omental wrap, Methylene blue color spongiography.

INTRODUCTION

The word "anastomosis" means joining two luminal structures end-to-end. Urethral anastomosis is usually done for traumatic stricture disease. The factors involved in making decision of urethral anastomosis include anatomical, etiological, pathological and patient demographics. The aim of anastomotic urethroplasty is to create a wide urethral lumen to initiate spontaneous normal voiding thus avoiding further instrumentation and damage to upper tracts. The results of anastomotic urethroplasty depend on the type, length and site of urethral stricture, surgical technique, previous surgery and urethral vascularity.[1-3] An adequate urethral mobilization without tension, an excision of scar tissue, and a precise mucosa approximation are the pillars of a successful anastomotic urethroplasty.[4] Failures after the anastomotic urethroplasty and other associated complications still pose considerable challenges to the reconstructive urologist. This chapter addresses the recent concepts, techniques, complications and indications of anastomotic urethroplasty.

INDICATIONS

Penile Urethra

Acute penile transection injury with a sharp weapon should be subjected for primary anastomosis. It is best avoided for other causes for the fear of chordee.

Bulbar Urethra

Anastomotic urethroplasty is preferred for traumatic bulbar strictures. Transection of the bulbar urethra is debatable for nontraumatic strictures due to vascular considerations.[5]

Posterior Urethra

Posterior anastomotic urethroplasty by a progressive perineal approach forms the mainstay of pelvic fractures and urethral distraction defects.

INVESTIGATIONS

History and Examination

From the history our attempt should be to get as much information about the etiology and the mechanism of urethral trauma. Also inquire about any past procedures and about his erectile functional status. Examination should aim at assessing the presence of any abdominal/perineal scars, site of the suprapubic catheter and any tell-tale signs of fistulae/abscess. Digital rectal examination is done to assess the overriding of the prostate.

Blood and Urine Tests

These include routine hematological and biochemical analysis with urine culture.

Uroflowmetry

It is used to assess preoperative status in bulbar strictures and all postoperative results.

Ultrasonography

It is used to look for upper tracts, degree of urinary retention and calculi.

Penile Doppler

It is done with intracavernosal papaverine injection to rule out and document vasculogenic erectile dysfunction.

Sonourethrography

It is useful in selected cases of bulbar strictures to know the extent of spongiofibrosis and planning surgical approach.

Retrograde and Micturating Cystourethrography

It helps to know the anatomy of the stricture or defect, for follow-up studies and documentation. It should be done in lateral position to avoid overlapping of the bulbar urethra. In pelvic fracture urethral distraction, it is imperative to do an "up-and-down-o-gram" taking special care that the bladder neck is open to judge exact length of the defect.[6,7]

Cystourethroscopy

It can be done intraoperatively to assess the extent and diameter of the stricture. Suprapubic cystoscopy, preferably with a flexible scope, can be more informative in posterior urethral injury to assess the proximal urethral stump and bladder neck. It is rarely done for diagnostic and follow-up purpose.

Computed Tomography Scan and Magnetic Resonance Imaging

These investigations are done only in complex and redo cases.

PREOPERATIVE PREPARATION AND ANESTHESIA

Apart from the routine preparations, all patients should be given preoperative prophylactic intravenous antibiotics and asked to paint the operative site with povidone-iodine scrub. The suprapubic catheter site is cleaned.

All types of anastomotic urethroplasty are done under regional anesthesia preferably spinal. General anesthesia may be preferred by some.[8]

Patient is given lithotomy position, preferably on the hydraulic (Allen) stirrups, which gives an advantage of intraoperative positioning, if needed. Care must be taken during painting and scrubbing the operative site so as not to induce penile erection.

OPERATIVE STEPS

Bulbar Anastomotic Urethroplasty

Through a vertical midline perineal incision, the bulbospongiosus muscle is divided in the midline. The dissection of the bulbospongiosus muscle from the urethra may be difficult at the site of injury due to fibrosis and adhesions.[9]

The bulbar urethra is mobilized from the corpora cavernosa. A dilator is passed through meatus into the urethra. A firm nodule is felt in the corpora spongiosa at the site of injury and the urethra is transected at this level.

The spongiofibrotic tissue **(Fig. 6.1)** is excised on the proximal and the distal end of the urethra till healthy urethral mucosa is encountered. The urethra is spatulated on opposite sides into normal pink urethra up to 1.5 cm[10] **(Fig. 6.2)**.

The anastomosis is performed with a single suture line of interrupted 4/0 polyglactin (vicryl) sutures posteriorly. Anteriorly a two layer anastomosis is done. The first layer picks up the urethral mucosa and can be continuous or interrupted. The second layer picks up the corpora spongiosa.[10,7]

A 14 F silicone Foley catheter is introduced into the bladder. The wound is closed in layers with absorbable sutures. Drains are seldom used and catheter is kept for 3–4 weeks.

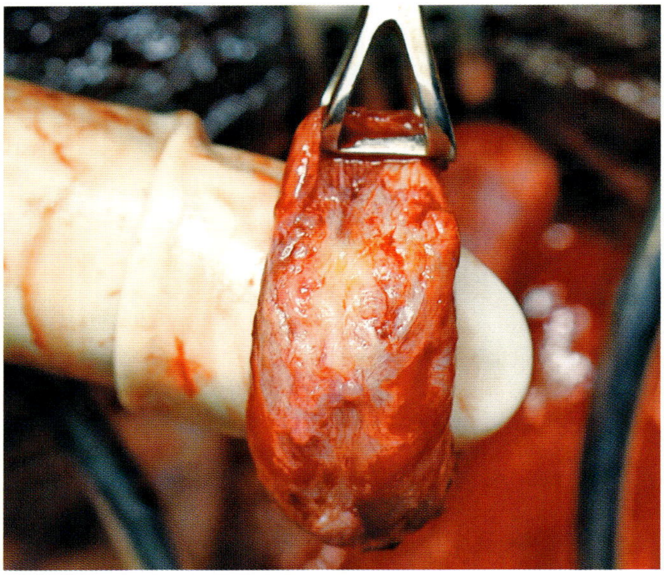

Fig. 6.1: The scar is visible at the distal urethral end as unhealthy and whitish tissue

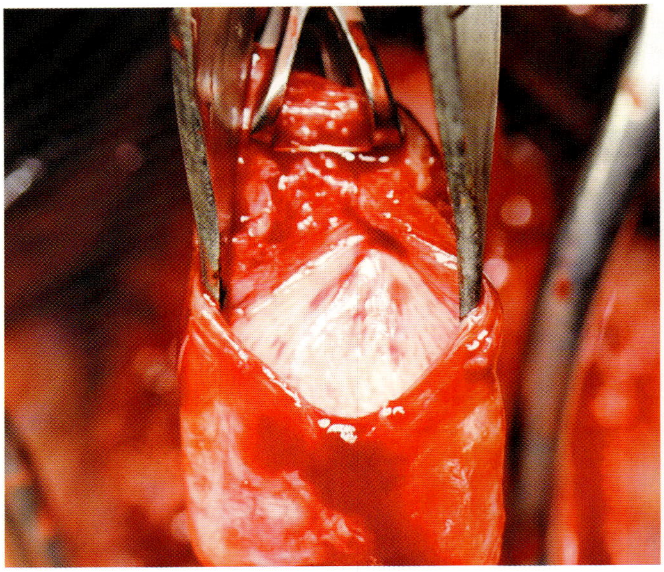

Fig. 6.2: After cutting the entire scar at the distal urethral end, a healthy pink mucosa is visible

Follow-up

First follow-up is at catheter removal when uroflowmetry is done. Further follow-up is at 3 months and 6 months.

Anastomotic Urethroplasty for Posterior Urethral Injury

Perineoabdominal Progression Approach

The surgery is progressively performed by following six steps depending upon length of the defect:

1. *Bulbar urethral mobilization*: Vertical midline perineal incision is preferred. Inverted 'Y' fork at bottom of the incision is usually not required. In case of a complex situation, if a perineal urethrostomy is anticipated then an inverted 'U' incision is preferred. A Turner Warwick ring retractor with six blades is applied.[11]

   The bulbospongiosus muscle is divided in midline. The dissection continues lateral to the corpora spongiosa. The spongiosa is lifted from the cavernosa by sharp dissection and circumflex vessels from cavernosa to spongiosa are coagulated **(Fig. 6.3)**.

   A 6 F feeding tube is passed around the mobilized urethra, which is manipulated to further dissect the urethra from cavernosa. This minimizes handling of spongiosa.

   The distal mobilization of the bulbar urethra is continued till the penoscrotal junction. Mobilization of the penile urethra may lead to chordee formation and

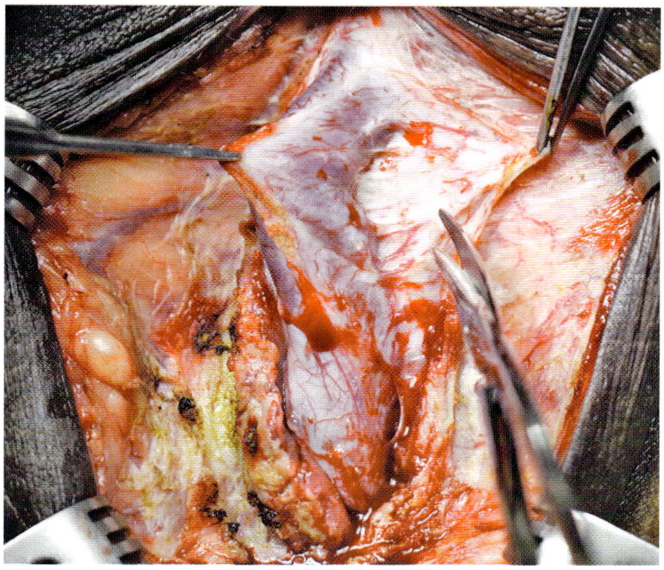

Fig. 6.3: Note that the bulbar urethra is retracted toward the patient's right with an atraumatic forceps and it is being separated from the corpora cavernosa with a sharp tenotomy scissors

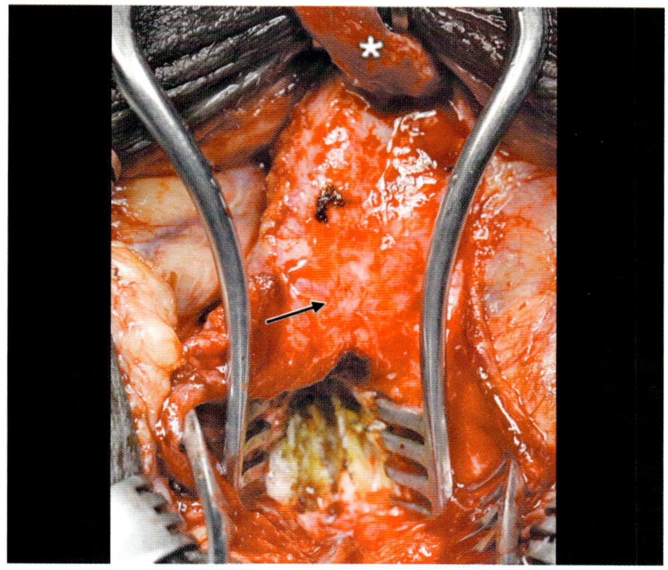

Fig. 6.4: Crural separation. Note the distal urethra (white star) is tucked away below the mastoid retractor. Two mastoid retractors are used to separate the crural bodies. An incision is made in the midline (arrow)

is avoided. Mobilization of the distal end of the bulbar urethra up to the suspensory ligament of the penis, as described by some authors, is difficult to perform as we do not dissect dorsal to the penis at its base.[11]

Proximal dissection of the bulbar urethra allows lifting of the bulb from the perineal body.[12] A mastoid retractor is placed inside the bulbospongiosus muscle and spread to allow the proximal bulb dissection. A Babcock forceps applied gently to the ventral spongiosa squeezes it and allows lateral and posterior dissection of the bulb under vision.

A urethral boogie (sound) is passed through the meatus and the tip is rotated laterally. If tip of the boogie is felt with a finger, the proximal dissection is sufficient. If the tip is not felt, more dissection proximally is needed.

Proximally the urethra is transected at the site of fibrosis. The bulbar urethra is opened and spatulated for 1.5 cm. A rigid 17-Fr cystoscope is passed through the suprapubic cystotomy into the prostatic urethra.

An incision is made in the perineum over the scar and cutting is performed under light of the endoscope. This maneuver prevents anastomosis to the false passage. The scar at apex of the prostatic urethra is completely excised avoiding aggressive dissection on posterolateral surface of the prostate near neurovascular bundles.

2. *Crural separation*: An incision is made in the midline avascular plane between the two corporal bodies by using Metzenbaum scissors, at a length of 3–4 cm **(Fig. 6.4)**. In redo cases, the crural separation may be difficult and any inadvertent opening of the corpora cavernosa is immediately repaired by a suture.[11]
3. *Inferior pubectomy*: A mastoid retractor is applied to spread the crura apart. Gentle dissection allows visualization of the dorsal penile vein **(Fig. 6.5)** which is retracted laterally; its collateral tributaries require coagulation with a bipolar current or ligation.

   An incision is made in the midline on the anterior aspect of the pubic symphysis. By using a diathermy probe, which is bent to 45° at the half-way point, the periosteum is elevated from the pubic bone laterally on either side. Inferior pubectomy is performed by using a Capener's gouge **(Fig. 6.6)** and a rongeur. Adequate size of the bone is excised providing enough space for surgical manipulation[9] **(Fig. 6.7)**.
4. *Supracrural rerouting*: If the tension persists at the two urethral ends then this step is followed. At the base of the penis, one side of the corpora cavernosa is dissected. A small pubectomy is necessary to make room for the urethra and its supracrural route. The surgeon's index finger should be able to go through the space smoothly without bony speckles and fibrous tissue. This maneuver allows the S-shape of the urethral route to be straightened out to give a tension-free anastomosis.[4]
5. *Total pubectomy using transpubic approach*: If tension persists after step four, this next step is followed. This

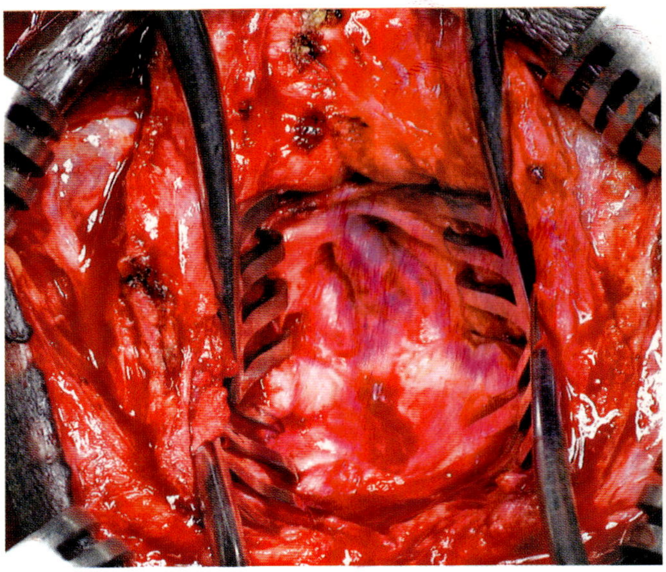

Fig. 6.5: Dorsal penile vein seen in the center

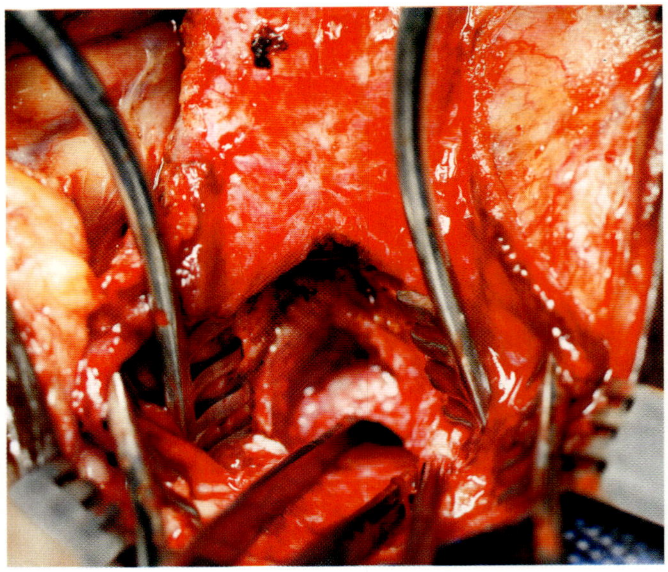

Fig. 6.7: After adequate inferior pubectomy, all the scar at the proximal urethral end is excised till the supple pinkish urethra is encountered. Note ends of the forceps in the proximal urethra

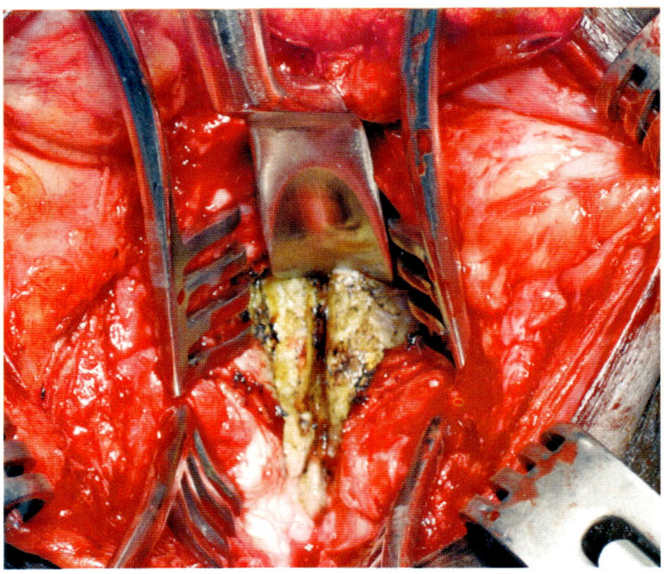

Fig. 6.6: An inferior pubectomy being done by using a Capener's gouge

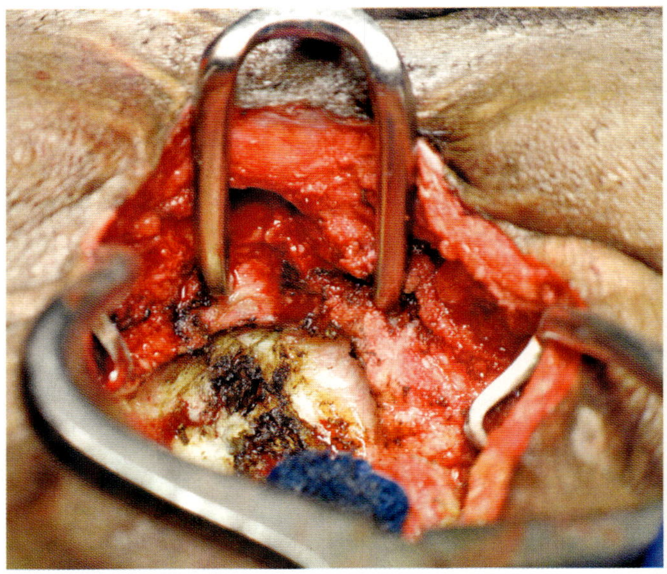

Fig. 6.8: Transpubic approach. The anterior surface of the pubic bone being exposed

may be necessary for complex, redo and pediatric cases with the classical "pie in the sky" bladder and extensive fibrosis. Through a midline infraumbilical incision, the retropubic space is dissected. The anterior surface of the bladder is gently dissected all around. The periosteum over the anterior surface of the pubic bone is incised **(Fig. 6.8)**, and a total pubectomy is performed with a Capener's gouge **(Fig. 6.9)** and rongeur or using a Gigli's saw. A retrograde boogie is passed through the bladder neck into the prostatic urethra. The firm and white scar at the prostatic apex is excised.

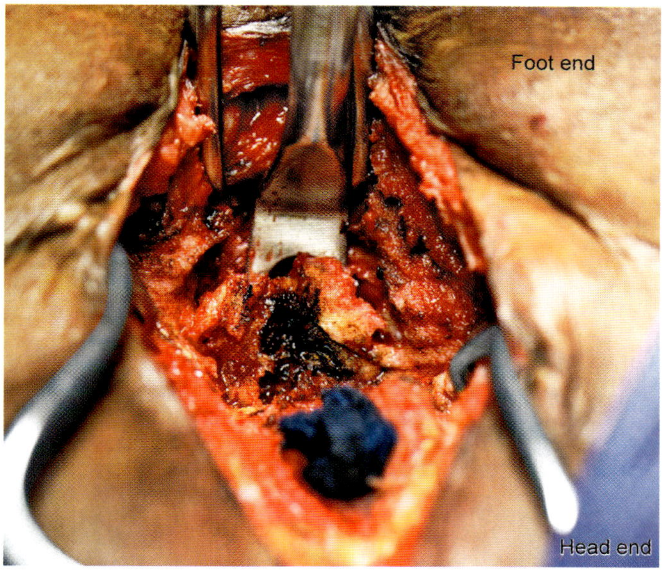

Fig. 6.9: A total pubectomy being performed with a Capener's gouge

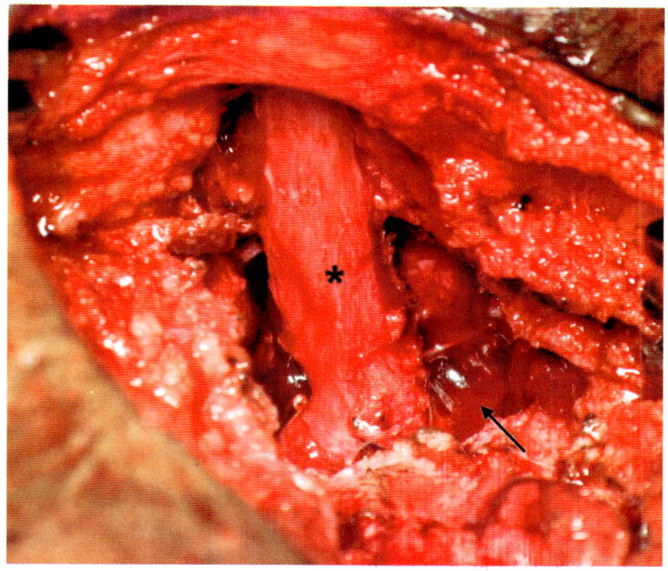

Fig. 6.10: Final appearance after the spatulated distal urethral end (star) is anastomosed to the prostatic apex (arrow) anteriorly

Six interrupted sutures are placed at positions 1, 3, 5, 7, 9, and 11 o'clock by using 4/0 polyglactin (vicryl) suture on a 16 mm 3/8th circle taper cut needle. All the sutures are placed on the mosquito forceps and parked with the ring retractor following a clock format. Care is taken to prevent entanglement of sutures. A 14-Fr Foley silastic catheter is placed across and the knots are tied after approximating the two urethral ends **(Fig. 6.10)**.

6. *Omental wrap*: The peritoneum is incised at the midline toward the umbilicus and omentum is mobilized. At this point, the patient may notice some discomfort under spinal anesthesia and general anesthesia may have to be supplemented. The omentum is wrapped around the anastomosis and fixed to itself with sutures **(Fig. 6.11)**. The omentum fills the dead space created by the pubectomy and keeps the anastomotic site supple. The peritoneum is closed leaving a small gap for the omentum. A 16-Fr Foley catheter is used as a suprapubic tube. Abdominal or perineal drains are rarely used. The abdominal and the perineal incisions are closed and a cross compressive perineal dressing is applied.

Postoperative Care and Follow-up

Patient is discharged on the 4th or 5th day of surgery. A pericatheter urethrogram is obtained 3 weeks postoperatively and the urethral catheter is removed after ruling out extravasation. The suprapubic catheter is removed a week later after satisfactory voiding is confirmed. Uroflowmetry is performed at the end of 3 months and annually thereafter.[8] When the symptoms of decreased force of stream are evident or maximum flow on uroflowmetry is less than 12 ml/sec, retrograde urethrography is repeated. If urethral narrowing is evident, then the urethroscopy is performed.[13]

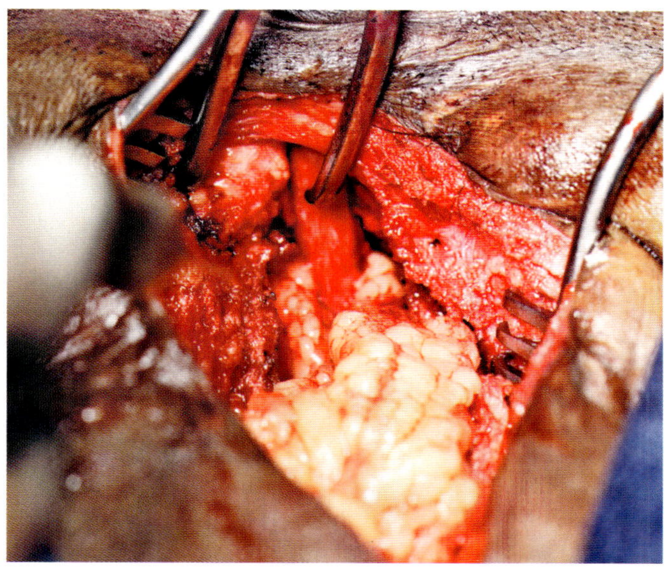

Fig. 6.11: Omentum is wrapped around the anastomosis

Augmented Anastomosis

If a patient has a long bulbar stricture with a very narrow lumen then it is not feasible to perform primary augmentation or primary anastomosis.[14] In such situations, augmented anastomosis is performed.[15,16] The concept is to excise this tight stricture and spatulate the urethra on both sides and anastomize the urethra to form a flat urethral plate. A buccal mucosa graft (BMG) is used as the patch of augmentation either on ventral or dorsal side. The BMG takes care of the gray urethra on both sides of the stricture. Ultimately, the tight stricture is excised and the remaining bulbar urethra is augmented with a rooftop configuration. This procedure is best suited for long bulbar strictures with a very narrow urethral plate, which is not suitable for direct augmentation. However, due to the recently evolving concept of nontransection of the urethra for nontraumatic strictures this procedure is fallen in debate.[17]

Operative Steps

With a midline vertical perineal incision, the bulbar urethra is mobilized and spatulated dorsally. The tight segment of the bulbar urethra is excised. A 1.5 cm wide and 6 cm long BMG is spread and quilted on the corpora cavernosa. The ventral urethral plate is reconstituted by anastomizing the proximal and distal urethral ends. The urethral plate is now flat and sutured to the BMG as in Barbagli technique.

ANASTOMOTIC URETHROPLASTY: CONCEPTS

Urethral Anatomy

Dual Vascularity

The male urethra derives its blood supply from two sources: (1) the antegrade supply from the bulbar arteries and the circumferential branches of the dorsal penile artery; and (2) the retrograde supply which arises from the glans penis through the cavernosal arteries.[18] The implication is that after transection and mobilization of the urethra at any given point the antegrade blood supply is compromised, while the retrograde supply is the only savior. Repeated mobilization after transection can lead to necrosis of long urethral segment causing primary repair difficult. Antegrade supply gets invariably compromised in strictures caused due to trauma, hence transection is rational in such events.[19]

Penile Urethra

It has limitations for anastomotic urethroplasty due to its fixation to the corpora cavernosa.[18,19] Extensive mobilization can lead to chordee. The bulk of spongiosa is less which may hamper a two-layer closure of the urethra.

Bulbar Urethra

It is best suited for end-to-end anastomotic urethroplasty due to the bulky spongiosa and muscle cover and a good margin for mobilization.[19] It can be mobilized up to the penoscrotal junction without the fear of chordee. However, transection of the bulbar urethra should be avoided in nontraumatic strictures due to the aforementioned reasons.

Posterior Urethra

In contrary to the previous belief that posterior urethral injury causes transection of urethra at the membranoprostatic junction, the recent finding is that it happens at the bulbomembranous junction. The decision and approach for anastomotic urethroplasty in posterior urethral injury depend upon the degree of prostatic apex displacement, past surgery, and duration from the actual injury and associated injury to the rectum.[13,20]

Urethral Extensibility

Alexsandro et al. analyzed macroscopically the normal, fresh cadaveric urethra from 25 men 6 months to 73 years old at death. They determined the penile, bulbar and membranous urethral length under maximal constant traction and the maximal stretched length without penile curvature at artificial erection. They defined urethral extensibility as the percentage of variation in initial length at rest and maximal constant traction length. They concluded that knowledge of the safe anatomical limit of urethral extensibility applied to reconstructive surgery may avoid complications and the necessity for more complex techniques. This limit should be approximately 75% of the maximal constant traction length or a gap-to-normal urethra ratio of 1:4.[21]

Technical Concepts

Adequate Urethral Mobilization

Dissection of the bulbar urethra up to the penoscrotal junction in posterior urethral trauma and mobilization of both ends during bulbar anastomotic urethroplasty helps in creating a tension-free anastomosis with better results. Progressive perineal approach and, if required, abdominoperineal approach is necessary to adequately mobilize the urethra for improved results.[6,22]

Complete Scar Excision

Scar excision is the most important determinant of postoperative results after anastomotic urethroplasty. It is imperative to excise the entire scar between the two ends of the urethra so that anastomosis is done between two supple mucosal ends.[20,22]

Adequate Urethral Spatulation

Both proximal and distal urethral ends need to be adequately spatulated. The location of the spatulation depends upon the site of anastomosis. Spatulation helps to create a wide anastomosis and avoids narrowing after healing.[4]

Surgical Skill and Expertise

Recurrent surgical insult to the urethra leads to loss of urethral length making further procedures difficult, thus yielding unsatisfactory results. Hence, the first intervention should be done at a center with good surgical experience, skill and expertise. The urethral handling should be gentle and integrity of the tissue planes should be maintained.

COMPLICATIONS OF ANASTOMOTIC URETHROPLASTY

Intraoperative and Perioperative

Uncontrolled Bleeding

The uncontrolled bleeding from the dorsal vein of the penis or the bulbar arteries can be troublesome. It can be prevented by identification and pre-emptive ligation of the vein. The arterial bleeding can be controlled easily by momentary packing of the defect, which helps in easy identification and cauterization of the individual arteries.

Injury to the Rectum

An injury to the rectum is possible during posterior urethral reconstruction, especially in redo cases associated with extensive fibrosis. This can be prevented by doing a bimanual dissection using left index finger into the rectum. It is best prevented by early anticipation which is possible with good training and experience.

In case of rectal injury, the defect should be closed in layers with an absorbable suture. If required, diverting colostomy should be done to protect the urethral anastomosis. Drains are necessary after such event.

Inability to Complete the Anastomosis

Rarely it is impossible to get the two ends together in spite of adequate urethral mobilization. In such circumstances, perineal urethrostomy should be done and referral to a reconstructive urologist should be considered.

Perurethral Catheter Displacement

Spontaneous catheter displacement after surgery is not uncommon. Gentle single attempt to replace the Foley should be done. If this fails we have two options: (a) Guided catheterization using a glide wire under C-arm Fluoroscopy; (b) Do a urethroscopy/cystoscopy using a smaller caliber scope and very minimal saline pressure/flow so as not to cause any stress on the suture line at the anastomotic site. Then pass a wire through the scope in the bladder and then thread the catheter over the wire (make the normal catheter into a council tip catheter by cutting the tip bit by bit till lumen is seen).

Pubic Osteomyelitis

It happens rarely after inferior pubectomy during posterior anastomotic urethroplasty. It is managed with bed rest, antibiotics and analgesics.

Others

Wound infections and hematomas should be drained and supplemented with intravenous antibiotics. Catheter blockage should be prevented by advising adequate hydration and flushing. Rarely the use of medications to prevent penile erection is required. Catheter related epididymo-orchitis should be managed with scrotal support and antibiotics.

Postoperative

Anastomotic Site Leak

Usually, it happens in redo cases with difficult anastomosis. We routinely confirm this by doing a pericatheter retrograde urethrogram before catheter removal. In case of a leak, it is advisable to retain the catheter for a week. Most of the leaks stop after a week or two. Seldom repeat surgery is required for a persistent anastomotic site leak.

Recurrent Stricture

Short recurrent stricture after bulbar anastomotic urethroplasty can be managed with gentle single step under-vision dilatation or an optical urethrotomy. Recurrence after posterior anastomotic urethroplasty can be managed by optical or laser urethrotomy. Eventually redo anastomotic urethroplasty is required in these cases.[22,23]

Erectile Dysfunction

This is an issue after posterior anastomotic urethroplasty. Impotence is noted in 30% of patients with short dislocations and up to 70% of patients with long dislocations. It is important to document the preoperative erectile function status by doing a penile Doppler. It can be prevented by avoiding dissection at the posterolateral aspect of the posterior urethra.[7,24]

Urinary Incontinence

It is seen in 5% of patients. Concomitant injury to the bladder neck in pelvic fracture can lead to incontinence after posterior anastomotic urethroplasty. It is best anticipated during the micturating cystourethrogram by carefully observing the passive descent of the contrast into the prostatic urethra through the open bladder neck. It is prudent to caution the patient before surgery about this problem. It can be managed by doing a bladder neck repair or subsequent placement of artificial urinary sphincter.

Penile Shortening or Chordee

Extensive penile urethral mobilization should be avoided to bridge the gap. This can result in chordee and penile shortening. The penile urethra should not be mobilized beyond the level of the suspensory ligament.

OUTCOMES OF ANASTOMOTIC URETHROPLASTY

Perineal end-to-end urethroplasty is an excellent procedure for anterior as well as posterior urethral stricture repair.[25] It is the standard of care for posterior urethral distraction defects after pelvic fractures. Due to the recently evolving concepts about the urethral vasculature, end-to-end urethroplasty for bulbar urethral strictures is getting limited to traumatic strictures due to the debate on urethral transection for nontraumatic strictures.[26] We prefer not to transect the bulbar urethra for nontraumatic strictures. Exceptions, like short obliterative bulbar strictures, are still amendable to anastomotic repair. The success rate of anastomotic urethroplasty is about 90–95% in primary cases. The exact incidence of redo cases is not known; however, the success rate is less in our experience and it reduces further with every intervention.[7,23,24]

Complex Situations

Anastomotic urethroplasty is challenging in pediatric age group. The anatomy of posterior urethral injury is different and associated with a greater incidence of bladder neck injury. Anastomotic urethroplasty in this age group should be done only at an experienced center.

Anastomotic urethroplasty is seldom required in females with urethral injuries due to pelvic fractures. The data is, however, very scanty. It is done preferably by the abdominoperineal approach.[27]

ANASTOMOTIC URETHROPLASTY IN NONTRAUMATIC BULBAR URETHRAL STRICTURES (ESPECIALLY THE VERY SHORT SEGMENT ONES)

For traumatic bulbar urethral stricture transection of the urethra, excision of the scar and end-to-end spatulated anastomosis of two normal ends of the urethra is standard of practice.

There is an ongoing debate whether to transect or not the bulbar urethra for nontraumatic urethral stricture.

There is no standard definition of short strictures.

Traumatic Bulbar Strictures

In traumatic bulbar strictures, the accident circumferentially crushes the urethra so as to cause a "functional transection." The proximal to distal urethral blood supply is disconnected due to the circumferential spongiofibrosis or scar. Transection is performed as the vascular continuity is anyway lost. We have normal urethra on both sides of the trauma.

The urethra is usually transected at the site of injury, where one can feel the firm fibrous nodule. After transection, the scar or spongiofibrosis on both sides of the urethra is excised. Suppose we excise 1 cm urethra. Then the opposite ends of the urethra are spatulated for 1.5 cm. The total shortening of the urethra is 2.5 cm. Both ends of the urethra are normal. The success rate of anastomotic urethroplasty for traumatic bulbar urethral strictures is around 90%. In 10% patients when the urethroplasty fails, one can attempt single direct visual internal urethrotomy and if it fails redo surgery is necessary. This involves retransection of the obliterative urethral stricture leading to further shortening of the urethra and may lead to chordee. The incidence of impotence after transection of the bulbar urethra is around 10% and may be temporary or permanent.

Nontraumatic Bulbar Strictures (Short Segment)

In nontraumatic bulbar strictures, the urethra on both sides of the stricture may not be normal. Anastomosis of these not so normal ends may lead to higher failure rate. If we choose to perform augmentation urethroplasty with oral mucosa patch, we will maintain continuity of the urethral blood supply. There is less chance of impotence, if we perform ventral onlay BMG urethroplasty as compared to anastomotic urethroplasty. The success rate of this patch urethroplasty is around 85%. So in 15% patients when it fails, the restricture is not obliterative as in transection cases. One can perform dorsal onlay BMG urethroplasty.

If the patient has hypospadias or severe meatal stenosis, the retrograde urethral blood supply may be inadequate if we transect the bulbar urethra and may lead to distal bulbar urethral ischemia.

There are certain situations where the nontraumatic strictures are associated with a very narrow urethral plate. In such situations, a double faced buccal mucosa may be applied both dorsally and ventrally without transection.

Methylene Blue Color Spongiography

Author introduced his new concept of methylene blue (MB) color spongiography. This test is still under investigation and may require further refinement. It is a simple technique where, at the beginning of surgery, we inject MB in the glans near the meatus. The stricture is opened ventrally. The MB is expected to travel from the glans into the proximal corpora spongiosa.

If MB is seen traversing proximal to the stricture in the spongiosal tissue, it means that spongiofibrosis is not significant and the blood supply from distal end is intact, and such strictures are best managed by augmentation than transection.

If MB does not traverse across the stricture proximally indicating significant spongiofibrosis, these strictures are best managed by transection and anastomosis.

EDITORIAL COMMENTS

Dr Rajesh Gulia

We have 18% of the world population, 1% of the world vehicle population but 6% of the world accidents. About 100,000 die on the road every year and many more injured. Economic loss amounts to ₹ 550 crores (approximately 12.5 billion dollars), an amount that equals our defense budget. According to WHO predictions, if a concerted effort is not made to improve the services by 2020, there will be 147% increase in road traffic accident deaths in India.[28] So we have a large population of patients with posterior urethral injuries and the potential to be the world leaders in urethroplasty.

Still in 2012, we have a shortage of trained urologists doing complex urethral reconstructive surgery. A patient of pelvic fracture urethral disruption defect is referred to the nearest secondary hospital where railroading is still done, and everybody has seen the outcomes of railroading, both in short-term and long-term.

As in the management of certain other surgical problems, this too has come back a full circle, but with improved modifications. Nowadays instead of immediate, we are talking about early endoscopic alignment in posterior urethral trauma. This is nothing, but controlled under vision endoscopic railroading. This requires highly trained endourologists, and a two urology team approach, one approaching transurethrally, the other entering suprapubically.

During the progressive perineal approach for posterior urethral distraction injuries, it has been seen that a majority of cases can be tackled via the perineal route alone. Only in complex redo cases we need to resort to a transpubic approach. Transpubic approach has its own set of problems with patients coming back with ugly bulges and hernia of all types which are not easy to manage. Also, all said and done, pubic symphysis is important in rotational stability of the pelvis. Complete pubectomy leads to increased stress on the sacroiliac joints and can lead to chronic pain later on. Also a host of muscles from the lower extremity are attached to it apart from all important rectus abdominis. It is better to be more aggressive in your inferior pubectomy than to resort to a transpubic approach. Even if in certain situations total pubectomy is required we prefer to do a superior pubectomy, whenever possible, as this leaves the important inferior pubic ligament that contributes to anterior pelvic stability.

REFERENCES

1. Azoury BS, Freiha FS. Excision of urethral stricture and end-to-end anastomosis. Urology. 1976;8(2):138-40.
2. Bellinzoni P, Rigatti P. Comparison of surgical techniques: resection and termino-terminal anastomosis. Arch Ital Urol Androl. 2002;74(3):117-8.
3. Brandes SB, Smith J, Virgo K, et al. Adult anterior urethral strictures: a national practice patterns survey. J Urol. 2001;165:53.
4. Koraitim MM. Post-traumatic posterior urethral strictures: preoperative decision making. Urology. 2004;64(2):228-31.

5. Da Silva EA, Schiavini JL, Santos JB, et al. Histological characterization of the urethral edges in patients who underwent bulbar anastomotic urethroplasty. J Urol. 2008;180(5):2042-6. Epub 2008.
6. Rosen MA, McAninch JW. Stricture excision and primary anastomosis for reconstruction of the anterior urethral stricture. In: McAninch JW (Ed). Traumatic and Reconstructive Urology. Philadelphia: WB Saunders; 1996. p. 565.
7. Santucci RA, Mario LA, McAninch JW. Anastomotic urethroplasty for bulbar urethral stricture: analysis of 168 patients. J Urol. 2002;167(4):1715-9.
8. Wright EJ, Webster GD. Urethral stricture and disruption. In: Graham JS (Ed). Glenn's Urologic Surgery, 5th edition. Philadelphia: Lippincott-Raven; 1998. p.425.
9. Andrich DE, Mundy AR. What is the best technique for urethroplasty? Eur Urol. 2008;54(5):1031-41.
10. Jezior JR, Schlossberg SM. Excision and primary anastomosis for anterior urethral stricture. Urol Clin North Am. 2002;29(2):373-80.
11. Crane C, Santucci RA. Surgical treatment of post-traumatic distraction posterior urethral strictures. Arch Esp Urol. 2011;64(3):219-26.
12. Morey AF, Kizer WS. Proximal bulbar urethroplasty via extended anastomotic approach—what are the limits? J Urol. 2006;175(6):2145-9; Discussion 2149.
13. Mundy AR. Transperineal bulbo-prostatic anastomotic urethroplasty. World J Urol. 1998;16(3):164-70.
14. Eltahawy EA, Virasoro R, Schlossberg SM, et al. Long-term follow-up for excision and primary anastomosis for anterior urethral strictures. J Urol. 2007;177(5):1803-6.
15. El-Kassaby AW, El-Zayat TM, Azazy S, et al. One-stage repair of long bulbar urethral strictures using augmented Russell dorsal strip anastomosis: outcome of 234 cases. Eur Urol. 2008;53(2):420-4.
16. Guralnick ML, Webster GD. The augmented anastomotic urethroplasty: indications and outcome in 29 patients. J Urol. 2001;165(5):1496-501.
17. Andrich DE, Mundy AR. Non-transecting anastomotic bulbar urethroplasty: a preliminary report. BJU Int. 2012; 109(7):1090-4.
18. Yiee JH, Baskin LS. Penile embryology and anatomy. Scientific World Journal. 2010;29(10):1174-9.
19. Akman Y, Liu W, Li YW, et al. Penile anatomy under the pubic arch: reconstructive implications. J Urol. 2001;166(1): 225-30.
20. Koraitim MM. On the art of anastomotic posterior urethroplasty: a 27-year experience. J Urol. 2005;173(1): 135-9.
21. Da Silva EA, Sampaio FJ. Urethral extensibility applied to reconstructive surgery. J Urol. 2002;167(5):2042-5.
22. Koraitim MM. Failed posterior urethroplasty: lessons learned. Urology. 2003;62(4):719-22.
23. Mangera A, Chapple C. Management of anterior urethral stricture: an evidence-based approach. Curr Opin Urol. 2010;20(6):453-8.
24. Gupta NP, Mishra S, Dogra PN, et al. Outcome of end-to-end urethroplasty: single-center experience. Urol Int. 2009;82(2): 179-82.
25. Gupta NP, Mishra S, Dogra PN, et al. Does a previous end-to-end urethroplasty alter the results of redo end-to-end urethroplasty in patients with traumatic posterior urethral strictures? Int J Urol. 2008;15(10):885-8.
26. Barbagli G, Palminteri E, Bartoletti R, et al. Long-term results of anterior and posterior urethroplasty with actuarial evaluation of the success rates. J Urol. 1997;158(4):1380-2.
27. Keegan KA, Nanigian DK, Stone AR. Female urethral stricture disease. Curr Urol Rep. 2008;9(5):419-23.
28. Madan VS. Road Traffic Accidents: Emerging Epidemic. Indian Journal of Neurotrauma (IJNT1). 2006;3(1):1-3.

7

CHAPTER

Bulbar Oral Graft: Buccal Mucosal Graft, Urethroplasty

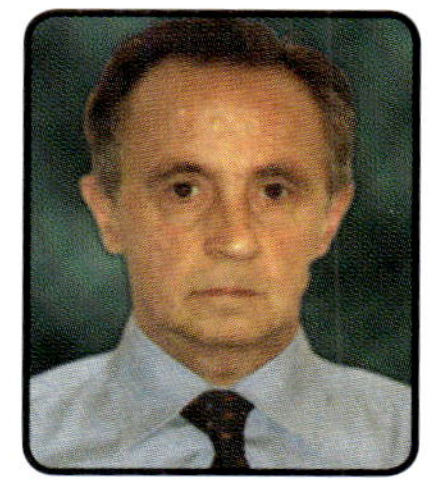

Guido Barbagli

Guido Barbagli, Salvatore Sansalone, Giuseppe Romano, Massimo Lazzeri

Chapter Outline

Abstract

This chapter on the use of buccal mucosal graft (BMG) is written by Professor Guido Barbagli himself. After Kasaby, it was he who successfully used the BMG in various positions—dorsally (DOG), ventrally (VOG) and laterally. Described in detail with diagrams are the various steps as he performs it. This chapter also has diagrams drawn by the master himself. Also mentioned is the latest nerve sparing bulbar urethroplasty, where attention is given to minimal dissection and mobilization so as to preserve the sexual and ejaculatory function. The postoperative care and follow-up are also detailed by the master himself.

Keywords

Oral mucosal graft, Buccal mucosal graft (BMG), Dorsal onlay graft (DOG), Ventral onlay graft (VOG), Nerve sparing bulbar urethroplasty, Fibrin glue, Grooved silicon catheter, Augmented anastomotic repair (Webster's), Ice bag, Voiding cystourethrography.

INTRODUCTION

The current surgical approach to the uncomplicated bulbar urethral stricture began in 1993 when El-Kasaby et al. described the repair of penile and bulbar urethral strictures by using an oral mucosa graft.[1] In 1996, Morey and McAninch described reconstruction of the bulbar urethra, suggesting suturing the oral graft to ventral surface of the urethra.[2] In 1996, Barbagli et al. described dorsal free graft urethroplasty, suggesting suturing the graft to dorsal surface of the urethra, over albuginea of the corpora cavernosa.[3] In 2001, Guralnick and Webster described augmented anastomotic urethroplasty as an evolution of dorsal onlay graft urethroplasty.[4] One-stage oral mucosal graft urethroplasty, using these three techniques, represents the most widespread method for the repair of strictures in the bulbar urethra due to its highly vascular spongiosum tissue.

Location of the graft on the dorsal versus ventral urethra surface has become a contentious issue since Barbagli et al. described, in 1996, the technique of dorsal onlay graft urethroplasty.[3,5] Wessells suggested a list of the technical advantages of bulbar ventral onlay urethroplasty.[6] Armenakas emphasized that ventral graft placement, requiring less urethral dissection and mobilization, is technically easier.[7]

Success with bulbar oral mucosal grafts has been high with dorsal[5,8-11] or ventral[2,6,7,12] graft location, and different graft positions have shown no difference in success rate.[13-15] Barbagli et al. showed that placement of the grafts on the ventral, dorsal or lateral surface of the bulbar urethra offered the same success rates (83–85%), and stricture recurrence was uniformly distributed in all patients.[14]

Recently, we developed a new muscle and nerve sparing bulbar urethroplasty avoiding full opening of the bulbospongiosum muscle, thus better preserving ejaculatory function.[16] The selection of a surgical technique for bulbar urethra reconstruction, in addition to respecting status of the genitalia tissue and components, must also be based on proper anatomic characteristics of the bulbar urethra, to ensure graft take and survival. Furthermore, sexual function can be placed at risk by any surgery on the genitalia, thus dissection must avoid interference with the neurovascular supply to the penis and genitalia. The bulbar urethroplasty using grafts should not compromise penile length or cause penile chordee and certainly should not untowardly affect penile and genitalia appearance.

PREOPERATIVE INVESTIGATIONS

Preoperative tests include urine culture, retrograde and voiding urethrography, urethral ultrasonography and urethroscopy. The patient's clinical history, and site and length of stricture are carefully examined to better define the characteristics the oral mucosal graft should have.

PATIENT PREPARATION

The patient is intubated through the nose, allowing the mouth to be completely free. Two surgical teams work simultaneously at the donor and recipient site, with each having its own set of surgical instruments including suction and bipolar cautery equipment. The mouth retractor is provided with its own light, so by using this instrument just one assistant is sufficient for harvesting of the oral mucosa **(Fig. 7.1)**. The oral graft is taken from the cheek according to our standard technique.[17]

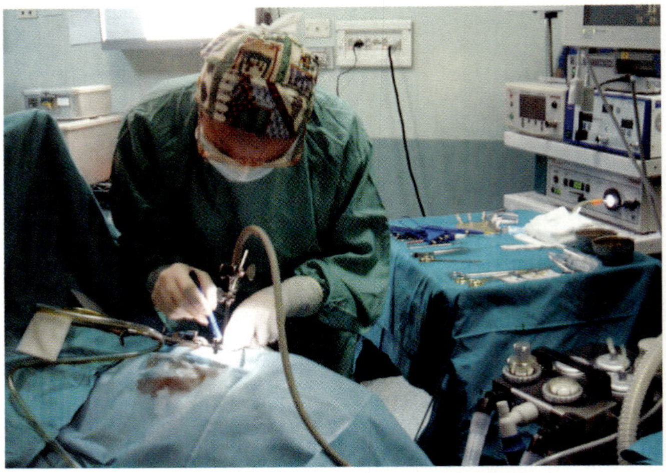

Fig. 7.1: One assistant is sufficient for harvesting of the oral graft using mouth retractor with its own light

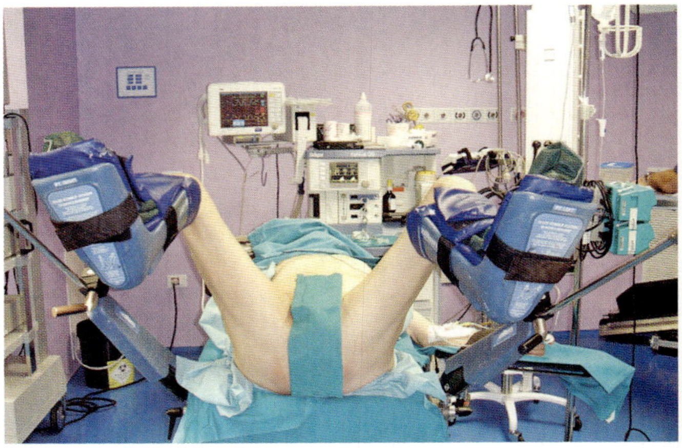

Fig. 7.2: The simple lithotomy position

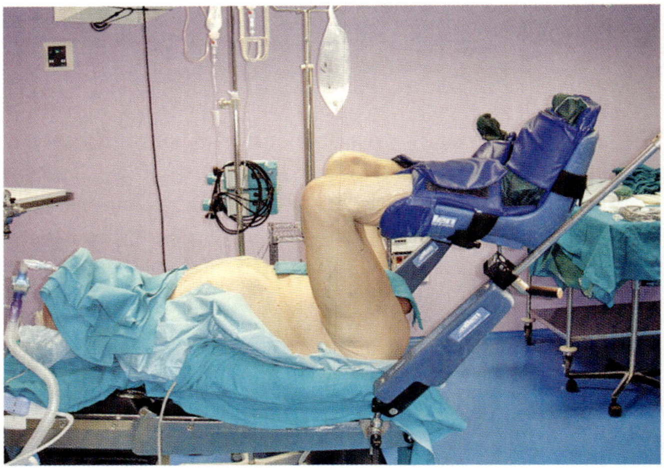

Fig. 7.3: The patient's lower extremities are suspended by his feet within the boots of the Allen's stirrups

The patient is placed in a simple lithotomy position **(Fig. 7.2)**. His calves are carefully placed in Allen stirrups and the lower extremities are then suspended by his feet within the boots of the stirrups **(Fig. 7.3)**. Proper positioning ensures that there is no pressure on any aspect of the calf muscles and no inward boot rotation, so as to avoid perineal nerve injury **(Fig. 7.4)**. In obese patient or in patient with leg vascular diseases, sequentially inflatable compression sleeves are used **(Fig. 7.5)**. The skin of the suprapubic region, scrotum and perineum is shaved, and this region is prepared, draped and appropriately disinfected using chlorhexidine. Preoperatively urethroscopy is performed by using 7 Fr rigid ureteroscope **(Fig. 7.6)**. A sensor 3 Fr

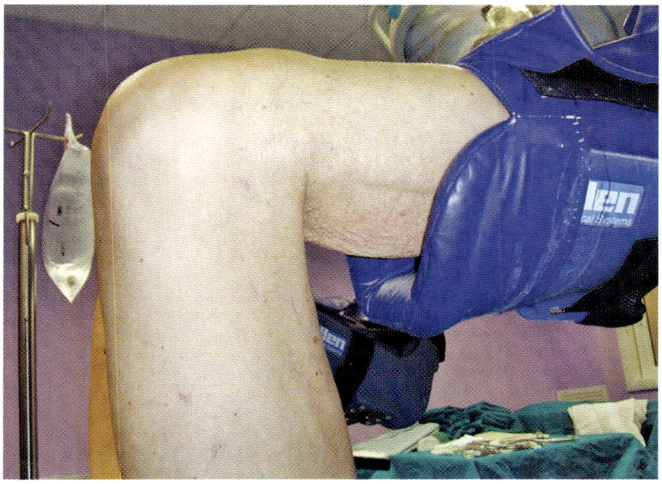

Fig. 7.4: Proper positioning ensures that there is no pressure on any aspect of the calf muscles

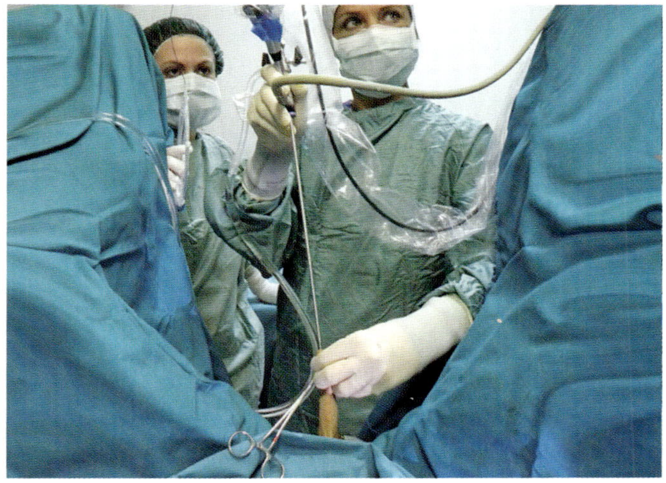

Fig. 7.6: Urethroscopy using 7 Fr rigid ureteroscope

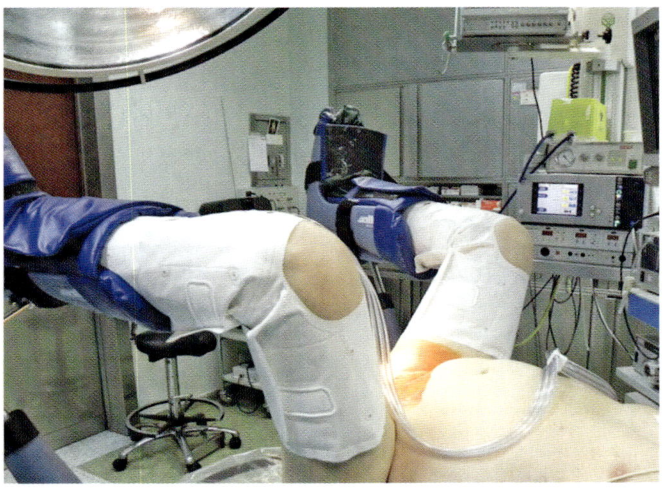

Fig. 7.5: Sequentially inflatable compression sleeves

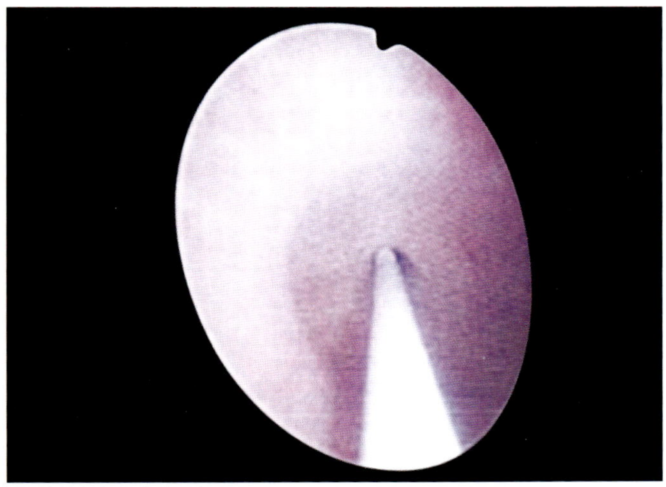

Fig. 7.7: Sensor 3 Fr guidewire inserted through the stenosis

guidewire is inserted through the urethra into the bladder **(Fig. 7.7)**. Methylene blue is injected into the urethra **(Fig. 7.8)**. The distal site of the stenosis is identified by inserting a 16 Fr plastic rounded tip Nelaton catheter **(Fig. 7.9)**. The distal site of the stenosis is then outlined in the perineal area **(Fig. 7.10)**.

VENTRAL ORAL MUCOSAL GRAFT URETHROPLASTY

Patient Selection

The ventral onlay oral mucosal graft bulbar urethroplasty is suggested in all patients presenting nontraumatic urethral strictures in the proximal bulbar urethra, ranging from 1 cm to 5 cm in length **(Fig. 7.11)**. This technique may also be used in patients with repeated failed urethrotomy or previous failed bulbar urethroplasty.

Surgical Technique

A midline perineal incision is made. A plastic ring retractor with plastic hooks is put in place. The bulbospongiosum muscle is separated from the corpus spongiosum of the bulbar urethra **(Figs 7.12A and B)**. This step is made at 12 o'clock using delicate smooth scissors leaving lateral margins of the muscle and central tendon of the perineum

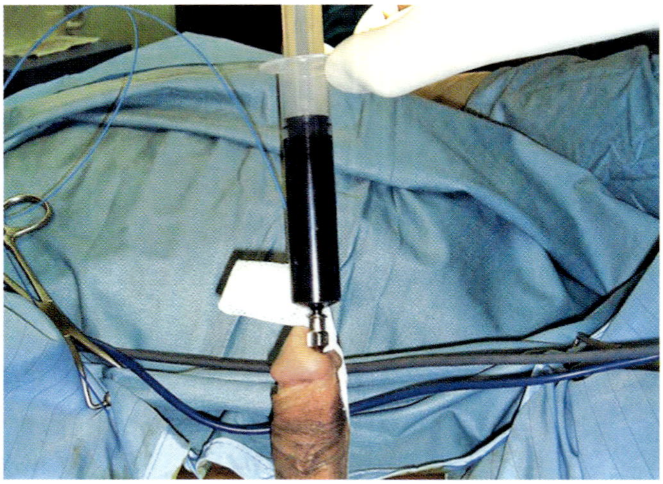

Fig. 7.8: Methylene blue injected into the urethra

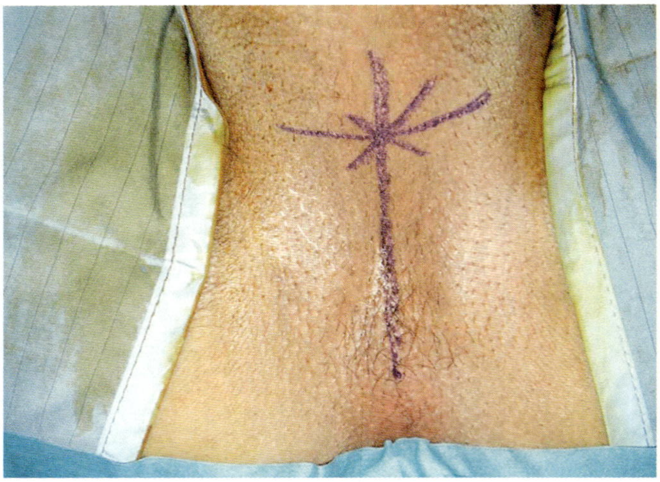

Fig. 7.10: The distal site of the stenosis is outlined

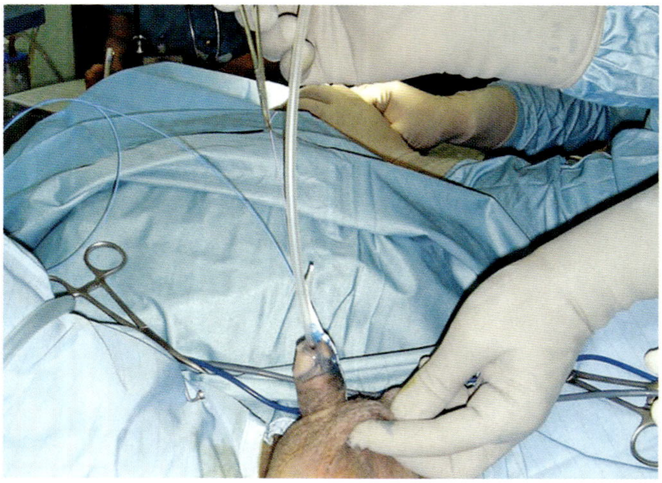

Fig. 7.9: The distal site of the stenosis is identified by inserting a 16 Fr Nelaton catheter

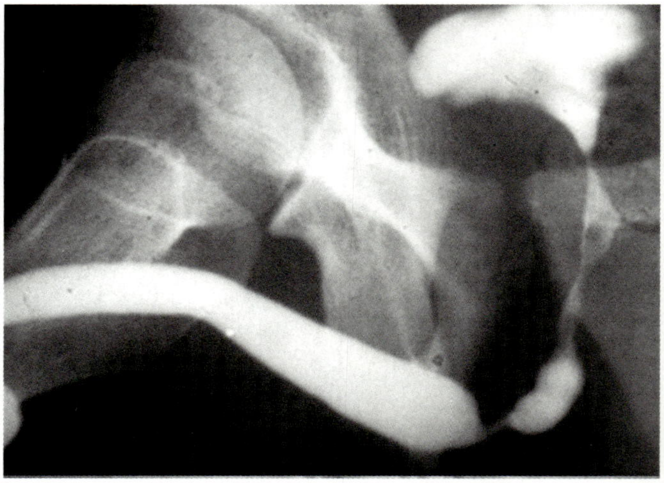

Fig. 7.11: Retrograde urethrography showing proximal bulbar urethral stricture

intact **(Figs 7.13A and B)**. The bulbospongiosum muscle is pulled down by using two small Farabeuf retractors **(Figs 7.14A and B)**. The ventral urethral surface is fully exposed **(Figs 7.15A and B)**. The corpus spongiosum is ventrally opened for 2 cm distally and proximally to the stenosis, and the nasal speculum is inserted into the proximal urethral opening **(Figs 7.16A and B)**. The scarred white mucosal ring is incised as far as the pink mucosa is identified, near the verumontanum **(Figs 7.17A and B)**. This incision should be limited to the urethral mucosa and does not involve the underlying spongiosum tissue, so as to avoid bleeding. The proximal urethral opening is inspected by using a nasal speculum to see the verumontanum. The needle used for a 5-0 polyglactin suture is modified by the surgeon into a J-shaped needle **(Fig. 7.18)**. This needle is passed through the spongiosum tissue in front up to the verumontanum **(Figs 7.19A and B)**. Using this technique, three stitches are made at 5, 6 and 7 o'clock **(Fig. 7.20)**. The oral mucosal graft is trimmed to its appropriate size, according to length and width of the urethrotomy. The two ends of graft are sutured to the proximal and distal apices of the urethrotomy and running 6-0 polyglactin suture

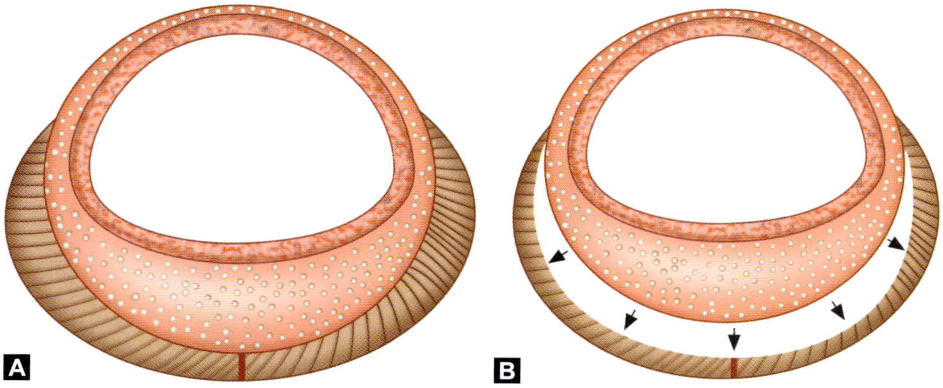

Figs 7.12A and B: (A) Anatomical relationship between the bulbospongiosum muscle and the corpus spongiosum; (B) The bulbospongiosum muscle is separated from the corpus spongiosum

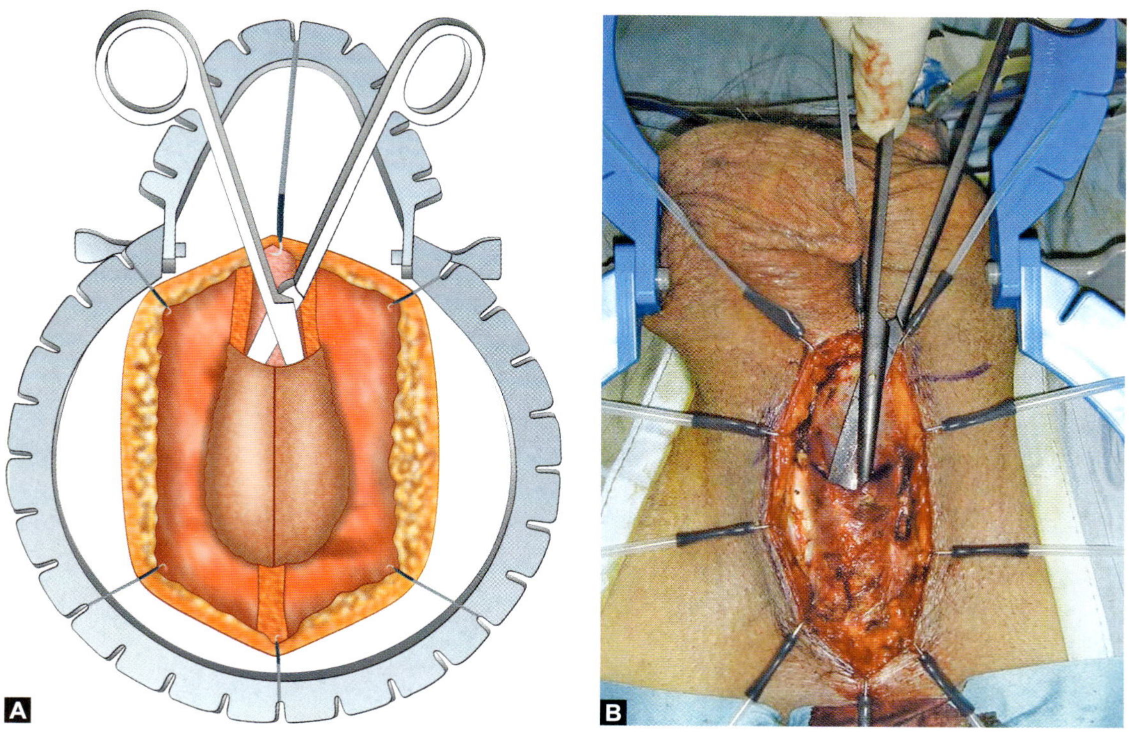

Figs 7.13A and B: The bulbospongiosum muscle is separated from the corpus spongiosum at 12 o'clock by using smooth scissors

is used to complete a watertight anastomosis between left margin of the graft and left margin of the urethral mucosal plate **(Figs 7.21A and B)**. The stitches previously placed at 5 and 6 o'clock in front up to the verumontanum, are passed into the proximal oral mucosal graft edge **(Figs 7.21A and B)**. Using this step, the oral mucosa graft is pushed very deeply inside the healthy urethral mucosa near the verumontanum, where the mucosa is not involved in the scarring process. The stitch previously placed at 7 o'clock in front up to the verumontanum is passed into the proximal oral mucosal graft edge **(Fig. 7.22)**. A Foley 16 Fr grooved silicone catheter is inserted. The graft is

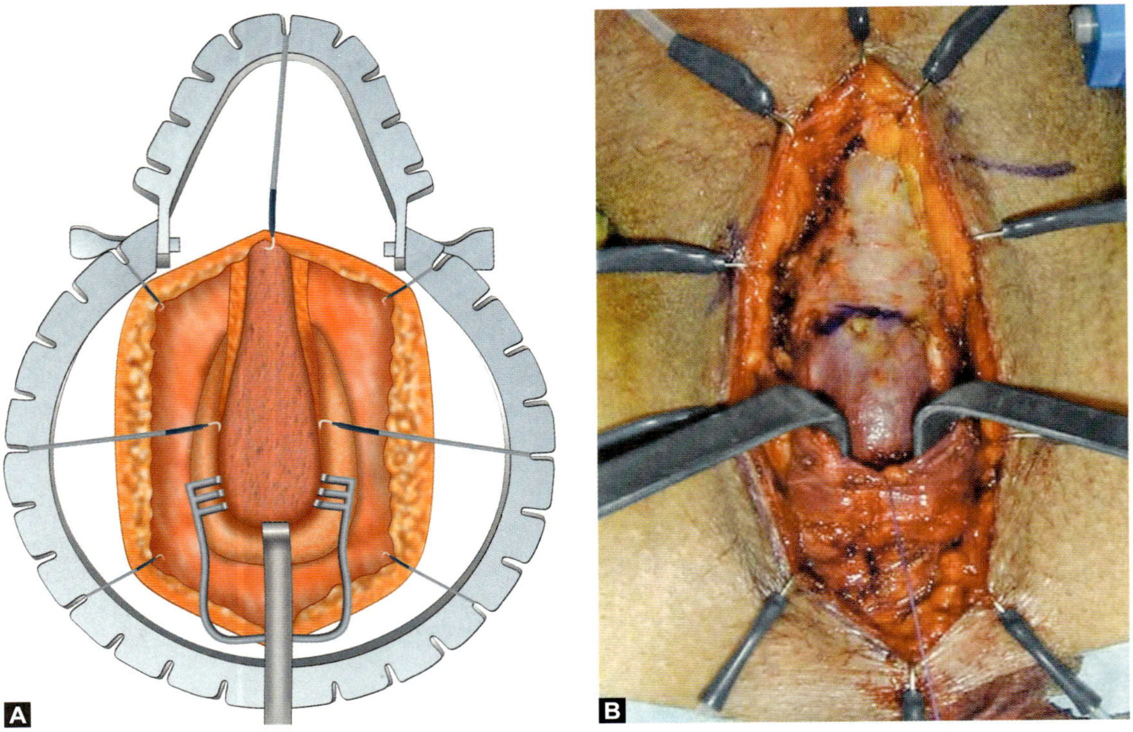

Figs 7.14A and B: The bulbospongiosum muscle is gently pulled down

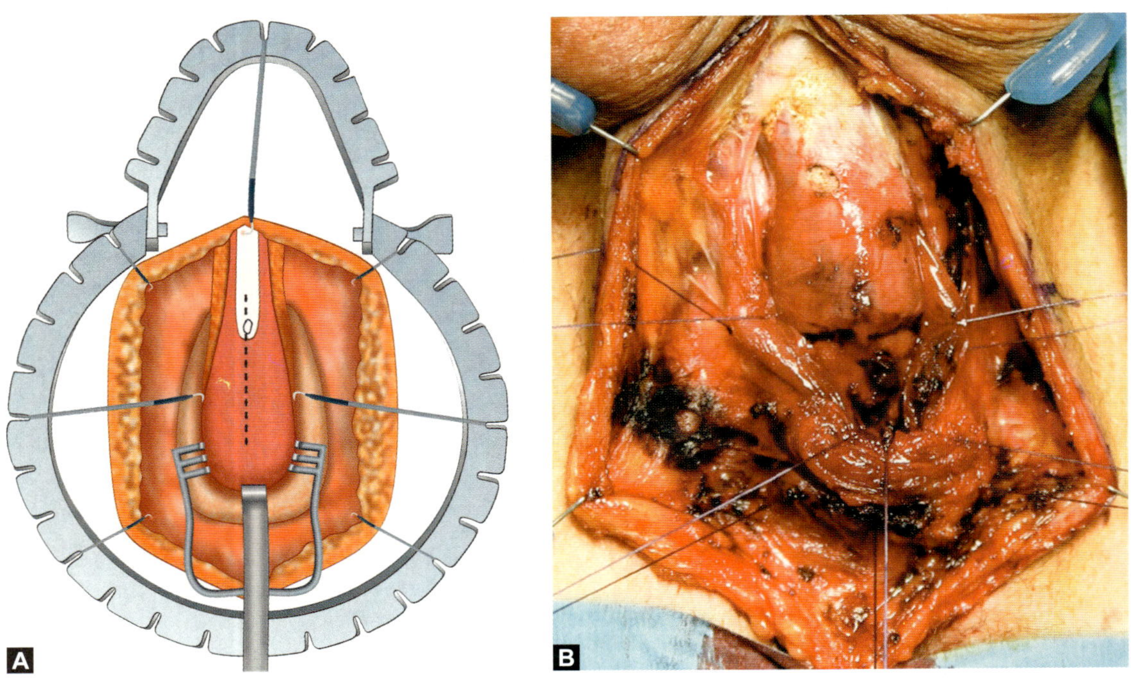

Figs 7.15A and B: The ventral urethral surface of the bulbar urethra is exposed

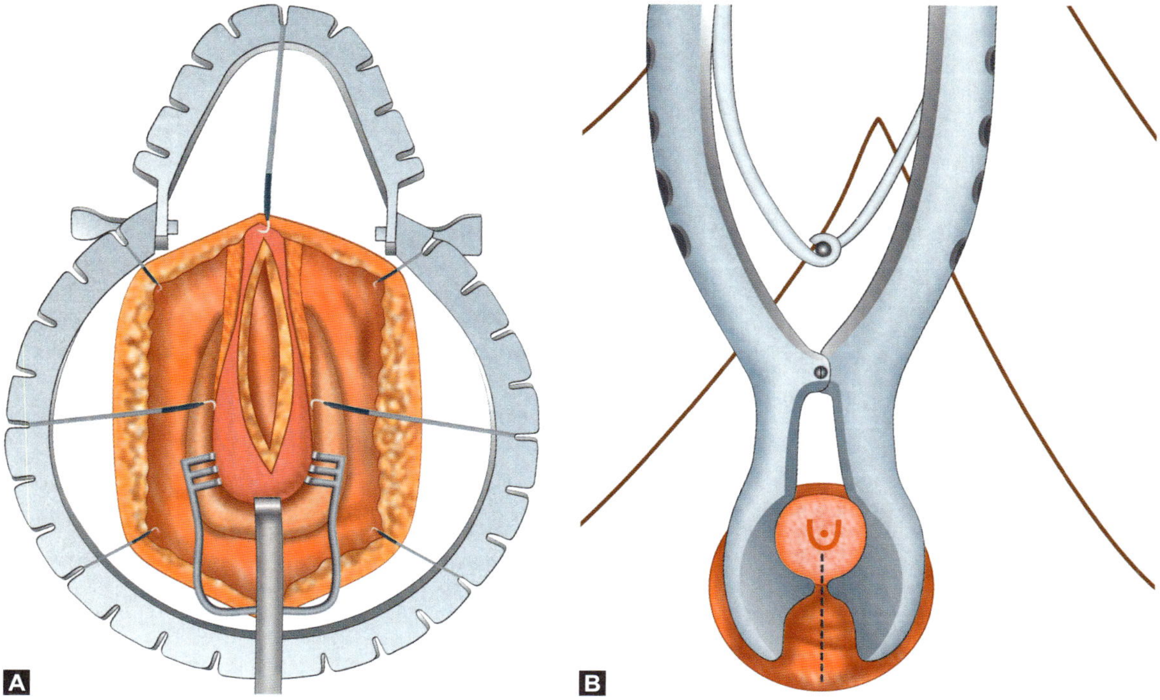

Figs 7.16A and B: (A) The corpus spongiosum is ventrally opened; (B) The nasal speculum is inserted into the proximal urethral opening, and the incision of the mucosa at 6 o'clock is outlined

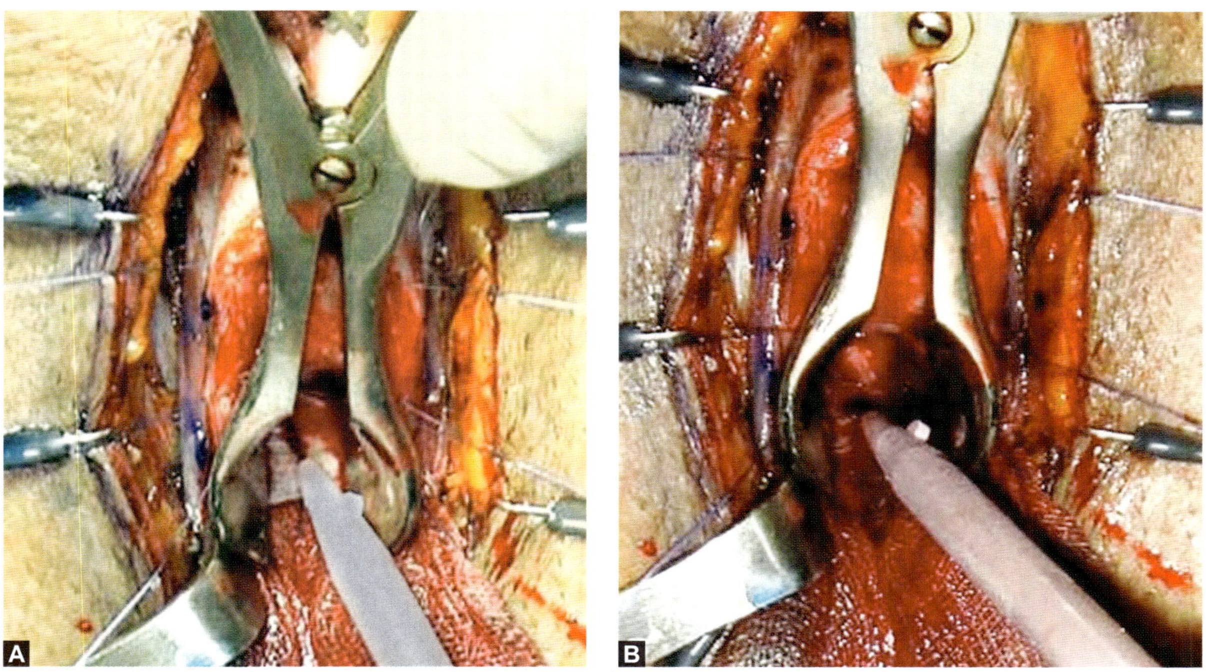

Figs 7.17A and B: (A) The scarred white mucosal ring is incised at 6 o'clock; (B) The pink urethral mucosa is identified in front up to the verumontanum

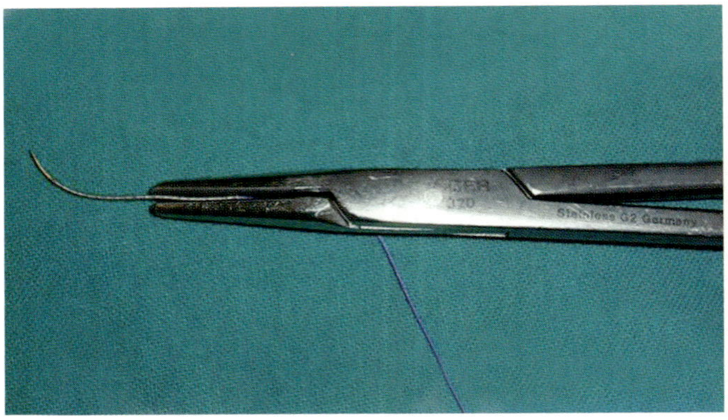

Fig. 7.18: The J-shaped needle

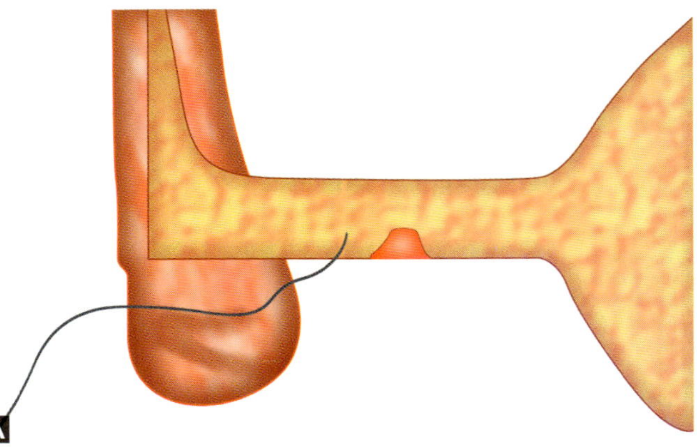

A

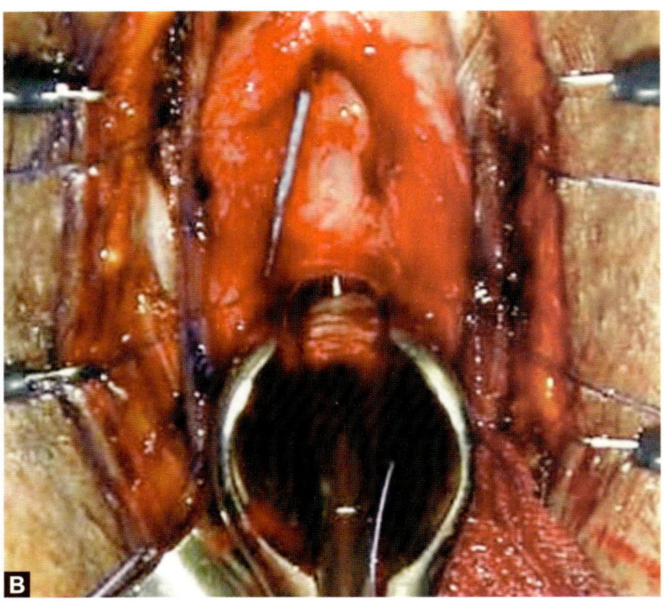

B

Figs 7.19A and B: The J-shaped needle is passed through the spongiosum tissue in front up to the verumontanum

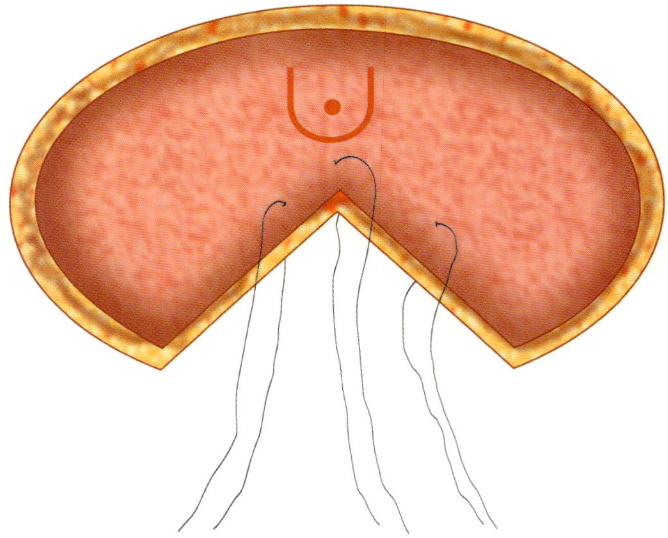

Fig. 7.20: Three stitches are made at 5, 6 and 7 o'clock in front up to the verumontanum

rotated over catheter and running 6-0 polyglactin suture is used to complete a watertight anastomosis between right margin of the graft and right margin of the mucosal urethral plate **(Figs 7.23A and B)**. The spongiosum tissue is closed over the oral mucosal graft using interrupted 5-0 polyglactin suture **(Figs 7.24A and B)**. Fibrin glue (2 ml) is injected over suture line of the corpus spongiosum **(Figs 7.25A and B)**. The bulbospongiosum muscle is picked up to cover the spongiosum tissue. The perineal fat and the skin are closed with interrupted absorbable sutures. A drain is unnecessary. The catheter is left in place for 3 weeks.

Results

The results of ventral oral mucosal graft urethroplasty are fully reported in the literature in large series of patients from different institutions.[2,6,7,12] In authors' center, from May 1999 to June 2010, a total of 219 patients with a median age of 38 years (range 14–80) underwent ventral oral mucosal graft urethroplasty. Of 219 patients, treatment of 187 (85.4%) was successful and 32 (14.6%) were failures. Average follow-up was 43 months (range 12–139). All data is available at: www.urethralcenter.it.

Alternative to this Procedure

- End-to-end anastomosis
- Dorsal onlay technique.

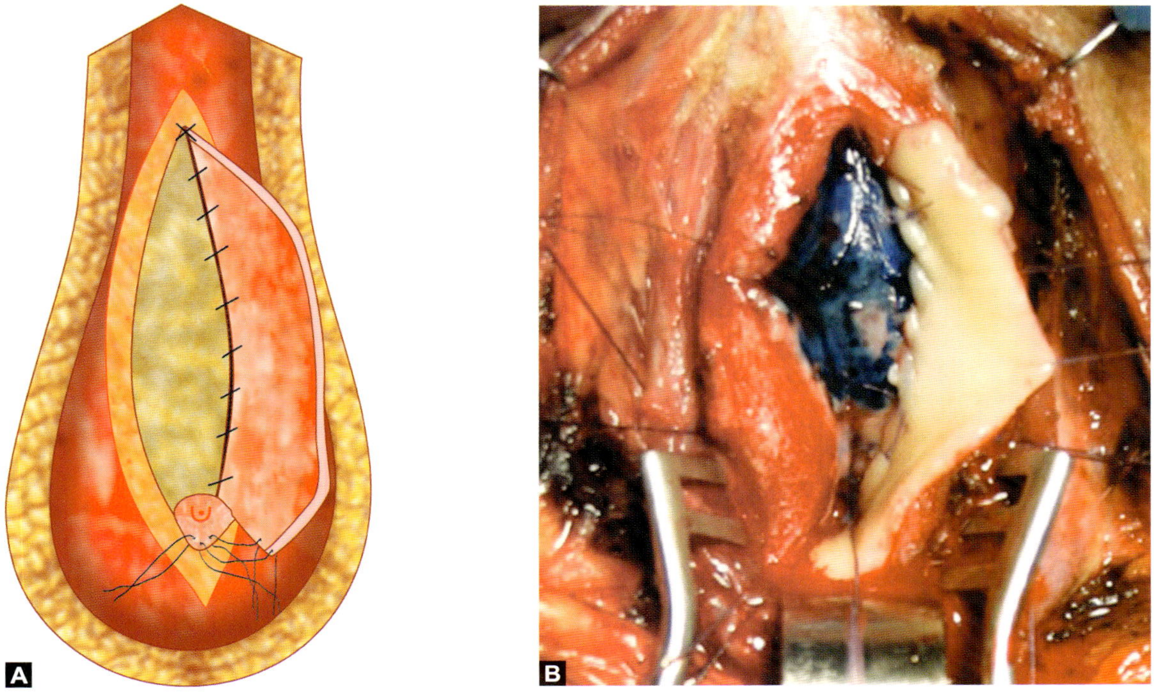

Figs 7.21A and B: Running suture is used to complete the anastomosis between margin of the graft and the urethral plate. Three stitches placed at 5 and 6 o'clock in front up to the verumontanum are passed into the proximal oral mucosal graft edge

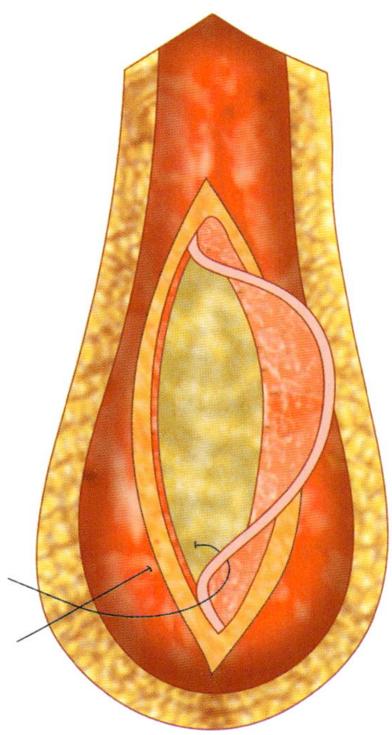

Fig. 7.22: The stitch placed at 7 o'clock in front up to the verumontanum is passed into the proximal oral mucosal graft

DORSAL ORAL MUCOSAL GRAFT URETHROPLASTY

Patient Selection

The dorsal onlay oral mucosal graft bulbar urethroplasty is suggested in all patients presenting nontraumatic urethral strictures in the distal bulbar urethra of any length, including patients with panurethral strictures **(Fig. 7.26)**. This technique may also be used in patients with repeated failed urethrotomy or previous failed bulbar urethroplasty.

Surgical Technique

A midline perineal incision is made. A plastic ring retractor with plastic hooks is put in place. The bulbar urethra is dissected from corpora cavernosa only along the left side, starting from the distal tract where muscles are absent, leaving the bulbospongiosum muscle and central tendon of the perineum intact **(Figs 7.27A and B)**. Along the right side, the urethra remains attached to the corpora cavernosa for its full length, thus preserving its lateral vascular blood supply. On the left side, the urethra is partially rotated and lateral urethral surface is underlined **(Figs 7.28A and B)**.

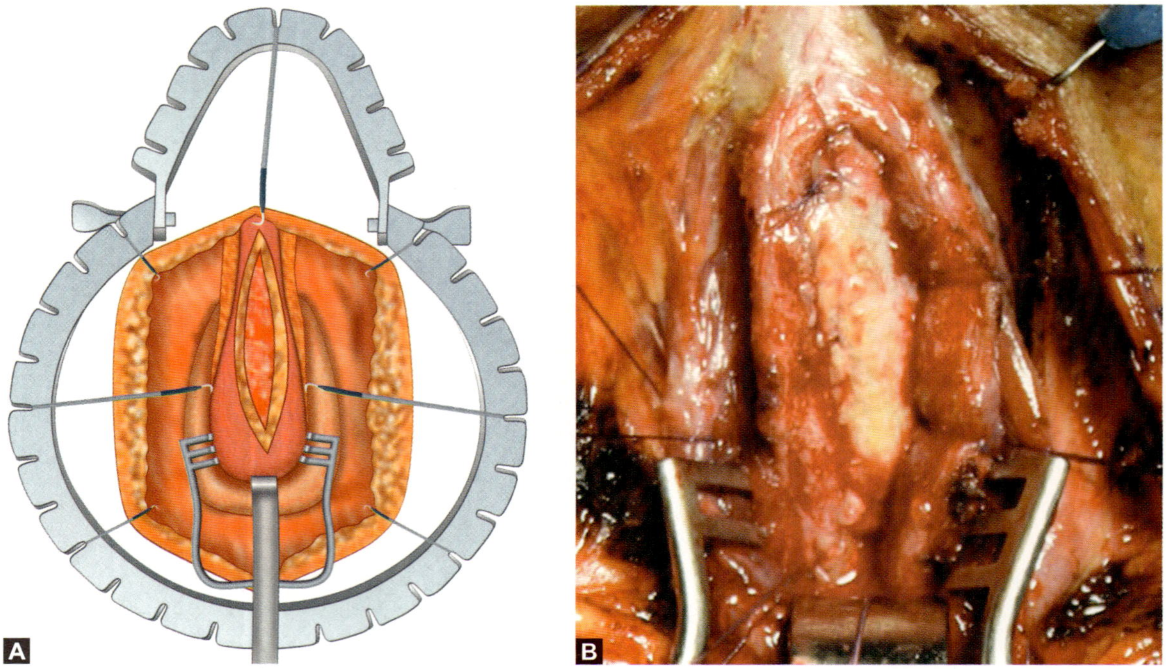

Figs 7.23A and B: The graft is rotated over catheter and a running suture completes anastomosis between margin of the graft and the urethral plate

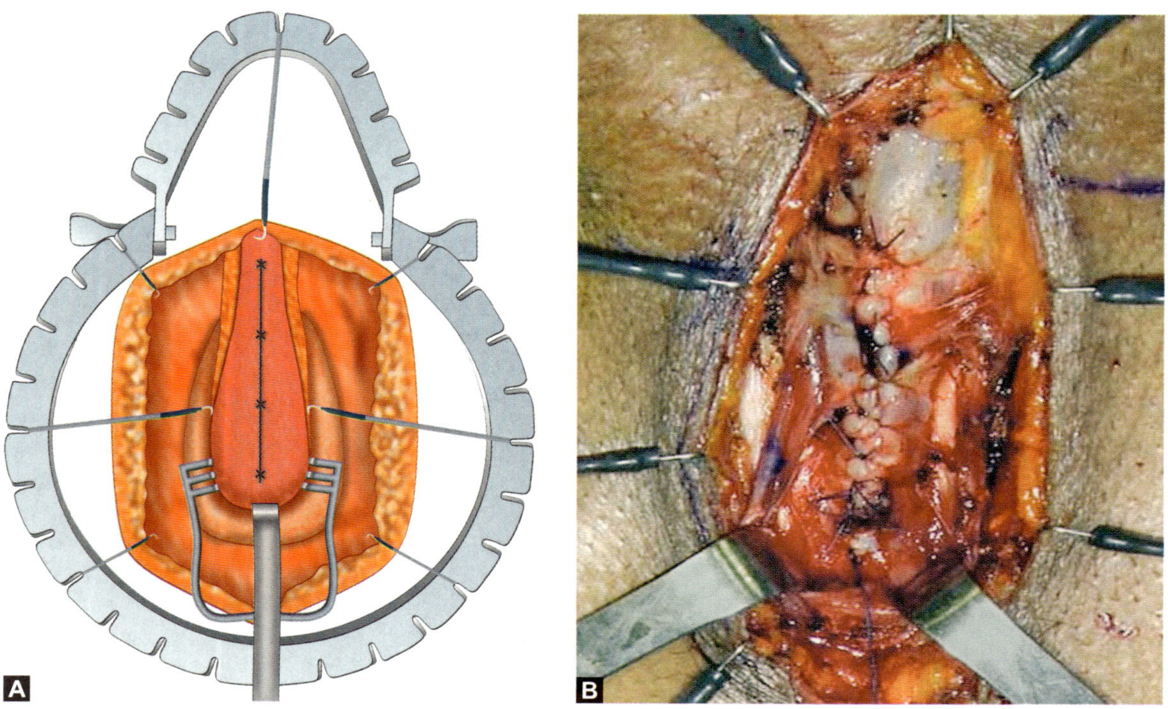

Figs 7.24A and B: The corpus spongiosum is closed over the oral graft

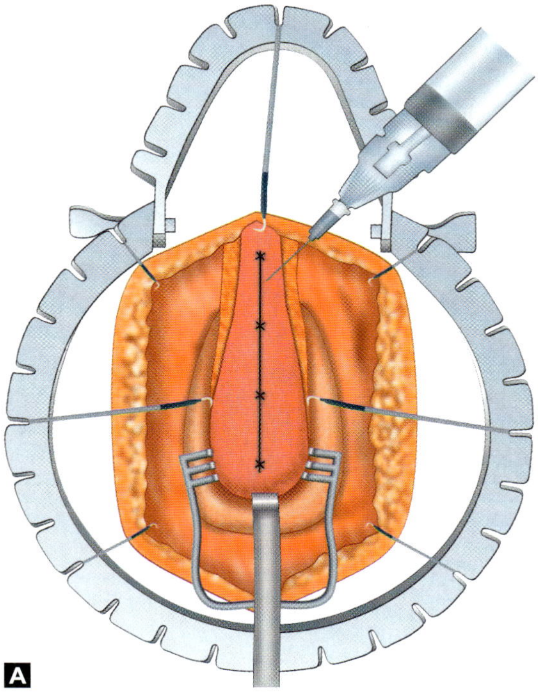

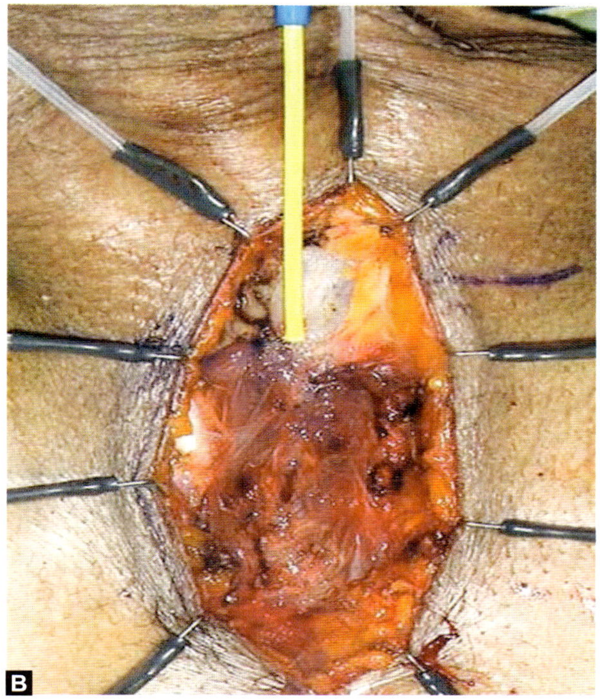

Figs 7.25A and B: Fibrin glue (2 ml) is injected over the corpus spongiosum

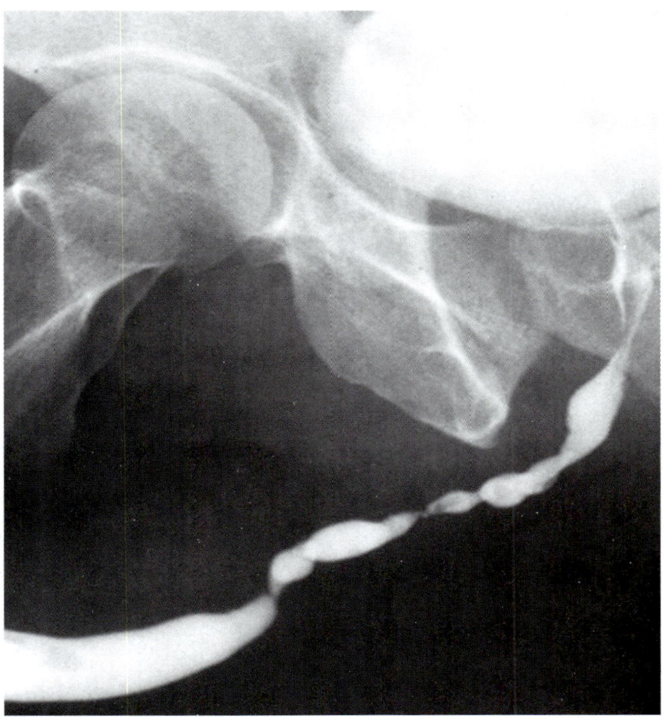

Fig. 7.26: Long urethral stricture extending in the distal part of the bulbar urethra

The distal extent of the stenosis is identified, the dorsal urethral surface is incised along the midline and the urethral lumen is exposed. The stricture is then incised along its entire length by extending the urethrotomy distally and proximally **(Figs 7.29A and B)**. Once the entire stricture has been incised, length and width of the remaining urethral plate is measured. Fibrin glue (2 ml) is injected over the corpora cavernosa and the oral mucosal graft, trimmed to an appropriate size according to length and width of the urethrotomy, is spread fixed over the tunica albuginea **(Figs 7.30A and B)**. The two apices of the graft are sutured to the proximal and distal apices of the urethrotomy **(Figs 7.31A and B)**. A Foley 16 Fr grooved silicone catheter is inserted, and the right margin of the oral graft is sutured to left margin of the urethral mucosal plate **(Figs 7.32A and B)**. The bulbar urethra, with the intact bulbospongiosum muscle, is rotated to its original position over the graft **(Figs 7.32A and B)**. Interrupted 4-0 polyglactin sutures are used to stabilize the urethral margins onto corpora cavernosa over the graft on left side. At end of procedure, the graft is completely covered by the urethra, then by the muscles, and 2 ml of fibrin glue are injected over the suture line **(Figs 7.33A and B)**. The perineal fat and the skin are closed with interrupted absorbable sutures. A drain is unnecessary. The catheter is left in place for 3 weeks.

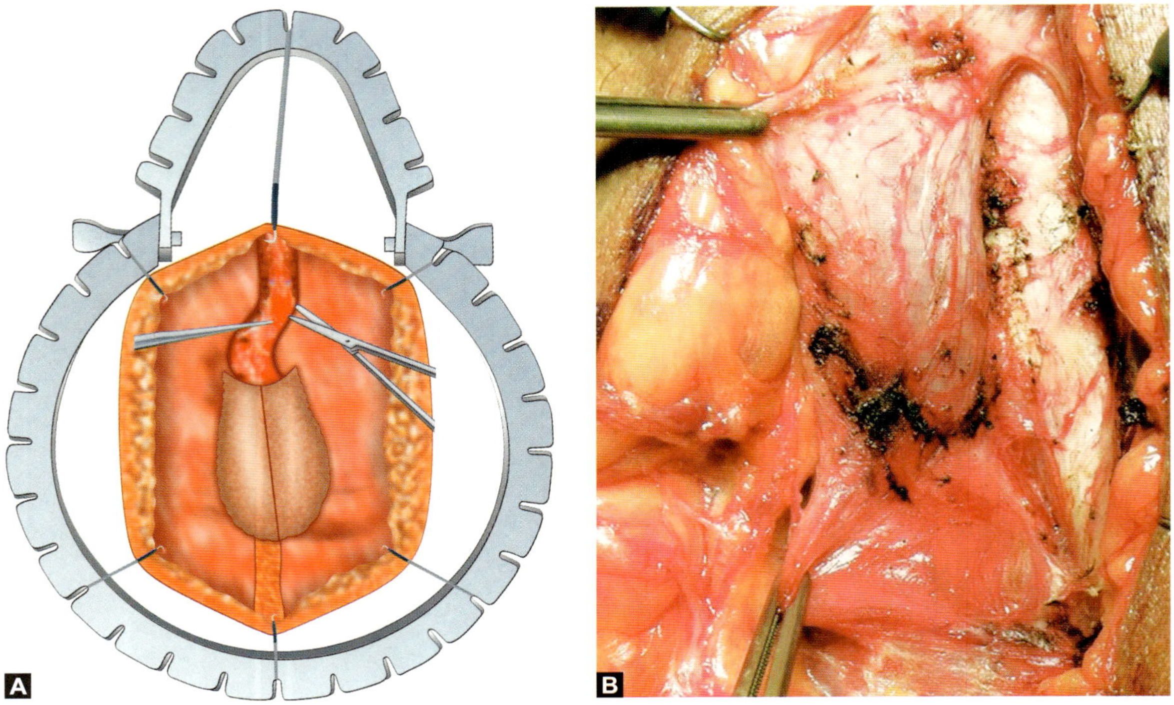

Figs 7.27A and B: The bulbar urethra is dissected from corpora cavernosa along the left side, starting from the distal tract

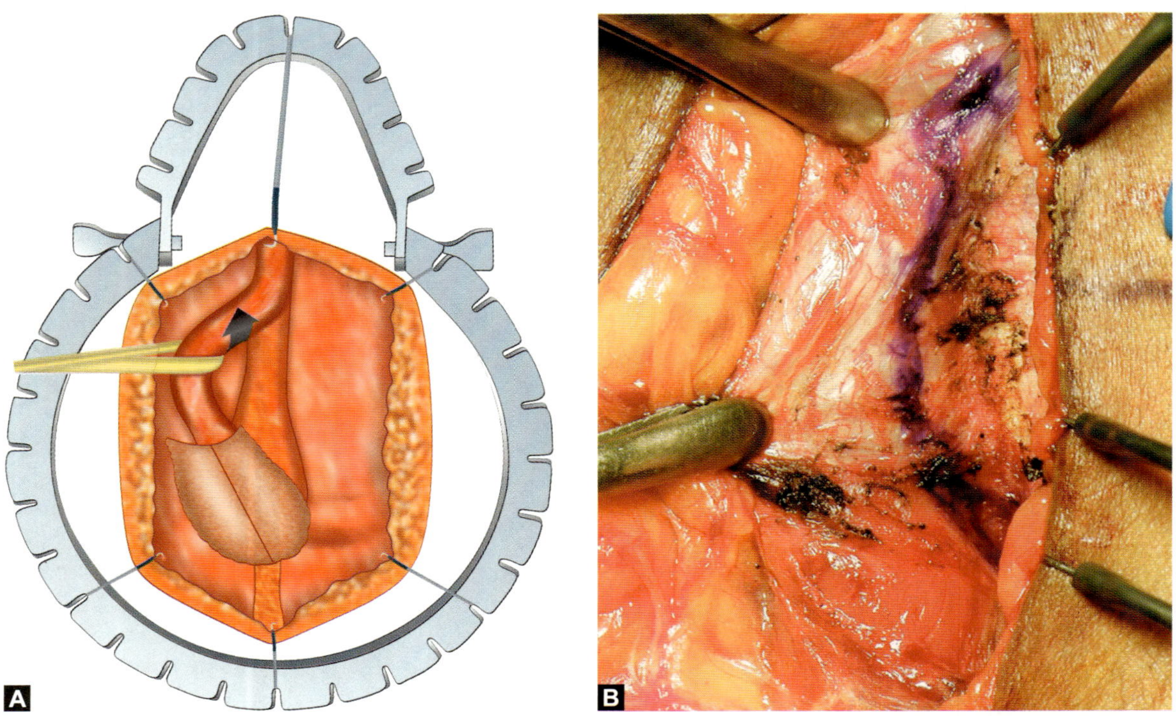

Figs 7.28A and B: The urethra is rotated and the dorsolateral urethral surface is underlined

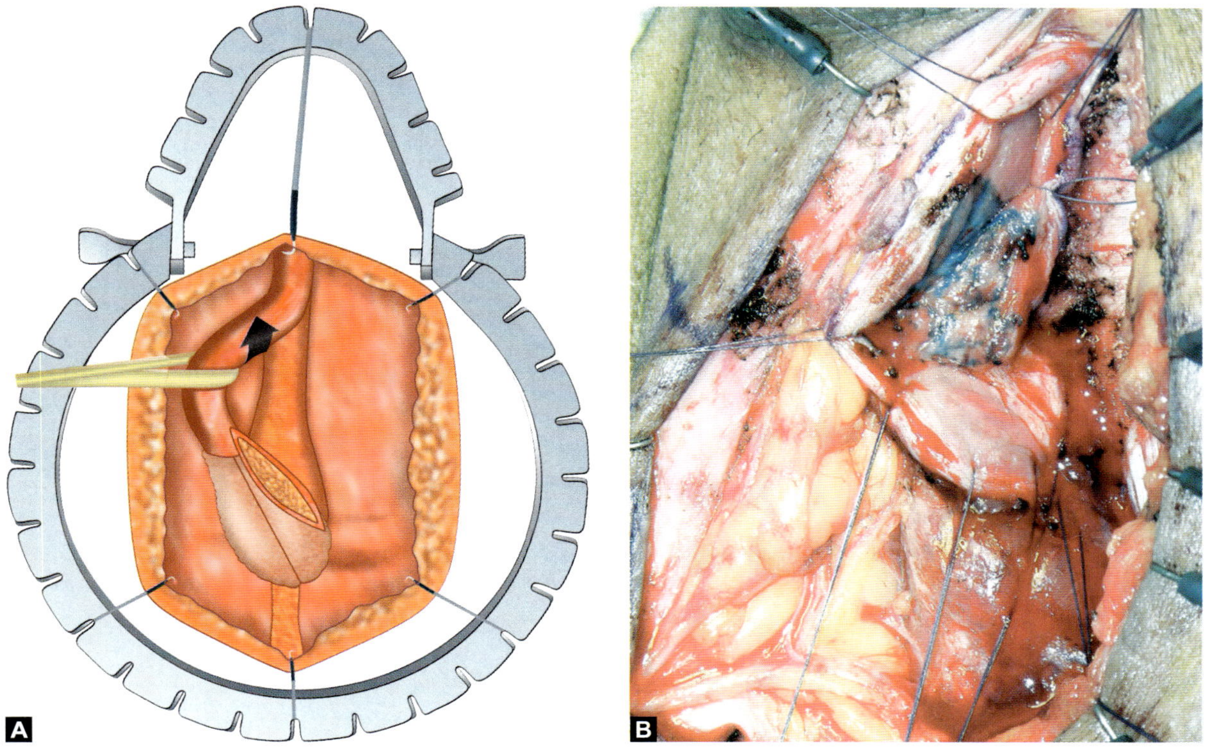

Figs 7.29A and B: The stricture is opened along its entire length

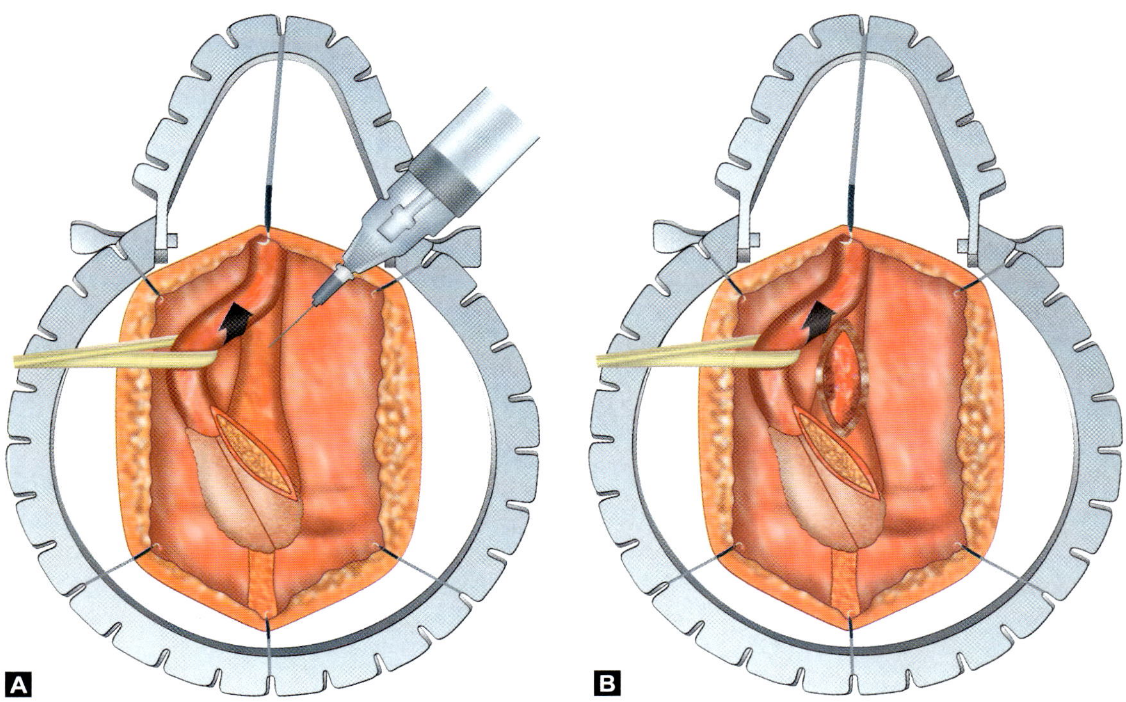

Figs 7.30A and B: Fibrin glue (2 ml) is injected over the corpora cavernosa, and the oral mucosal graft is fixed over the tunica albuginea

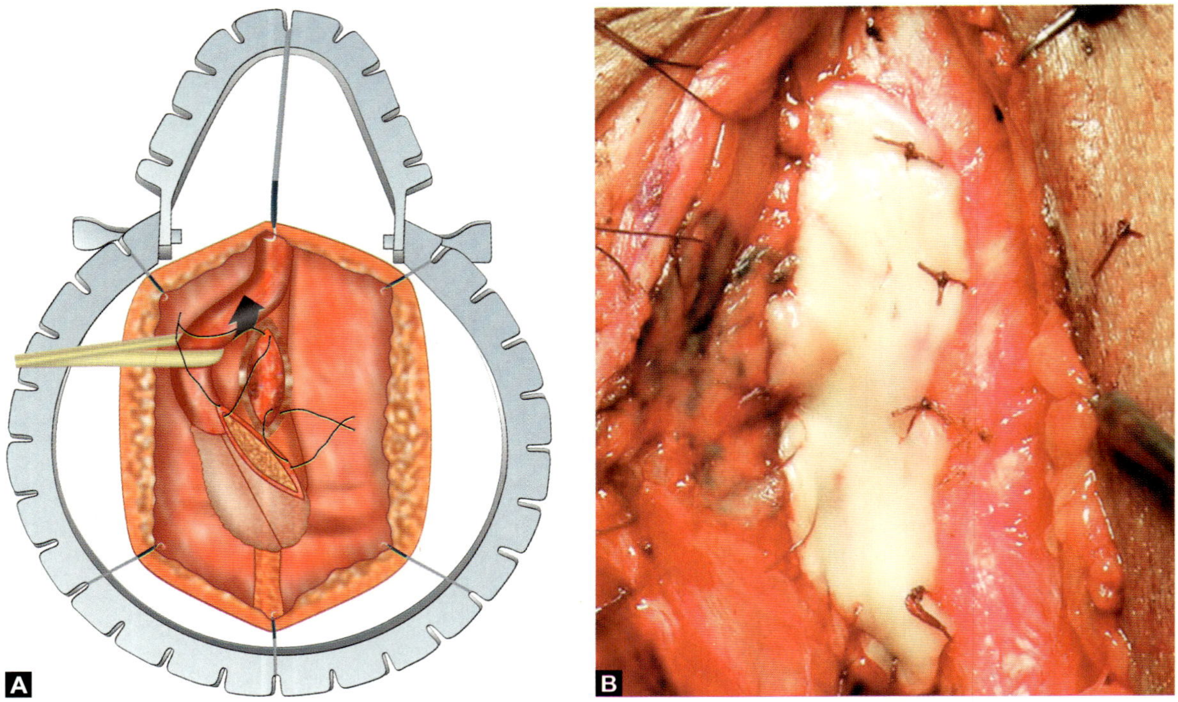

Figs 7.31A and B: The apices of the graft are sutured to the proximal and distal apices of urethrostomy

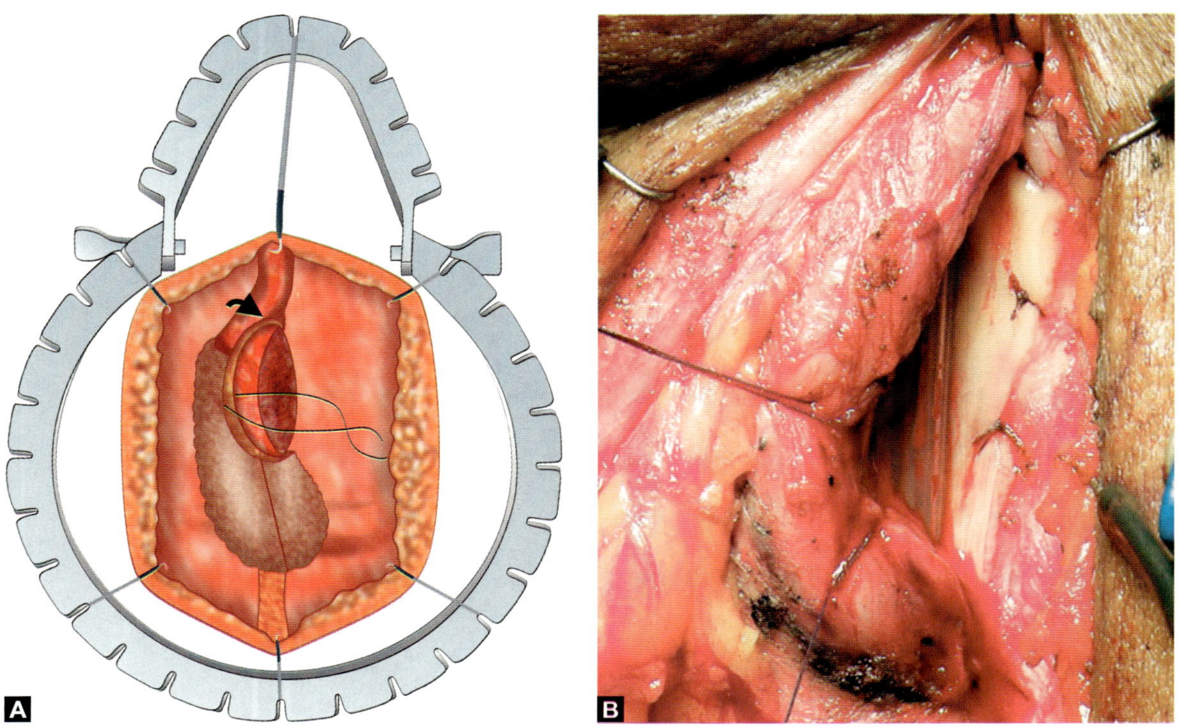

Figs 7.32A and B: The margin of oral graft is sutured to the urethral mucosal plate, and the urethra is rotated to its original position

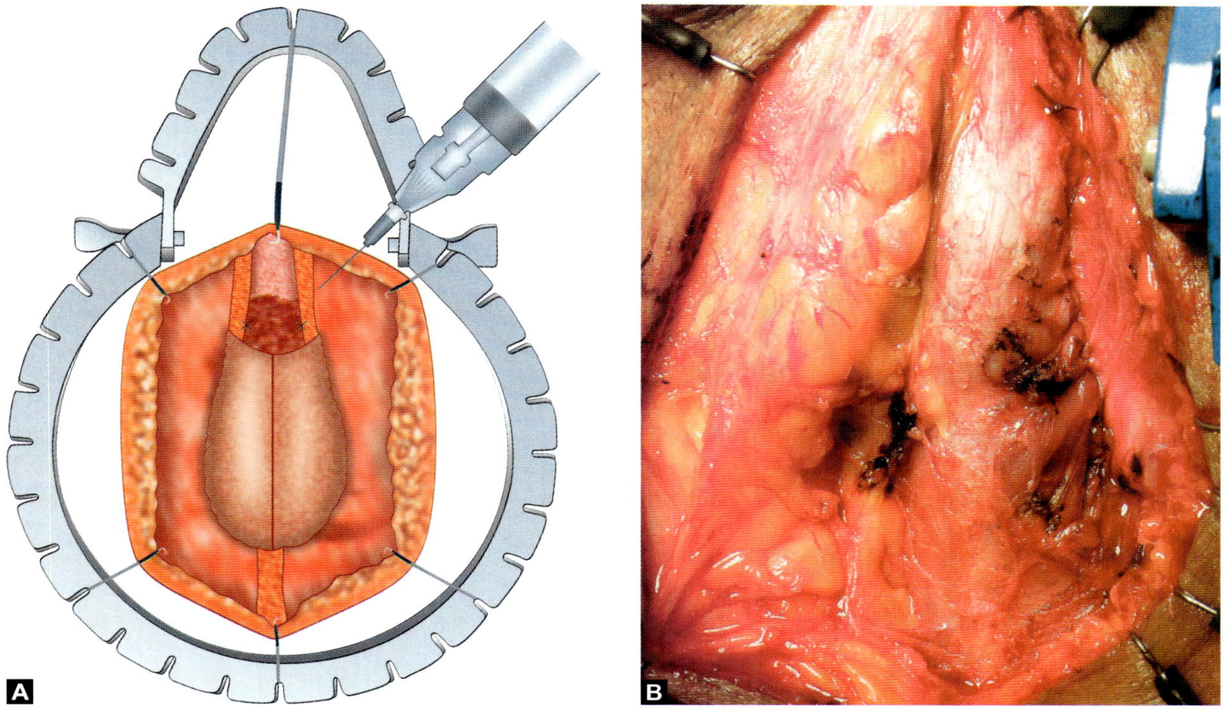

Figs 7.33A and B: Fibrin glue (2 ml) is injected over the suture line

Results

The results of dorsal graft urethroplasty are fully reported in the literature in large series of patients from different institutions.[5,8-11] In authors' center, from October 1998 to June 2010, a total of 27 patients with a median age of 39 years (range 24–77) underwent dorsal oral mucosal graft urethroplasty. Of 27 patients, treatment of 20 (74.1%) was successful and 7 (25.95) were failures. Average follow-up was 69 months (range 12–146). All data is available at: www.urethralcenter.it.

Alternative to this Procedure

Penile fasciocutaneous circular flap.

AUGMENTED ANASTOMOTIC REPAIR USING ORAL GRAFT

Patient Selection

The augmented anastomotic repair, using an oral graft, is suggested in patients presenting traumatic urethral strictures ranging from 2 cm to 5 cm in the distal or proximal bulbar urethra **(Fig. 7.34)**. This technique may

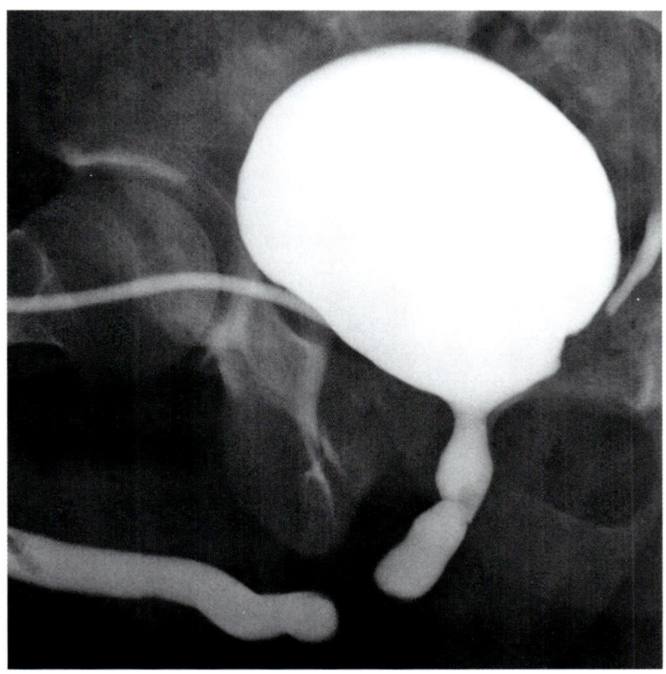

Fig. 7.34: Traumatic long bulbar urethral stricture

also be used in patients with repeated failed urethrotomy or previous failed bulbar urethroplasty.

Surgical Technique

A midline perineal incision is made. A plastic ring retractor with plastic hooks is put in place. The bulbospongiosum muscle is opened at the midline. The distal site of stenosis is identified and marked, and the bulbar urethra is circumferentially dissected from the corpora cavernosa **(Figs 7.35A and B)**. The bulbar urethra is completely transected at level of the stenosis **(Figs 7.36A and B)**. The scar tissue involving the urethral mucosa and spongiosum tissue is carefully removed. The distal and proximal urethral edges are opened and spatulated along the dorsal surface **(Figs 7.37A and B)**. Fibrin glue (2 ml) is injected over the albuginea of the corpora cavernosa **(Figs 7.38A and B)**. The oral graft is glued to the corpora by fibrin glue **(Figs 7.39A and B)**. The distal and proximal apices of the graft are fixed to the distal and proximal mucosal edges. The distal urethra is pulled down and sutured to the right graft margin, and the proximal urethra is pulled up and sutured to the right graft margin **(Figs 7.40A and B)**. The left urethral mucosal margin is sutured to the oral mucosal graft. The distal and proximal urethral edges are sutured together in the ventral surface like in an end-to-end anastomosis **(Figs 7.41A and B)**. At the end of procedure, the oral graft should be completely covered by the urethra, and 2 ml of fibrin glue is injected over the suture line **(Figs 7.42A and B)**. The bulbospongiosum muscle is sutured at the midline. The perineal fat and the skin are closed with interrupted absorbable sutures. A drain is unnecessary. The catheter is left in place for 3 weeks.

Results

The results of augmented anastomotic repair are reported in the literature.[4,9] In authors' center, from January 2000 to October 2006, a total of 24 patients with a median age of 38 years (range 21–72 years) underwent augmented anastomotic repair. Of 24 patients, treatment of 18 (75%) was successful and 6 (25%) failed. Average follow-up was 80 months (range 50–107). All data is available at: www.urethralcenter.it.

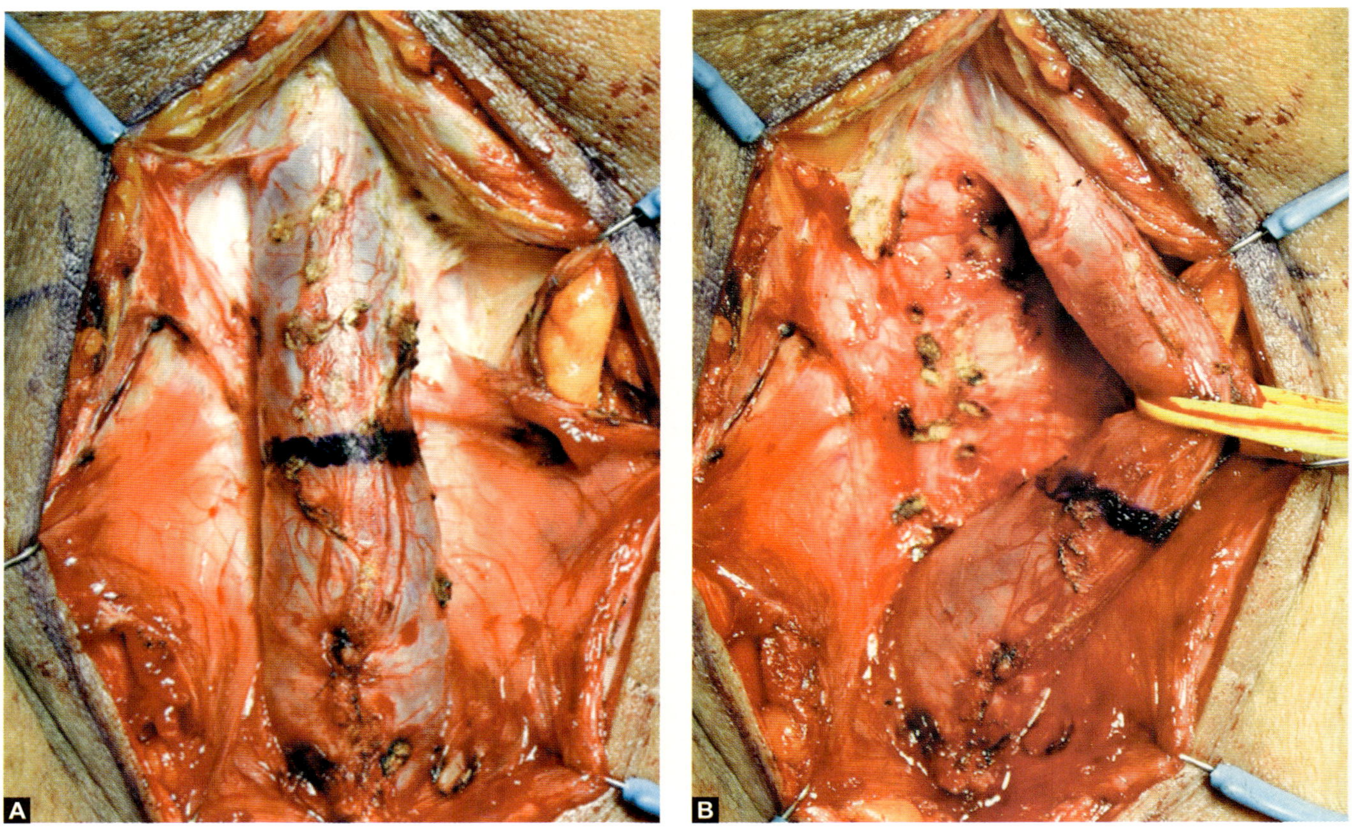

Figs 7.35A and B: (A) The distal site of stenosis is identified; (B) The bulbar urethra is dissected from the corpora cavernosa

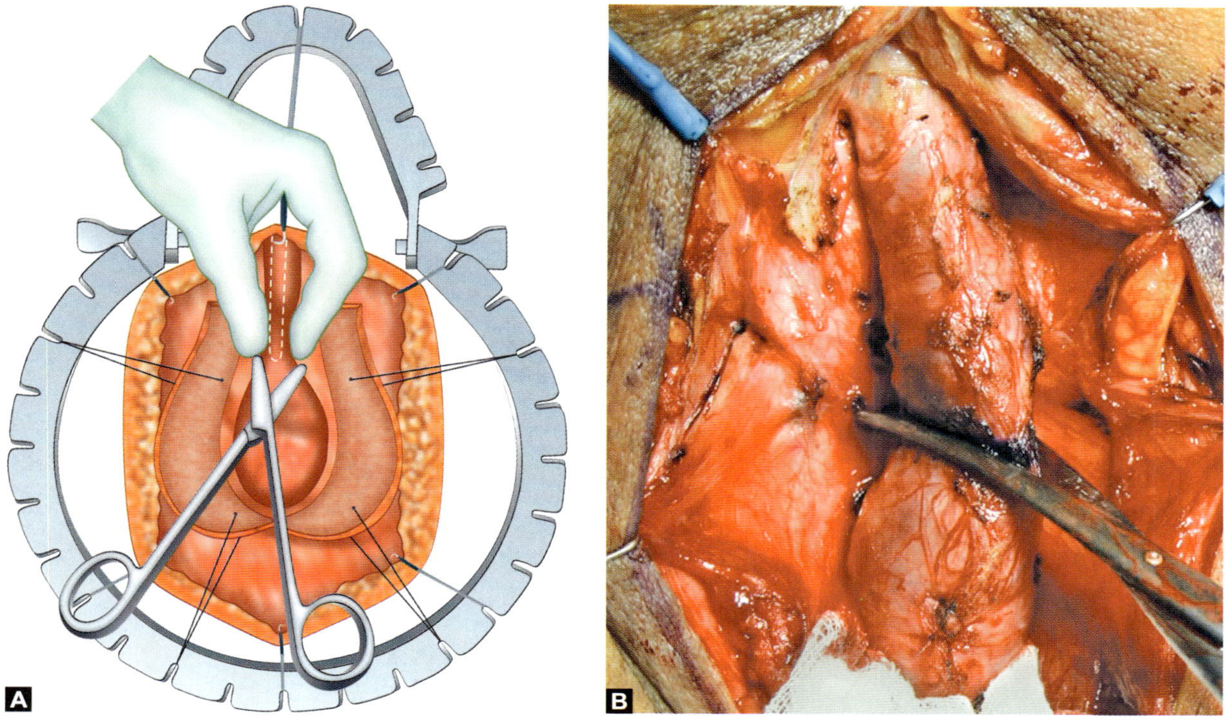

Figs 7.36A and B: The bulbar urethra is transected at the level of the stenosis

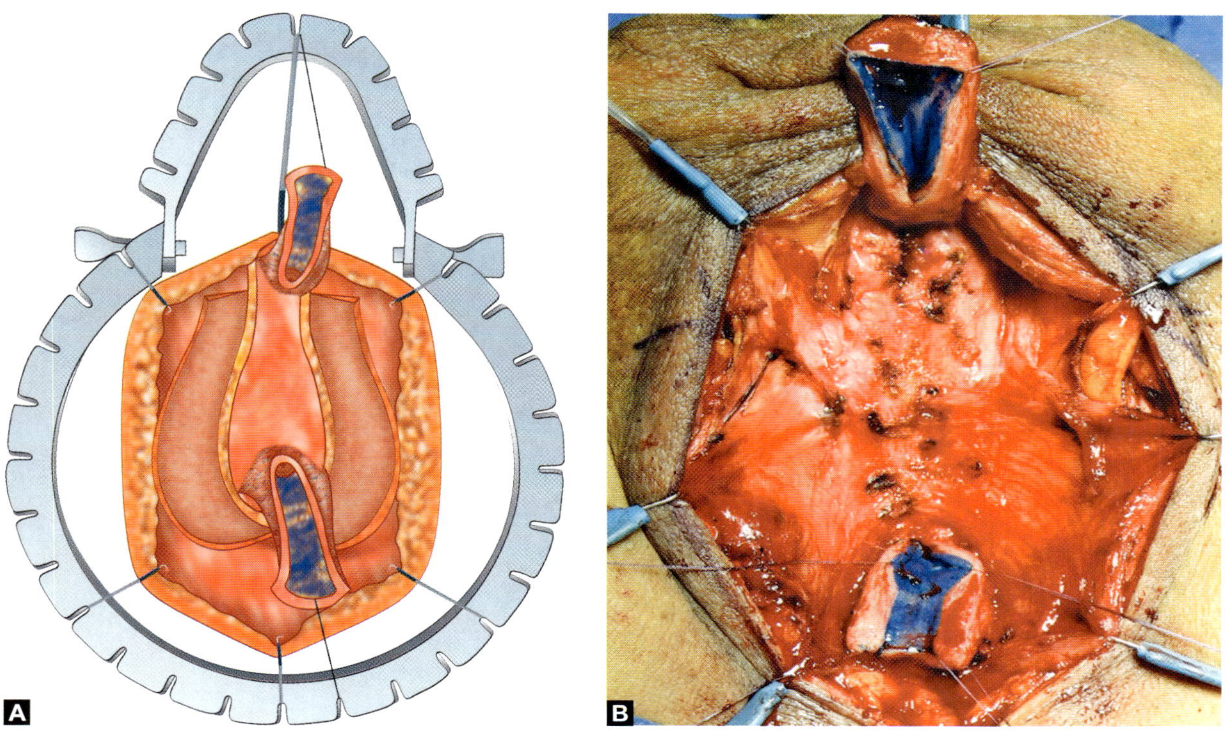

Figs 7.37A and B: The distal and proximal urethral edges are spatulated along the dorsal surface

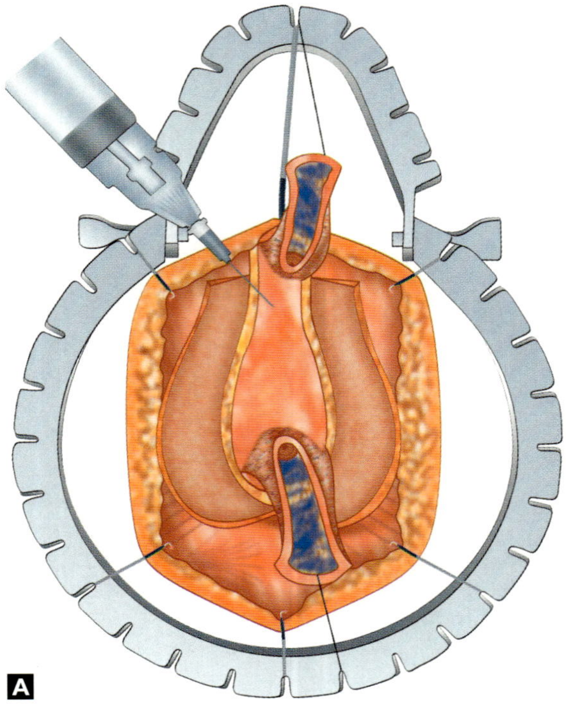
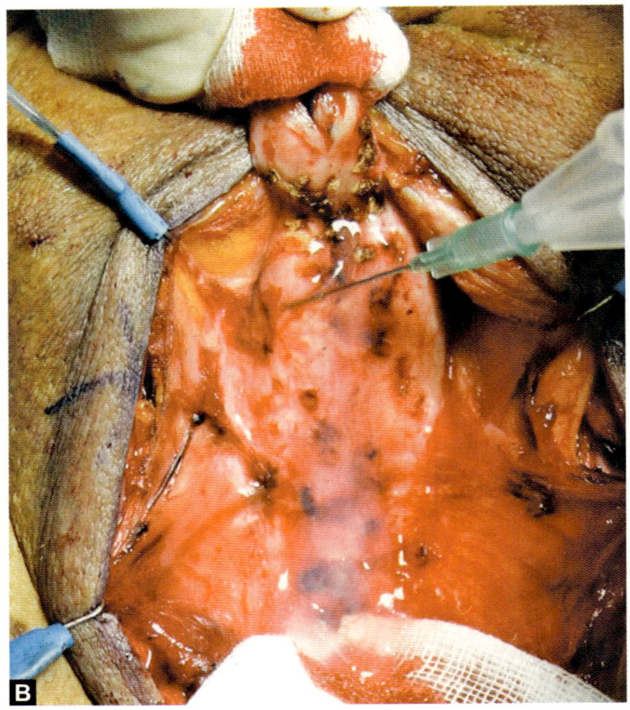

A B

Figs 7.38A and B: Fibrin glue (2 ml) is injected over the albuginea of the corpora cavernosa

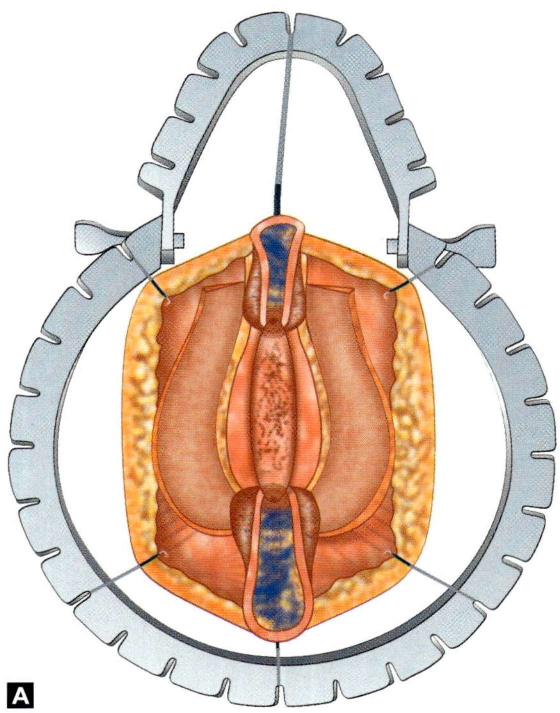
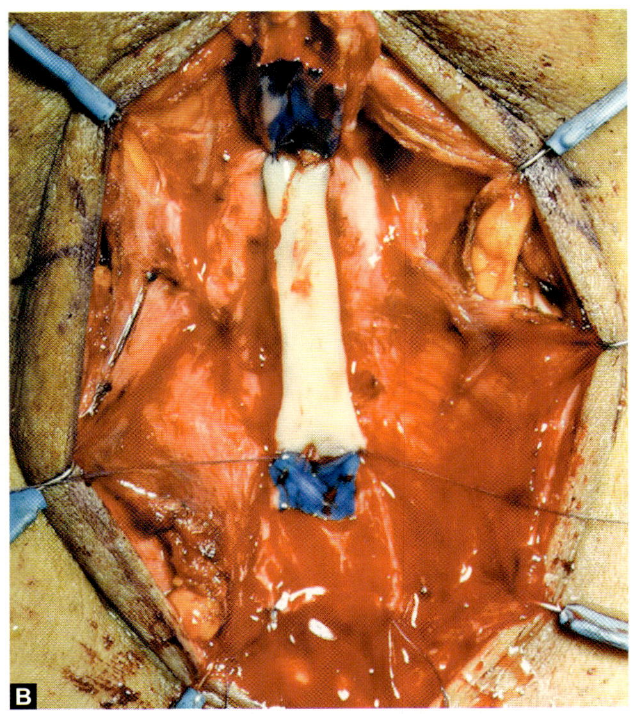

A B

Figs 7.39A and B: The oral graft is glued to the corpora

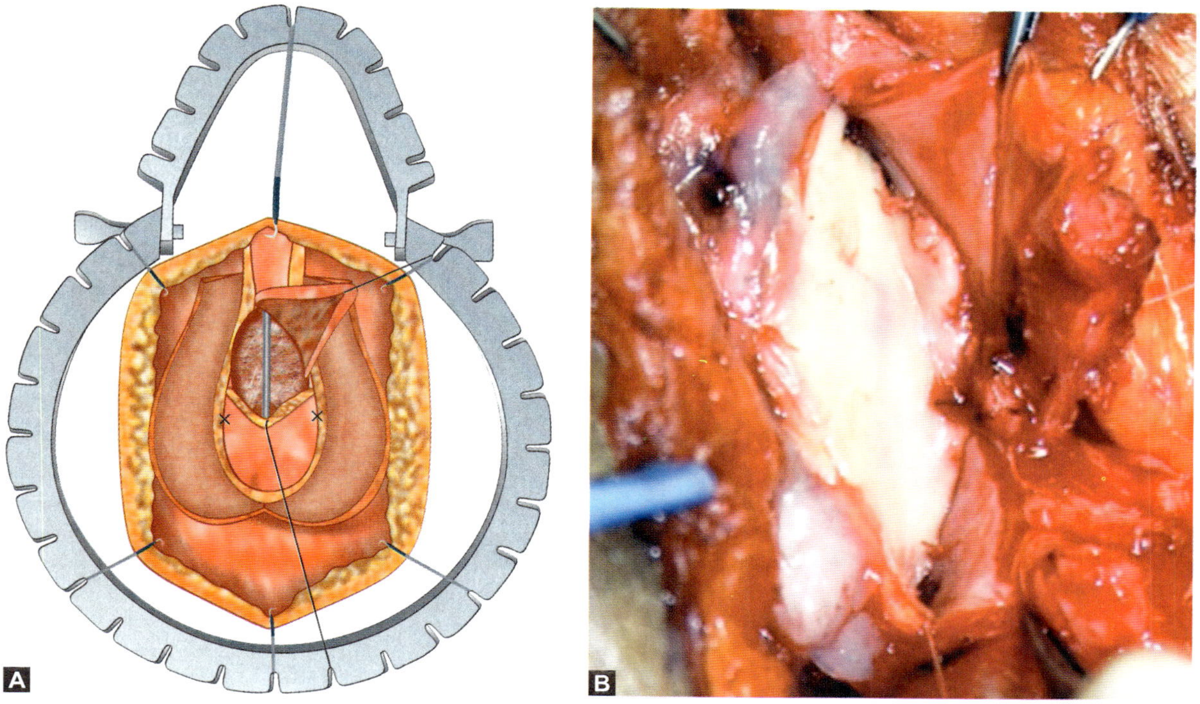

Figs 7.40A and B: The distal urethra is pulled down and the proximal urethra is pulled up

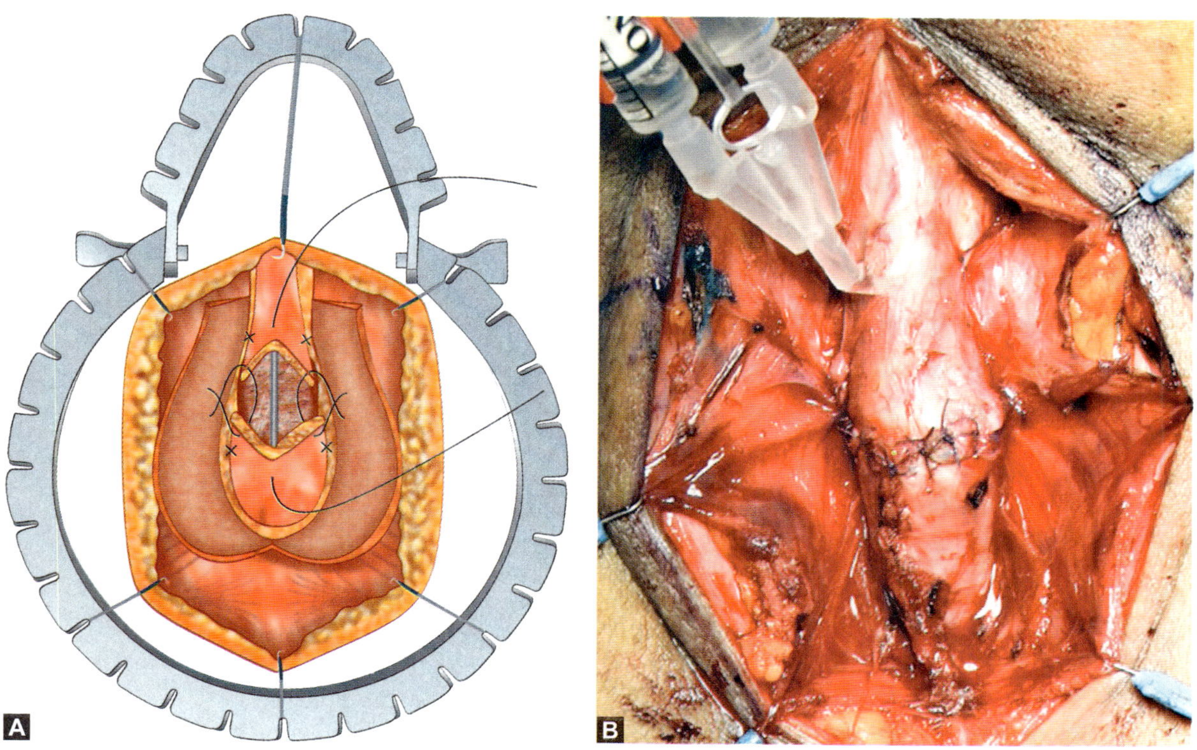

Figs 7.41A and B: The urethral mucosa is sutured to the oral mucosal graft. The distal and proximal urethral edges are sutured together in the ventral surface

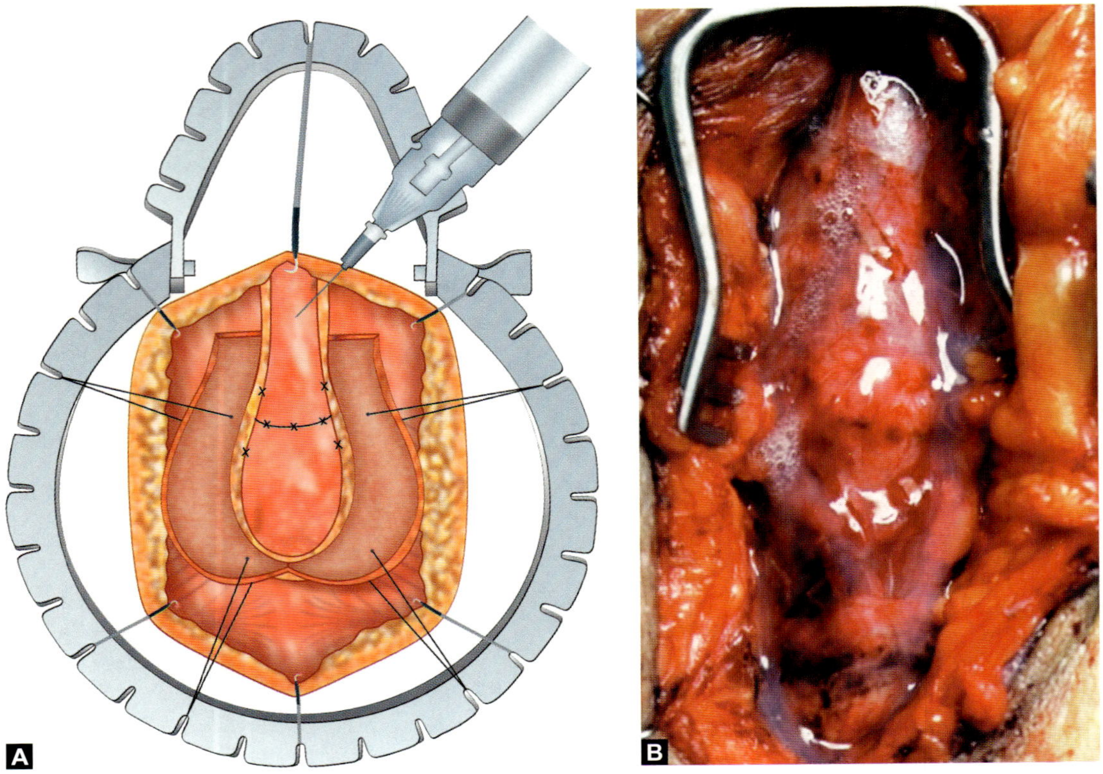

Figs 7.42A and B: Fibrin glue (2 ml) is injected over the suture line

Alternative to this Procedure

End-to-end anastomosis.

POSTOPERATIVE CARE AFTER BULBAR URETHROPLASTY USING AN ORAL GRAFT

An ice bag is applied to the cheek to avoid pain and hematoma. A clear liquid diet and ice cream is initially given and then advanced to a soft and regular diet. The patient ambulates on the 1st postoperative day and is discharged from the hospital 3 days after surgery. All patients receive postoperative broad-spectrum antibiotics and are maintained on oral antibiotics until the catheter is removed. Three weeks after surgery, the bladder is filled with contrast medium, the Foley catheter is removed and voiding cystourethrography obtained.

REFERENCES

1. el-Kasaby AW, Fath-Alla M, Noweir AM, et al. The use of buccal mucosa patch graft in the management of anterior urethral strictures. J Urol. 1993;149(2):276-8.
2. Morey AF, McAninch JW. When and how to use buccal mucosal grafts in adult bulbar urethroplasty. Urology. 1996;48(2):194-8.
3. Barbagli G, Selli C, Tosto A, et al. Dorsal free graft urethroplasty. J Urol. 1996;155(1):123-6.
4. Guralnick ML, Webster GD. The augmented anastomotic urethroplasty: indications and outcome in 29 patients. J Urol. 2001;165(5):1496-501.
5. Andrich DE, Leach CJ, Mundy AR. The Barbagli procedure gives the best results for patch urethroplasty of the bulbar urethra. BJU Int. 2001;88(4):385-9.
6. Wessells H. Ventral onlay graft techniques for urethroplasty. Urol Clin North Am. 2002;29(2):381-7.

7. Armenakas NA. Long-term outcome of ventral buccal mucosal grafts for anterior urethral strictures. AUA News. 2004;9:17-8.
8. Barbagli G, Palminteri E, Lazzeri M, et al. Interim outcomes of dorsal skin graft bulbar urethroplasty. J Urol. 2004;172 (4):1365-7.
9. Iselin CE, Webster GD. Dorsal onlay urethroplasty for urethral stricture repair. Word J Urol. 1998;16(3):181-5. Review.
10. Barbagli G, Selli C, di Cello V, et al. A one-stage dorsal free-graft urethroplasty for bulbar urethral strictures. Br J Urol. 1996;78(6):929-32.
11. Barbagli G, Palminteri E, Rizzo M. Dorsal onlay graft urethroplasty using penile skin or buccal mucosa in adult bulbourethral strictures. J Urol. 1998;160(4):1307-9.
12. Elliot SP, Metro MJ, McAninch JW. Long-term follow-up of the ventrally placed buccal mucosa onlay graft in bulbar urethral reconstruction. J Urol. 2003;169(5):1754-7.
13. Barbagli G, Guazzoni G, Lazzeri M. One-stage bulbar urethroplasty: retrospective analysis of the results in 375 patients. Eur Urol. 2008;53(4):828-33.
14. Barbagli G, Palminteri E, Guazzoni G, et al. Bulbar urethroplasty using buccal mucosa grafts placed on the ventral, dorsal or lateral surface of the urethra: are results affected by the surgical technique? J Urol. 2005;174(3): 955-7.
15. Abouassaly R, Angermeier KW. Cleveland clinic experience with buccal mucosa graft urethroplasty: intermediate-term results. J Urol. 2005;173:33.
16. Barbagli G, De Stefani S, Annino F, et al. Muscle- and nerve-sparing bulbar urethroplasty: a new technique. Eur Urol. 2008;54(2):335-43.
17. Barbagli G, Vallasciani S, Romano G, et al. Morbidity of oral mucosa graft harvesting from a single cheek. Eur Urol. 2010;58(1):33-41.

8

CHAPTER

Free Graft Urethroplasty by Ventral Sagittal Urethrotomy Approach

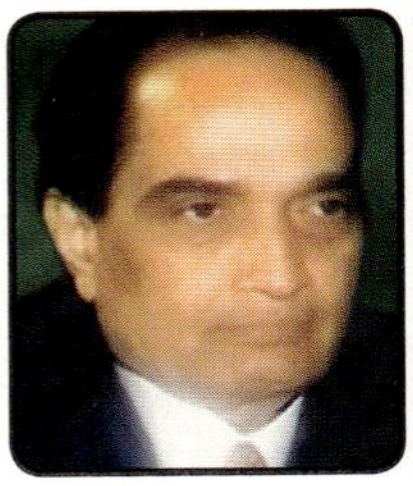

HS Asopa

HS Asopa, AL Vyas, GG Singhal

Chapter Outline

Abstract

Though this method is developed and perfected by Professor Asopa himself, he never calls this procedure by his name. Rather calls it as free graft urethroplasty by ventral sagittal urethrotomy approach. The basis is minimal dissection of the urethral plate to preserve its maximum nerve and blood supply. All this translates into better results. Also better preservation of sexual function. Practical steps and tips have been clearly described as to how Professor Asopa does it. Written by the master himself, it is a treat to go through this manuscript.

Keywords

Ventral sagittal urethrotomy, Tunica albuginea, Meshed free graft, Quilting of graft, Palminteri, Combined dorsal and ventral free graft urethroplasty, Bisected urethra, Dorsal free graft, Ventral free graft, Substitution urethroplasty, Circumflex vessels, Native urethral plate, Circumcoronal incision.

INTRODUCTION

The management of the anterior and posterior urethral strictures defers considerably. Although simple urethral dilatation and optical urethrotomy are commonly used procedures yet the long-term success remains always in doubt in the management of anterior urethral strictures. Simple stricture excision with primary spatulated anastomosis in bulbar urethral strictures is a common surgical treatment with long-term cure.[1]

The penile strictures, recurrent, multiple and long anterior urethral strictures need tissue substitution for cosmetic and long-term success. Presently buccal, preputial and penile skin are commonly used to substitute the urethra as free graft, which can be used dorsally, ventrally or both.[2]

Recently dorsal free graft has gained popularity and well accepted world over. Barbagli et al. (1996) described the dorsal free graft technique by mobilizing the strictured urethra and a dorsal stricturotomy.[3] Asopa et al. (2001) described dorsal free graft urethroplasty by ventral sagittal urethrotomy approach.[4] Since then this technique is well taken-up and practiced world over. This chapter describes the substitution urethroplasty for anterior urethral strictures by this technique. It can be further extended by combining a ventral free graft in refractory bulbomembranous strictures [as described by Palminteri et al. (2008)] with good results.

PREOPERATIVE EVALUATION

Every patient is evaluated by detailed history, physical examination, uroflowmetry, micturating cystourethrogram and retrograde urethrogram. In some cases urethroscopy is resorted to. Ultrasound examination and magnetic resonance imaging of stricture may be resorted to in difficult redo complicated cases where things are not amply clear.

SURGICAL TECHNIQUES

Dorsal Free Graft Urethroplasty by Ventral Sagittal Urethrotomy Approach in Penile Urethral Strictures

Patient is placed in supine position if the stricture is limited to the pendulous penile portion. Appropriate regional or general anesthesia is administered. Urethra is exposed by midline ventral penile incision. Methylene blue is injected (in the lumen of urethra) and 5 F feeding tube is placed in lumen of strictured urethra. Alternatively a guide wire is placed through the narrow lumen of strictured urethra with the help of urethroscopy. A 16 F Nelaton's catheter is introduced through the external urethral meatus to identify the distal site of stricture.

Step 1

Ventral urethrotomy is created to lay open the strictured portion on the urethra and extended for 1 cm, both proximally and distally into the healthy urethra **(Figs 8.1A and B)** after infiltrating 2% lignocaine with adrenaline diluted four times.

Step 2

Dorsal wall of the laid open strictured urethra is incised in the midline down to the tunica albuginea of the underlying corporal bodies (after infiltrating diluted lignocaine with adrenaline). The margins of incised dorsal urethra are dissected/excised from the tunica by sharp dissection without lifting the two halves of bisected urethra, to create an adequate elliptical raw area over tunica albuginea **(Fig. 8.1C)**. Medial margins of bisected urethra are anchored to underneath tunica using 5-0 polyglactin (vicryl) interrupted sutures **(Fig. 8.1D)**.

Step 3

A meshed free graft (defatted inner preputial or buccal mucosa or penile skin) is placed over raw area as dorsal inlay (the defatted surface facing the tunica) and anchored to the medial margins of bisected urethra, incorporating underlying tunica by using 5-0 polyglactin interrupted

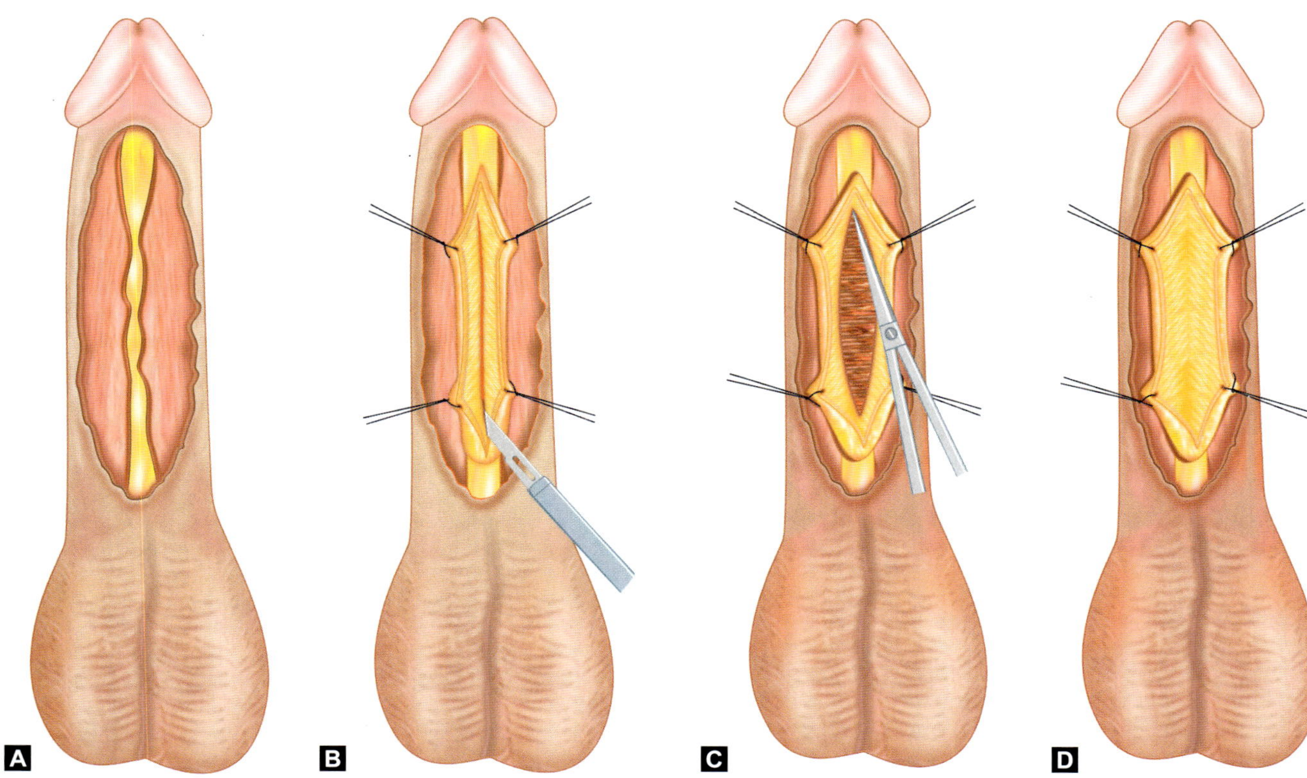

Figs 8.1A to D

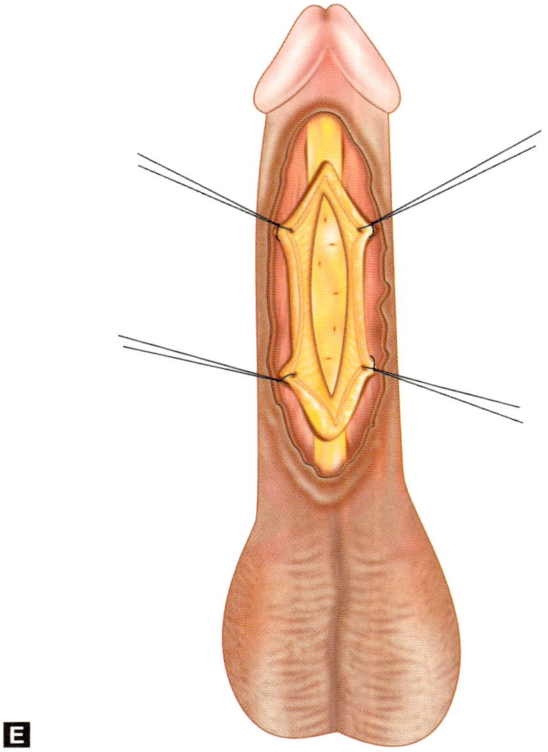

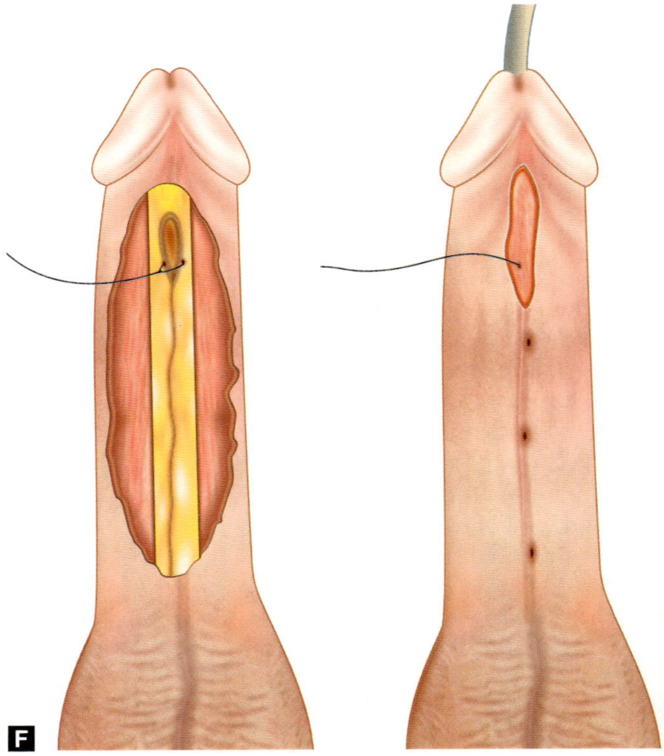

Figs 8.1E and F

Figs 8.1A to F: (A and B) Ventral urethrotomy is created to lay open the stricture; (C and D) Dorsal wall of the laid open strictured urethra is incised in the midline. Medial margins of bisected urethra are anchored to underlying tunica; (E) A meshed free graft is placed over the raw area and fixed to the margins as well as quilted to the underlying tunica; (F) Retubularization of the urethra with 4-0 vicryl and skin closure

sutures. The graft is further quilted to underlying tunica at several places **(Fig. 8.1E)**.

Step 4

Urethra is retubularized by continuous sutures of 4-0 polyglactin on an appropriate sized catheter **(Fig. 8.1F)**. Pressure dressing is done following layered wound closure.

Catheter is removed after 3 weeks. All patients are followed-up regularly, following surgery by uroflowmetry, and urethrogram is done when the Qmax (maximum flow rate) is less than 15 ml/min on uroflowmetry. Urethroscopy is done in selected cases.

Dorsal Free Graft Urethroplasty in Bulbar Urethral Strictures[5]

The patient is placed in lithotomy position. A midline perineal incision is made. Rest of the steps are same as described step-wise above and as illustrated in the **Figures 8.2A to G**.

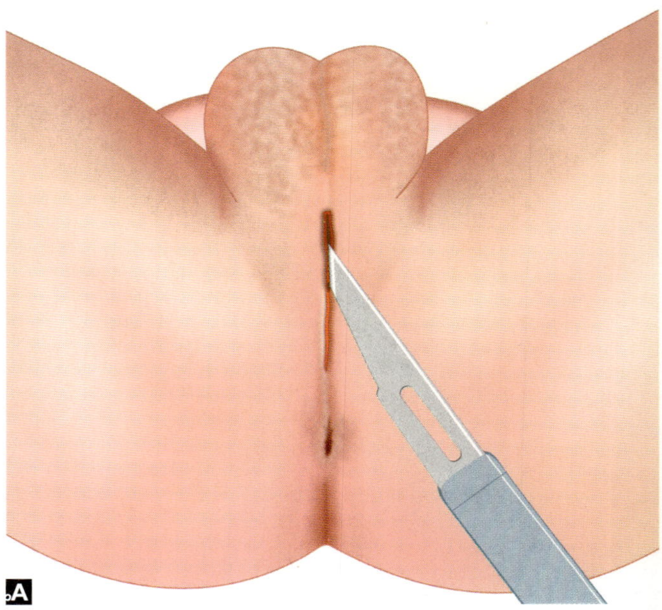

Fig. 8.2A

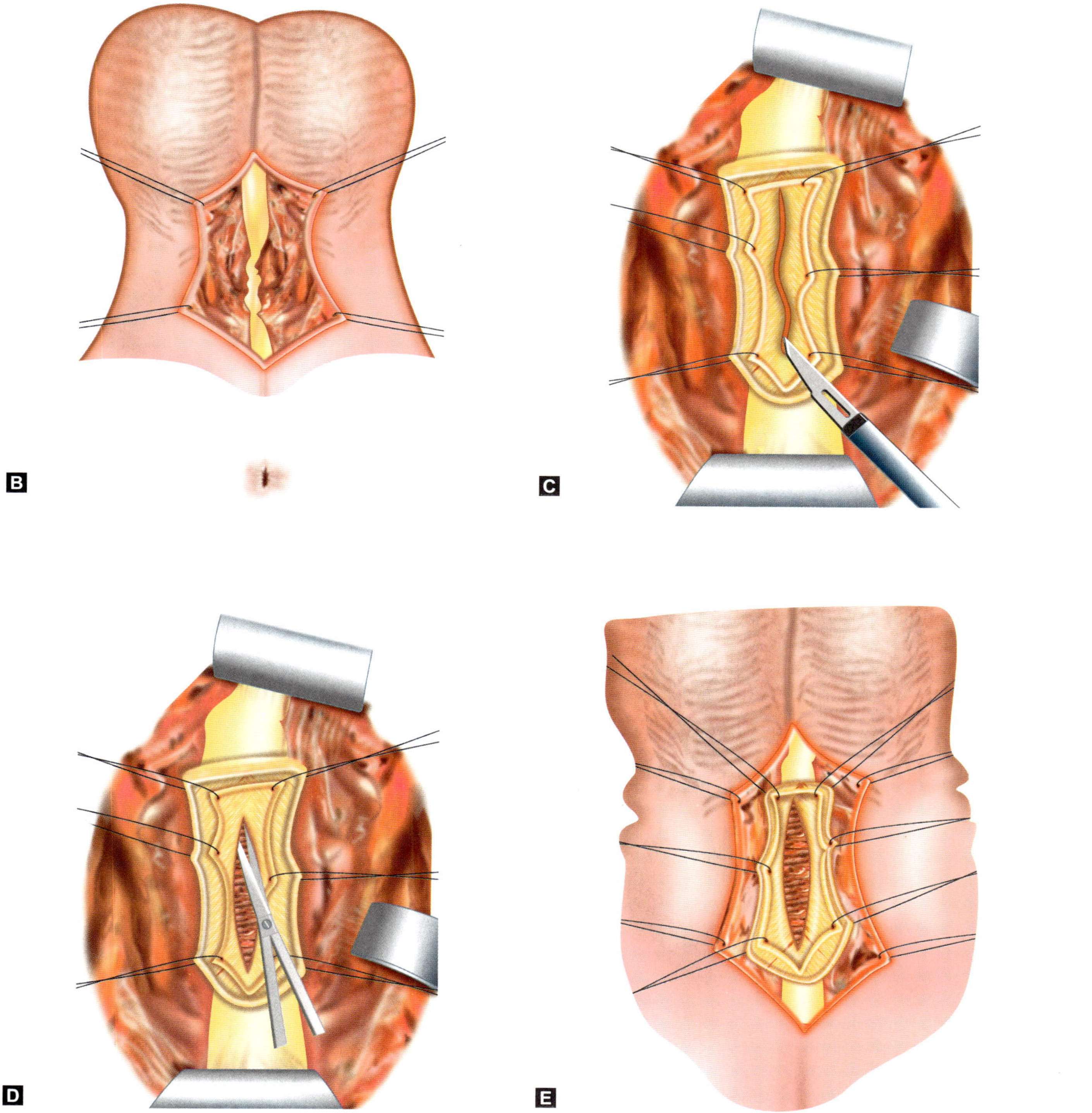

Figs 8.2B and E

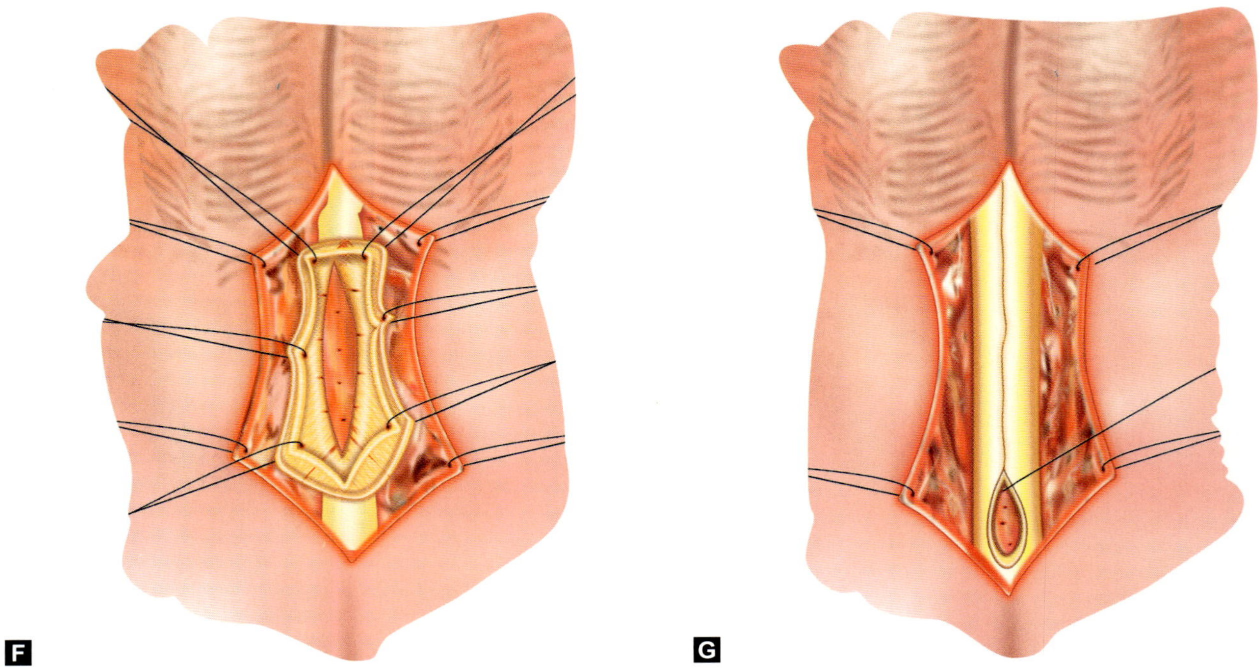

Figs 8.2F and G

Figs 8.2A to G: (A) Midline perineal incision; (B) The stricturous portion of the bulbar urethra is exposed; (C) After ventral urethrotomy and laying open of the stricture, a midline dorsal incision is given; (D) The midline dorsal incision is extended into healthy urethra on both sides; (E) Adequate raw area created as the graft bed. Note the medial margins of bisected urethra are fixed to the underlying tunica; (F) The free graft is placed on the raw area and fixed at margins as well as quilted to underlying tunica; (G) Retubularization of the urethra

Step 1

Midline perineal incision is given, the various fascial layers are cut in midline till bulbospongiosus is reached, which is incised in the midline (if required) to expose the stricturous portion of the bulbar urethra. A ventral urethrotomy is given and the stricturous part of the bulbar urethra is laid open. It is important to extend the incision into healthy urethra both proximally and distally **(Figs 8.2A to C)**.

Step 2

A midline dorsal incision is given in the stricturous part of the bulbar urethra and care is taken to extend it into healthy urethra both proximally and distally. Adequate raw area is created as the graft bed. If required, fibrous tissue may be excised bit by bit **(Figs 8.2D and E)**.

Step 3

The prepared buccal mucosa is placed on the raw surface and fixed on the margins as well as quilted to the underlying tunica **(Fig. 8.2F)**.

Step 4

The urethra is now retubularized starting from the proximal end. The wound is then closed in layers **(Fig. 8.2G)**.

Dorsal Free Graft Urethroplasty in Panurethral Strictures

Here also the basic steps are same as illustrated in **Figures 8.3A to E**. Patient is placed in the lithotomy position to enable approach to the bulbar urethra.

Step 1

Midline penile incision and ventral urethrotomy are given over some sort of guide in the urethra depending upon its calibre (glide wire/infant feeding tube/metal dilator) **(Fig. 8.3A)**.

Step 2

Liberal dorsal urethrotomy incision is given in **Figure 8.3B**.

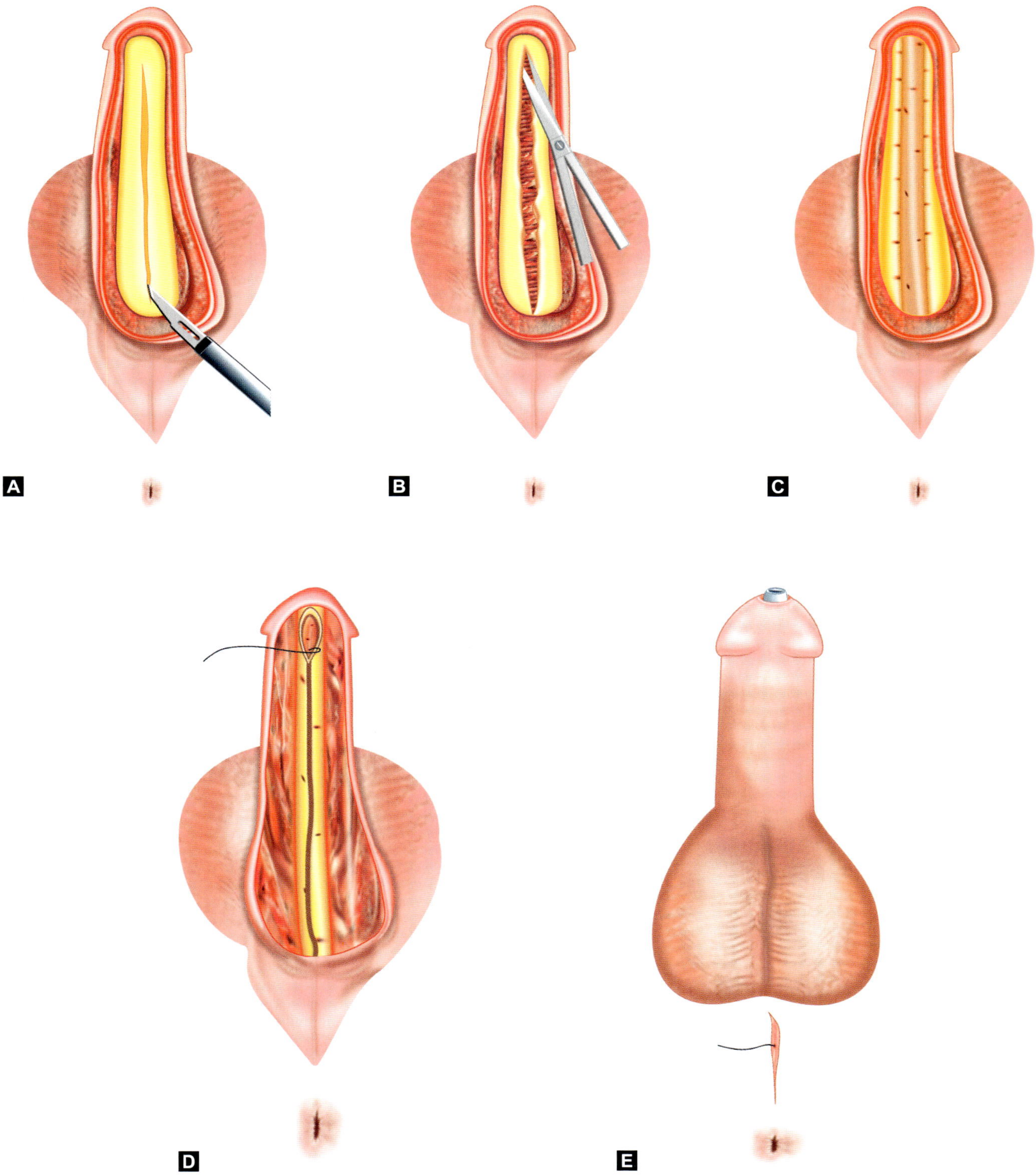

Figs 8.3A to E: (A) Ventral urethrotomy; (B) Dorsal urethrotomy; (C) Free graft placement and fixation as a dorsal inlay; (D) Retubularization of the urethra; (E) Wound closure in layers

Step 3

Buccal mucosal graft is placed with its raw surface on the underlying corpora and the mucosal surface facing the surgeon. It is then fixed to the underlying corpora using 5/8th curve 4'0 or 5'0 vicryl on a cutting needle **(Fig. 8.3C)**.

Step 4

The open urethra is now retubularized starting proximal to distal with continous absorbable suture with interlocking in between. The wound is then closed in layers **(Figs 8.3D and E)**.

Combined Dorsal and Ventral Free Graft Urethroplasty by Ventral Sagittal Urethrotomy Approach

Palminteri et al. (2008) described combined dorsal and ventral double buccal mucosa graft in bulbar urethral reconstruction.[6,7]

In tight bulbar and bulbomembranous strictures of varying length, authors have repaired these strictures by combining dorsal and ventral free graft urethroplasty (as suggested by Palminteri et al.) and thus preserved narrow urethral plate to obtain adequate urethral augmentation and to avoid sexual complications.

Surgical Technique

The strictured bulbar urethra is exposed by using ventral sagittal urethrotomy approach [(Asopa et al., 2001) dorsal free graft urethroplasty technique] with the aid of a guide wire and methylene blue, as described earlier and a dorsal free graft is applied **(Figs 8.4A to E)**.

Ventral Free Graft

Following dorsal augmentation, the second graft is sutured laterally to the right margin of bisected urethra, by running 5-0 chromic sutures (with epithelial surface facing toward the lumen). Indwelling catheter is inserted and graft is rotated and sutured laterally to the left margins of bisected urethra, by running 5-0 chromic sutures. Thus a neourethra is created by using dorsal and ventral free graft patches to the mucosal margins of bisected urethral plate. A few quilting stitches of 5-0 chromic catgut are given between ventral graft and corpora spongiosum. Finally fascia of corpora spongiosum is closed over the ventral graft with 4-0 running sutures **(Figs 8.4F to I)**.

Postoperative Assessment

It includes uroflowmetry and complete urine examination, every 4 monthly for 1st postoperative year and then annually thereafter. Urethrography and urethroscopy are performed for patients presenting a Qmax of less than 15 ml/sec.

RESULTS OF VENTRAL SAGITTAL URETHROTOMY APPROACH

In authors' series, 219 cases of long anterior urethral and multiple strictures ranging from 2 cm to full length were operated upon between January 1998 and July 2011 with follow-up from 6 months to 11.5 years. Urethroscopy was done in 12 cases, showing good take-up of graft and urethrogram showing normal caliber urethra in all cases after surgery. One patient developed temporary fistula which healed up spontaneously after 2 weeks of further catheterization. Twenty two cases developed restricture, six were controlled on dilatations done three times in 1 year and now voiding normally. Optical internal urethrotomy was done in 3 cases and 13 were operated, 4 by dorsal free buccal mucosal graft and 9 by ventral free graft. Uroflowmetry and calibration were done regularly following the surgery, which confirmed normal diameter of urethra with uroflow rate of more than 15 cc/sec. Of these, 129 patients had a follow-up of more than 1 year. Three patients with long penile stricture who had some chordee before surgery developed significant chordee after surgery, which had to be treated by dorsal plication.

Seventy seven patients of bulbar and bulbomembranous urethral stricture (1–5 cm long) have been treated by dorsal and ventral free graft urethroplasty by ventral sagittal urethrotomy approach with follow-up from 6 months to 6 years. All these patients have uroflow of 15–40 ml/sec (mean preoperative flow rate < 7 ml/sec). Three patients developed dense stricture and were managed by perineal urethrostomy after counseling.

COMMENTS

Substitution urethroplasty is the mainstay of treatment for long anterior urethral strictures, anterior and multiple urethral and penile strictures. Either skin or mucous membrane graft or vascularized graft from genital area has been used for several years. Free graft when used as a patch ventrally in penile urethral stricture is easy to perform but is without support of spongiosa ventrally, leading to pooling of urine, ballooning and restricturing making these less reliable in long-term. Free extragenital full thickness or partial thickness skin graft fares the worst.[8] It was believed that vascularized genital skin flap in one-stage or two-stages would fare well because of its own blood supply. Vascularized inner preputial or penile skin islands, when used as a tube, have the same fate due to ballooning and pooling of urine in proximal

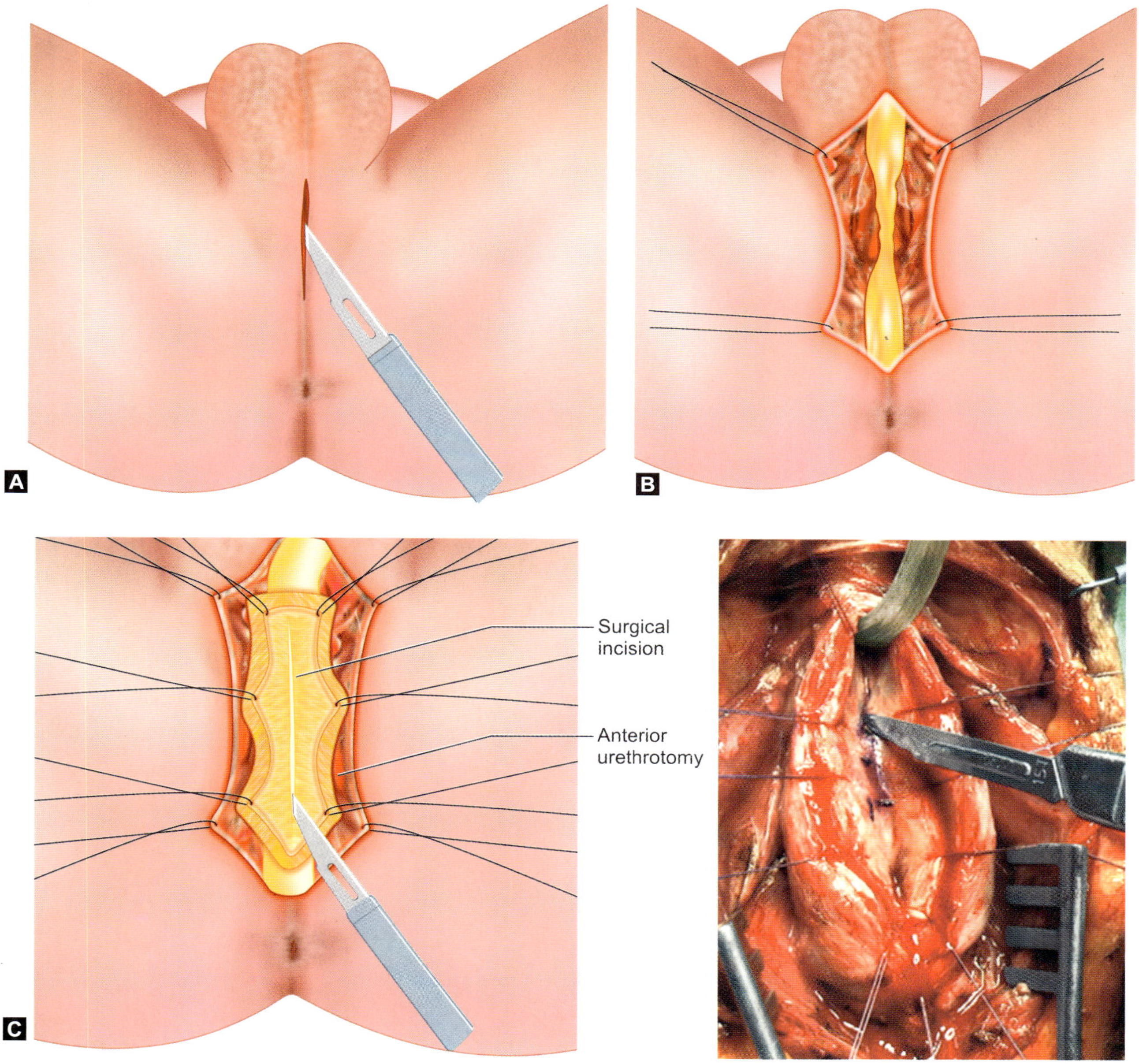

Figs 8.4A to C

anterior urethral strictures. Recent introduction of a technique, which places the free graft dorsally over the tunica after mobilizing the strictured urethra and a dorsal stricturotomy has found favor as it eliminates the outpouching and ballooning of the graft, because it is supported by corporal bodies (Barbagli).[3,9] In the present approach the urethra is not mobilized. Even long urethral strictures can be managed and approach is easy. The two halves of the urethra derive their blood supply from circumflex vessels and perforating vessels,[10,11] and these are preserved in this approach. In the approach in which the urethra is mobilized, these vessels are severed, thus compromising the vascular supply to the native urethral plate.

Dorsal and ventral graft urethroplasty technique in nonobliterative bulbar urethral strictures is an alternative to aggressive anastomotic urethroplasty as it provides enlarged urethral lumen, preserves vascularity and nerve supply, thus improving urinary flow and better ejaculatory sensations.

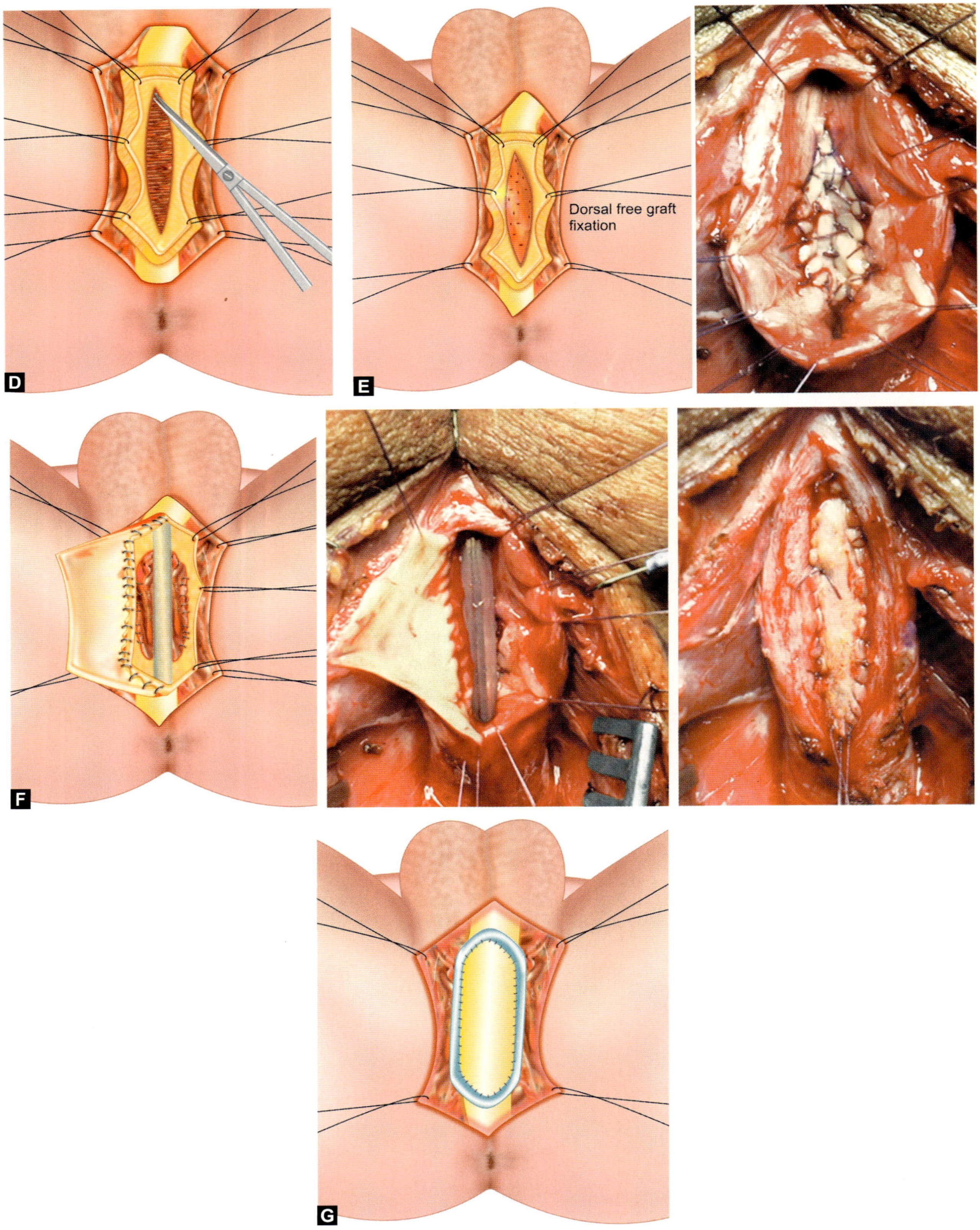

Figs 8.4D to G

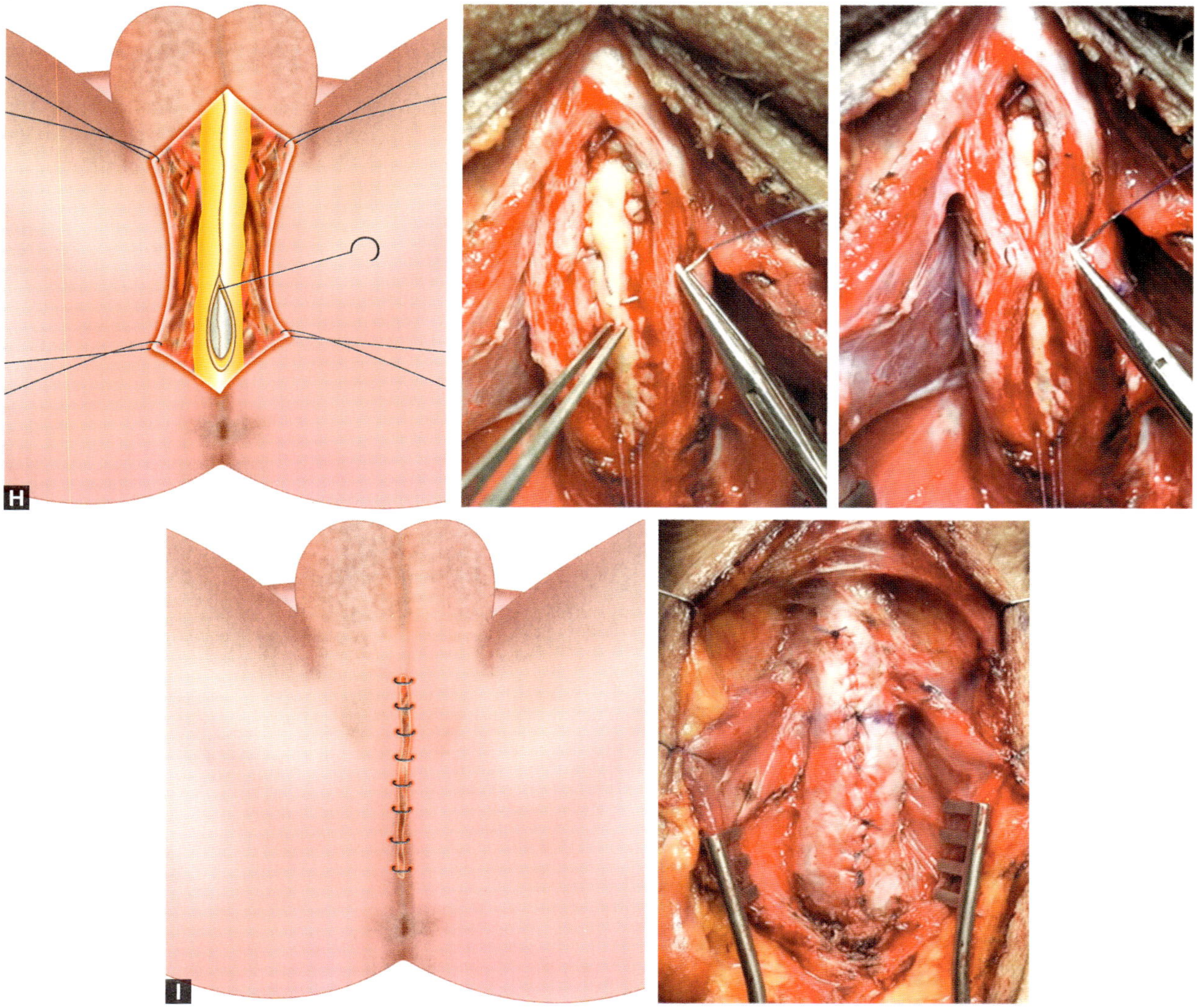

Figs 8.4H and I

Figs 8.4A to I: (A) Midline perineal incision for exposing the stricture of bulbar urethra; (B) Exposed strictured bulbar urethra; (C) Dorsal midline urethrotomy in ventrally laid open urethra; (D) Mobilization of bisected urethra from the tunica (without lifting two halves of the bisected urethra); (E) Anchoring and quilting of dorsal free graft; (F) Suturing of ventral free graft; (G) Completed dorsal free graft-ventral free graft; (H) Bulbospongiosa closed over ventral free graft taking few bites through the graft in between, as quilting sutures; (I) Completed dorsal and ventral graft urethroplasty

The present study only suggests an alternative approach to apply the free grafts. It is easier to perform as the scarred urethra is not mobilized. The patients who required dorsal placation had a full length penile urethral stricture with marked spongiofibrosis and mild chordee preoperatively. Patients with periurethral abscess and fistula were also dealt with, by staged procedures.

Advantages

- Easy to learn and does not require extensive training
- Can be done by circumcoronal or midline perineal incision, thus minimizes the risk of fistula and provides good esthetic outcome
- Respect of penile shaft components

- Flexibility to use preputial skin graft or oral mucosa
- As this technique requires no mobilization of urethra vascular and circumflex nerve supply is maintained
- Accurate sizing of graft minimizes pooling of urine and semen
- Dorsal and ventral graft technique provides better augmentation and thus wider lumen
- Provides good urinary flow and at the same time preserves ejaculatory sensations
- Dorsal and/or ventral free graft can be used in repeat procedure in cases of restenosis
- May be used in patients of strictures after hypospadias surgery
- Can be used in selected patients with strictures caused by lichen sclerosis or balanitis xerotica obliterans.

EDITORIAL COMMENTS

Dr Rajesh Gulia

Nowhere in the whole write-up has the author used the term "Asopa's urethroplasty". Very modest indeed. But we all know that the credit for this technique goes to Professor HS Asopa. The main strength of this technique lies in its simplicity. It follows the basic surgical principle of minimal tissue dissection to preserve maximal neural and vascular supply to the tissues undergoing handling. No wonder they are able to produce such excellent results (90% success). This is a very useful technique every urethral surgeon must have in his armamentarium.

Nowadays there is an ongoing debate on "to transect or not to transect" in nonobliterative bulbar urethral strictures. The combined dorsal and ventral free graft by the ventral sagittal urethrotomy approach is easy, fast and preserves the vascular and neural supply. This is important in preservation of the graft suture lines that give better outcome compared to situation in which the urethra is mobilized of the underlying tunica to make a dorsal urethrotomy. More important for the patient is that it preserves his natural ejaculatory action, which is a result of preserved bulbospongiosus muscle innervations. Also, the phenomena of cold or insensate glans is avoided, when the transection of bulbar urethra is avoided. All this translates into better preservation of sexual function, which nowadays patients are realizing and proactively questioning. That is why Professor Barbagli now talks of one-sided urethral mobilization off the tunica albuginea, to place the free oral buccal graft dorsally.

However, there are certain caveats I would like to re-emphasize to underline their unquestionable significance.

While giving a dorsal urethrotomy through the stricture, any fibrosis or unhealthy tissue in this area is also excised by sharp dissection. The end point being mild oozes from the raw bed.

The author's statement in step 4, "Urethra is retubularized by continuous sutures of 4-0 polyglactin on *an appropriate sized catheter*", requires further elaboration. It may not be prudent to place a large sized catheter thinking that it will act as a better splint in giving an adequate caliber urethra. In fact it proves to be counterproductive. It hinders drainage of the natural urethral secretions, which then become inspissated and predisposes to infection and disruption of the urethral closure suture line.

Following the retubularization of urethra, attempt is made to mobilize surrounding dartos fascia to cover the urethral suture line. Some surgeons have even described covering the urethral closure with tunica vaginalis flap. So far I have not had any strong compulsion to use it. More often than not I am able to put a second layer of dartos fascia. Having said this, these layers do not undermine the importance of a sound suture line. Further preparing a tunica vaginalis flap does entail an extra dissection time.

One must also be very careful, while applying pressure dressing lest it leads to pressure ischemia of the urethra resulting in disastrous consequences. Adequate fluffy layers of sterile cotton must be placed before any sticking plaster is applied. This provides as a cushioning space for the resultant postoperative tissue edema, without compromising on the vascularity.

REFERENCES

1. Andrich DE, Mundy AR. Urethral strictures and their surgical treatment. BJU Int. 2000;86(5):571-80.
2. Venn SN, Mundy AR. Early experience with the use of buccal mucosa for substitution urethroplasty. Br J Urol. 1998;81(5):738-40.
3. Barbagli G, Selli C, Tosto A, et al. Dorsal free graft urethroplasty. J Urol. 1996;155(1):123-6.
4. Asopa HS, Garg M, Singhal GG, et al. Dorsal free graft urethroplasty for urethral stricture by ventral sagittal urethrotomy approach. Urology. 2001;58(5):657-9.
5. Iselin CE, Webster GD. Dorsal onlay graft urethroplasty for repair of bulbar urethral stricture. J Urol. 1999;161(3):815-8.

6. Palminteri E, Manzoni G, Berdondini E, et al. Combined dorsal plus ventral double buccal mucosa graft in bulbar urethral reconstruction. Eur Urol. 2008;53(1):81-9.
7. Palminteri E, Berdondini E, Shokeir AA, et al. Two-sided bulbar urethroplasty using dorsal plus ventral oral graft: urinary and sexual outcomes of a new technique. J Urol. 2011;185(5):1766-71.
8. Webster GD, Brown MW, Koefoot RB Jr, et al. Suboptimal results in full thickness skin graft urethroplasty using an extra penile skin donor sites. J Urol. 1984;131(6):1082-3.
9. Barbagli G, Lazzeri M. Penile urethral stricture reconstruction–flap or graft? J Urol. 2011;186(2):375-6.
10. Mundy AR. The long-term results of skin inlay urethroplasty. Br J Urol. 1995;75(1):59-61.
11. Barbagli G. Editorial comment on: Dorsal buccal mucosal graft urethroplasty for anterior urethral stricture by Asopa technique. Eur Urol. 2009;56(1):205-6.

CHAPTER 9

Penile Fasciocutaneous Flap: McAninch Procedure

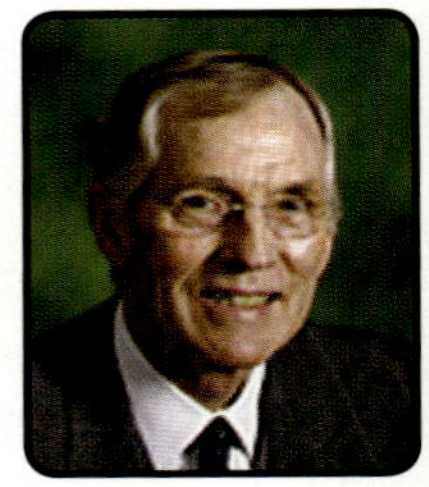

JW McAninch

BA Erickson, JW McAninch

Chapter Outline

Abstract

A difficult problem of long segment anterior urethral stricture is dealt very meticulously by McAninch himself describing the way he carries out the McAninch procedure. First detailing the anatomy of the flap he describes how he harvests the flap. A rule of thumb is that if hair follicles are seen on the undersurface of the skin, the surgeon is too superficial and must leave more tissue with the skin. This is a useful procedure where buccal graft cannot be taken. A must tool in the armamentarium of any urethral surgeon.

Keywords

Long segment anterior urethral stricture, Distal circular penile fasciocutaneous flap, McAninch, Tunica dartos pedicle, Buck's fascia, Tunica albuginea, Superficial dartos, Suspensory ligaments, Penoscrotal junction, Circumferential flap, Flap rotation, Skin necrosis, Postvoid dribbling.

INTRODUCTION

Long-segment anterior urethral stricture disease is a difficult problem for which the distal penile fasciocutaneous flap can often be a suitable solution. The flap, described originally by McAninch in 1993, is unique in its ability to provide 13–15 cm of nonhirsute and reliably well-vascularized penile skin that can be used in the entire anterior urethra.[1] Local skin flaps differ from grafts (i.e. buccal mucosa) in their ability to be transferred with their blood supply intact. This makes them especially useful in situations where surrounding blood supply may be questionable in its ability to support the neovascularization of a free graft. This chapter describes the anatomy, rationale, surgical procedure, outcomes and alternatives to the distal penile fasciocutaneous flap for long-segment urethral stricture disease.

FLAP ANATOMY

The McAninch flap is a true fasciocutaneous flap, relying on the underlying Buck's fascia to support the tunica dartos pedicle, which provides the supporting blood supply to the tissue.[1,2] **Figure 9.1** highlights the anatomical relationships of multiple fascial planes of the penis, which are crucial to understand before performing a successful graft harvest.[3]

Buck's Fascia

Buck's fascia has two distinct superficial and deep layers (lamella), which are best defined when they split dorsally to envelop the neurovascular bundle and ventrally to cover the corpus spongiosum. During graft harvest, both layers of Buck's fascia are lifted from the underlying tunica

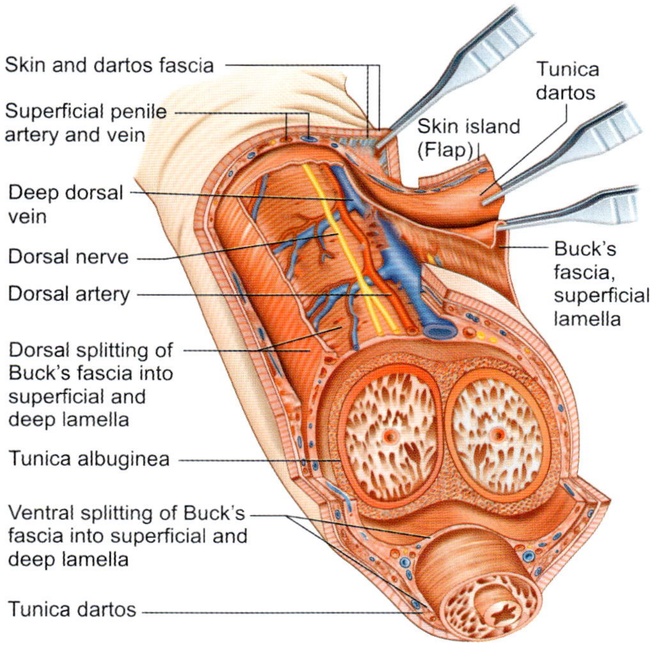

Fig. 9.1: Anatomical details of the skin island flap and the two plains that have to developed to raise a good skin island flap
Source: With permission from Buckley J, McAninch J. Distal penile circular fasciocutaneous flap for complex anterior urethral strictures. BJU Int. 2007;100(1):221-31.

albuginea, except at those areas where the fascia clearly splits, when only the superficial layer is taken. While the fascia itself does not carry its own blood supply, it is crucial that it is elevated with the dartos layer to provide support to the delicate vascular framework.

Dartos Fascia

The dartos fascia provides the vascular support to the fasciocutaneous flap and lies just superficial to Buck's fascia. Like Buck's fascia, the dartos fascia also consists of both the superficial and deep layers. The deep layer, which is known as the tunica dartos, is the true flap pedicle and contains all the necessary arterial and venous structures. This layer is devoid of fat, lies loosely over the underlying Buck's fascia and is continuous with Scarpa's fascia of the anterior abdominal wall. The superficial dartos layer lies immediate beneath the penile skin. This layer must be carefully separated from the dartos fascia during graft harvest and kept attached to the overlying skin so as to avoid skin necrosis of the remaining (nonflap) penile skin.

PATIENT SELECTION

The ideal candidate for the distal penile fasciocutaneous flap would be a patient with a long-segment (>5 cm) anterior urethral stricture. The absence of foreskin (circumcised patients) does not preclude patients from the procedure as we have found that nearly all patients will have sufficient redundant penile skin for closure. However, in rare cases where closure might not be possible, a split thickness skin graft to cover the defect would be appropriate.

Patients that are not suitable candidates for graft harvest would include those with significant balanitis xerotica obliterans or lichen sclerosus. Patients with prior hypospadias procedures in which a skin flap had already been utilized to form the neourethra must be evaluated on a case-by-case basis before the procedure is attempted. In the majority of these patients, however, alternatives should be explored.

SURGICAL TECHNIQUE

Patient Positioning

It is determined by the preoperative location of the stricture. In a purely penile stricture, the entire procedure can be performed in the supine position. If the stricture extends into distal bulbar urethra, we prefer to start the case by harvesting the graft in low lithotomy using Allen's stirrups and then reposition to high lithotomy during the stricture repair. If the stricture involves the proximal bulb, we first take the graft in supine position then, re-prepare and drape before repositioning to exaggerated high lithotomy with the candy cane stirrups.

Fasciocutaneous Flap Harvest

We begin by placing a 2-0 silk suture into the glans penis for traction. In circumcised patients, a 2–2.5 cm wide flap is marked out with the most distal mark generally made 2–3 mm from the glans margin **(Fig. 9.2)**.[3] It is imperative that the skin is fully stretched-out when making the marks, as it is a common mistake to make the graft too wide, leading to postoperative urethral sacculations and diverticula.

We incise the more proximal skin mark first down to, but not through, the level of the tunica dartos. The distal incision is then made to the level of Buck's fascia. The fascia is then lifted off the tunica albuginea circumferentially along shaft of penis down to level of the suspensory ligaments dorsally and the penoscrotal junction ventrally. Maximizing the amount of dissection at this step will make the eventual flap more mobile and easier to work with **(Fig. 9.3)**.[3]

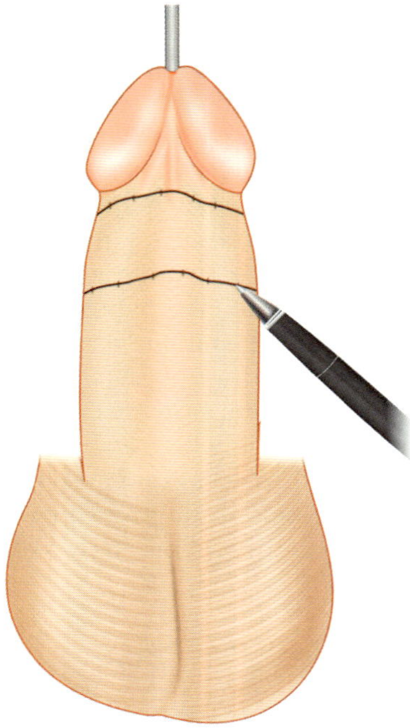

Fig. 9.2: Marking of the flap
Source: With permission from Buckley J, McAninch J. Distal Penile Circular fasciocutaneous flap for complex anterior urethral strictures. BJU Int. 2007;100(1):221-31.

We then return to the more proximal penile incision. A plane between the superficial dartos and tunica dartos is created, and this dissection is again taken down to the suspensory ligaments and penoscrotal junction. Great care must be taken to ensure the superficial dartos fascial layer that remains with the skin is thick enough to support it. In authors' experience, it is much easier to leave this layer too thin than to make it too thick, and skin necrosis will occur without an adequate blood supply **(Fig. 9.3)**.[3] A rule of thumb is that if hair follicles are seen on the undersurface of the skin, the surgeon is too superficial and must leave more tissue with the skin.

Once both the planes of dissection have been completed, we then split the graft ventrally to level of the penoscrotal junction with care to avoid any major flap vasculature (which can be easily seen) **(Fig. 9.4)**. This effectively converts the circumferential flap into a vertical strip, usually 13–15 cm in length. Stay sutures are placed at the lateral edges to assist with flap mobilization to varying locations of the urethra as necessary.[3]

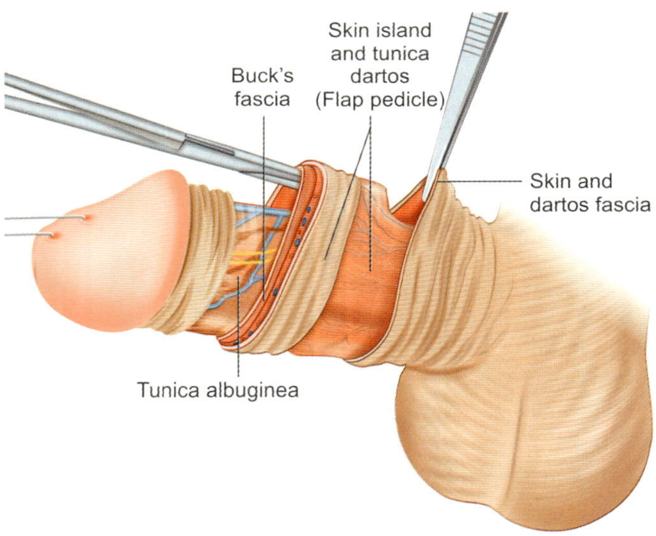

Fig. 9.3: Two planes along with the penis has to be degloved twice
Source: With permission from Buckley J, McAninch J. Distal Penile Circular fasciocutaneous flap for complex anterior urethral strictures. BJU Int. 2007;100(1):221-31.

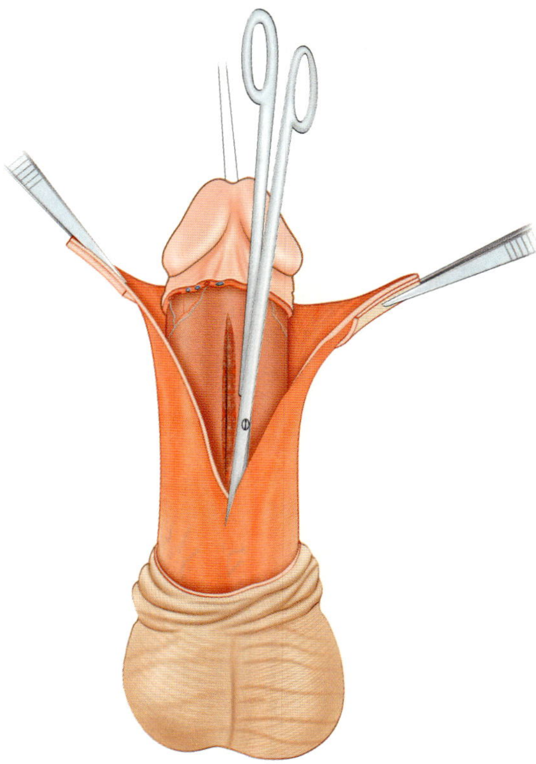

Fig. 9.4: The skin island flap incised in the midline
Source: With permission from Buckley J, McAninch J. Distal Penile Circular fasciocutaneous flap for complex anterior urethral strictures. BJU Int. 2007;100(1):221-31.

Stricture Exposure

Repositioning is based on the preoperative knowledge of stricture location or by our intraoperative ultrasound findings.[4] In purely penile urethral strictures, the procedure can be completed without the need for additional urethral exposure. In these situations we locate the most distal portion of the penile stricture using a 22 F red rubber catheter. An incision is made over the catheter to expose the urethral lumen and then extended proximally until normal diameter lumen is encountered **(Fig. 9.5)**.[3] The graft is then rotated from its dorsal position ventrally toward the urethra. In most cases, it does not matter if the flap is rotated clockwise or counterclockwise around the penis. However, the direction should be documented in operative note in the event of revision surgery to prevent damage to the pedicle.

In more proximally located strictures, a standard perineal incision is used to expose the bulbar urethra

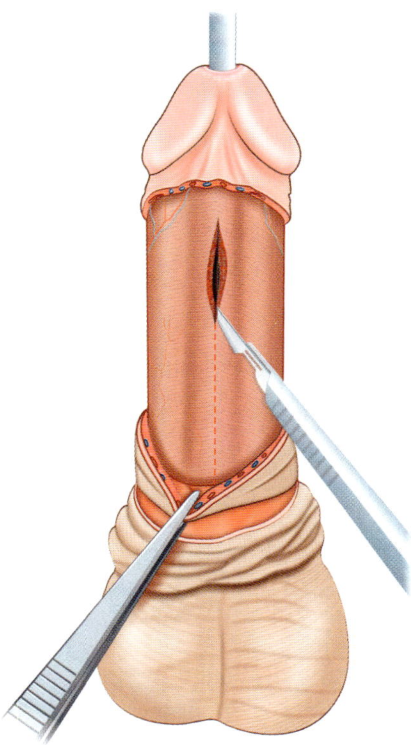

Fig. 9.5: The stricturous portion of the urethra being incised in the midline

Source: With permission from Buckley J, McAninch J. Distal Penile Circular fasciocutaneous flap for complex anterior urethral strictures. BJU Int. 2007;100(1):221-31.

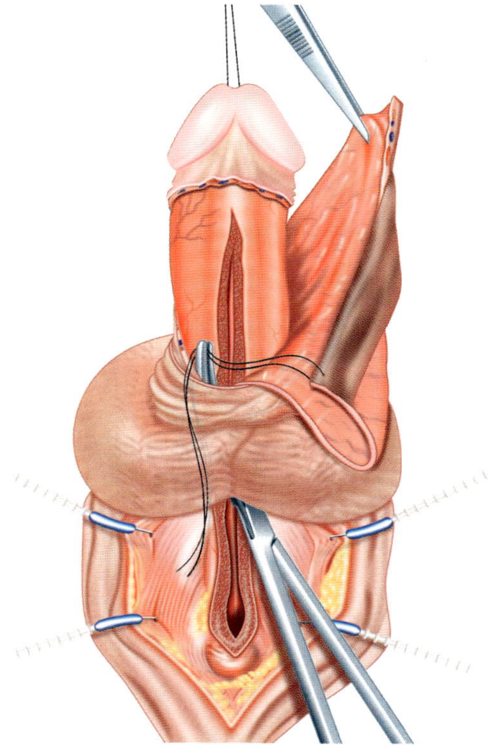

Fig. 9.6: The proximal end of the island flap being taken below the scrotal tunnel created between the penile and perineal incisions

Source: With permission from Buckley J, McAninch J. Distal Penile Circular fasciocutaneous flap for complex anterior urethral strictures. BJU Int. 2007;100(1):221-31.

(Fig. 9.6).[3] There is no need to split the scrotum in these situations. Rather, a tunnel between the perineal and penile incisions is created allowing for access to the entire anterior urethra. The flap can then be pulled through this tunnel for use anywhere along the length of the urethra as necessary **(Fig. 9.6)**.[3] The distal end of the stricture is again located with the 22 F red rubber catheter.

Anastomosis

We prefer to anastomose the graft to an existing urethral plate whenever possible as tubularization of the graft has a high failure rate (> 50%).[5] We first extend the ventral stricture urethrotomy 0.5 cm -1 cm, past the stricture both proximally and distally. The total length of the urethrotomy is then measured and the flap is tailored appropriately. It is advisable to excise only the epithelial layer during tailoring to preserve as much of the pedicle as possible. It should also be noted that the surgeon needs to account for very little graft contraction during the initial measurement unlike a graft procedure.

We begin by placing double-armed 5-0 polydioxanone (PDS) sutures at the proximal and distal portions of the flap, both of which are then secured to the urethra. If redundant flap material is noted at this point, it should be excised. Two additional interrupted 5-0 PDS sutures are then placed at each apex. We first secure the side of the flap that is closest to the pedicle so that we can more easily sew "inside" the urethra and not put undue strain on the pedicle **(Fig. 9.7)**.[3] Approximately every 2–3 cm along length of the urethra, we place 4-0 chromic suture so as to stabilize the flap during the anastomosis. A running 6-0 PDS suture is then used to secure first side of the flap to urethral plate, occasionally locking suture to prevent flap bunching. A 16 F catheter is then placed and contralateral side of the flap is secured to the urethra in a similar fashion using the running 6-0 PDS. All knots should be tied on outside of the urethral lumen when possible. The skin is then closed over the repair using interrupted 4-0 vicryl suture **(Fig. 9.8)**.[3]

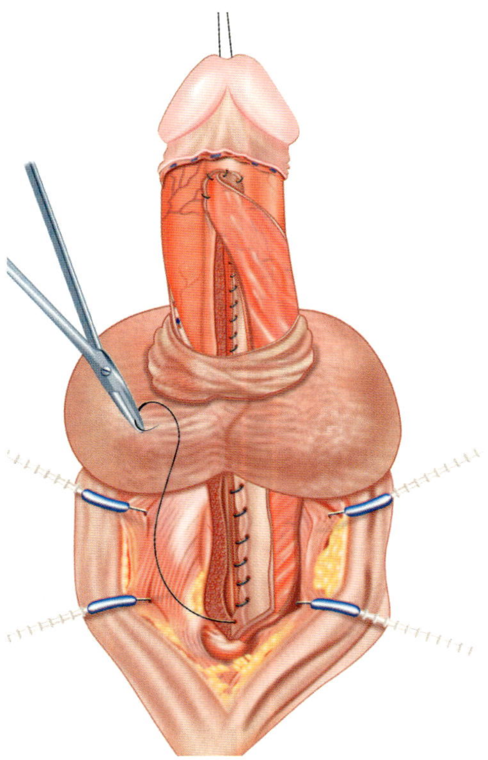

Fig. 9.7: The side of the open urethra closure to the flap is first sutured (suturing from inside)
Source: With permission from Buckley J, McAninch J. Distal Penile Circular fasciocutaneous flap for complex anterior urethral strictures. BJU Int. 2007;100(1):221-31.

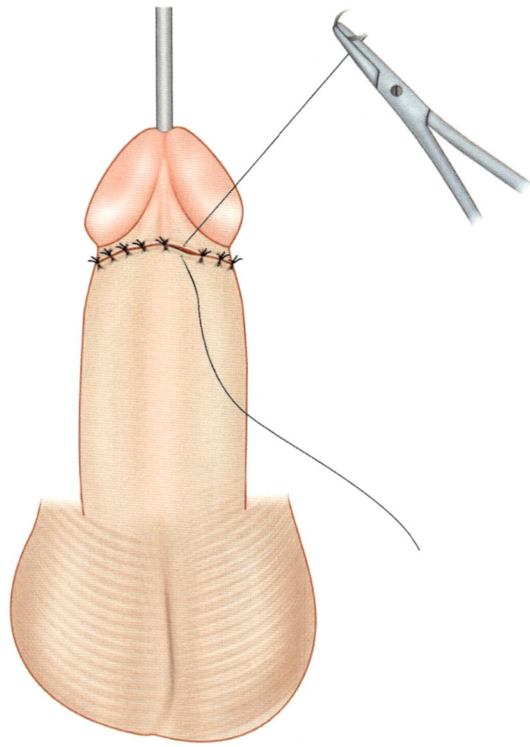

Fig. 9.8: The circumcoronal skin incision being closed
Source: With permission from Buckley J, McAninch J. Distal Penile Circular fasciocutaneous flap for complex anterior urethral strictures. BJU Int. 2007;100(1):221-31.

Special Circumstances

In some cases of panurethral stricture disease, the flap will not be long enough to repair the entire segment. In those cases, we have utilized two different techniques. In the bulbar urethra, a segment of the urethral plate (up to 2.5 cm) can be excised and reanastomosed, effectively decreasing total stricture length by length of the excised amount. It is advisable to excise the most narrowed segment, if this approach is attempted.[6] Alternatively, the flap can be augmented with a ventrally placed buccal graft. This graft can be sewn directly to the flap, and then be supported by the corpus spongiosum tissue. If this approach is used, it is advisable to always place the graft proximal to the flap, as the spongiosal tissue needed for coverage is more robust there.[6]

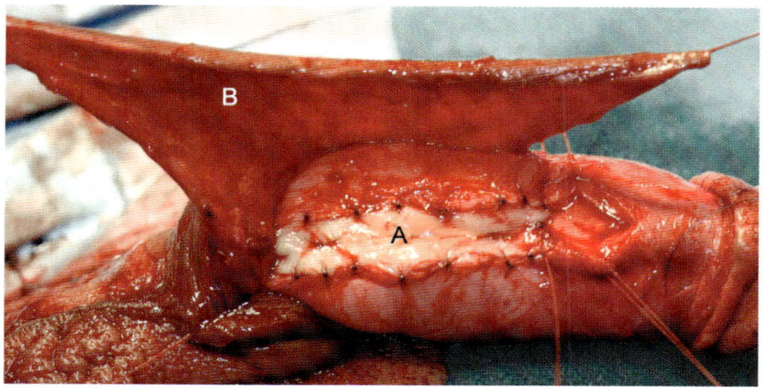

Fig. 9.9: The very narrow urethral plate in the penile area has been replaced by a buccal mucosal graft (A). (B) is the skin island flap

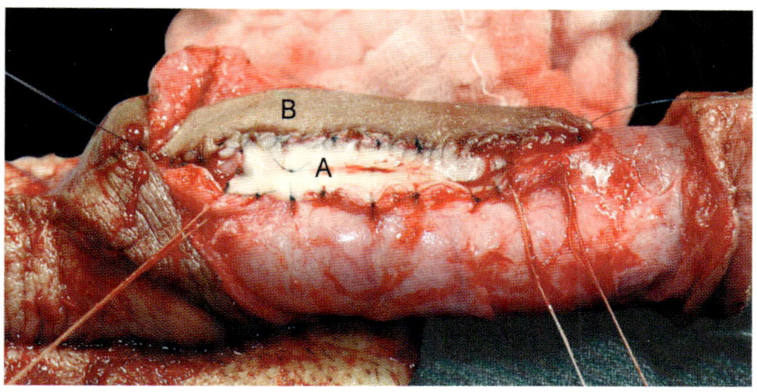

Fig. 9.10: The skin island flap (B) being sewn directly to the buccal mucosal graft (A) on one side

We have also encountered situations where the existing dorsal urethral plate is too narrow (< 5 mm) to accept a flap onlay. If this segment is in the bulbar urethra, an excision with primary anastomosis of the plate can generally be performed (segment is < 2 cm). In the penile urethra, however, primary anastomosis is not possible without risking significant chordee. In these cases **(Fig. 9.9)**, the dorsal plate can be replaced by a buccal mucosa graft and the flap can be sewn directly to the graft after being secured to the corporal bodies **(Fig. 9.10)**.[7]

Postoperative Care or Monitoring

We dress the incisions with Xeroform gauze and then cover with fluffs, securing everything with a scrotal support. We do not use a compression dressing (i.e. Coban) as this can compromise blood flow to both the penile skin and the flap. The catheter remains in place for a minimum of 3 weeks, at which time a voiding cystourethrography is performed to look for any urinary extravasation. All patients receive perioperative broad-spectrum antibiotics (cephalosporin and aminoglycoside) because most of them have a history of recurrent urinary tract infections, and their bladders and urethras are usually colonized. They are discharged on suppressive nitrofurantoin and continue this while the catheter is in place.

All patients are evaluated at 3 months and 12 months with a retrograde urethrogram and uroflowmetry. Follow-up is then done yearly with uroflowmetry. Those with new voiding symptoms and/or low maximum flow rates (< 15 ml/sec) are evaluated further with a retrograde urethrogram.

OUTCOMES

In 2008, authors evaluated 159 patients with urethral stricture disease that underwent fasciocutaneous flap repair at their institution between 1985 and 2006.[8] They noted overall success rates of 95%, 89%, 84% and 79% at 1, 3, 5 and 10 years follow-up, respectively. Multivariate analysis revealed that smoking [hazard ratio (HR) 4.0], prior hypospadias repair (HR 4.4) and long stricture length (7–10 cm, HR 7.0) were independent predictors of failure. In nearly all patients, recurrence was at the anastomosis of the flap to the normal urethra and not within the flap itself. Many initial failures were repaired with a single direct visual internal urethrotomy (DVIU) with good long-term results.

COMPLICATIONS

Postoperative complications specific to this procedure include penile skin necrosis (4.5%) and lower extremity neurovascular compromise (6%).[9] Fortunately, all of our patients that experienced significant skin necrosis healed by secondary intention alone after dressing the area daily with saline soaked gauze. However, a skin graft could have been used had they not healed with conservative measures. All of our neurologic complications occurred early in the series and were all due to excessive (> 5 hours) time in the high lithotomy position. With our above described intraoperative repositioning techniques, our lithotomy times are now rarely over 3 hours and we have not had any more of these complications.

Other postoperative patient complaints that deserve mentioning include postvoid dribbling and ventral tethering of the penis with erections. The postvoid dribbling can be reduced with appropriate tailoring of the graft during the original operation, but is sometimes unavoidable with loss of the bulbocavernosus muscle function. In these cases, we will simply teach the patients how to aggressively milk their urethra after voiding. Ventral tethering with erections occurs more frequently with more proximal placement of the flap. In all cases, this improved with time, presumably after the pedicle had time to stretch and accommodate the erectile length.

Stricture recurrences are usually found at the anastomosis of the normal urethra with the flap, both proximally and distally. If the stricture is less than 2 cm in length, we have found a single aggressive DVIU to be very successful.[8] Otherwise, repeat urethroplasty with dorsal or ventral onlay of buccal mucosa is usually implemented, and can generally be performed without disturbing the original flap.

ALTERNATIVES TO THE McANINCH FLAP

The advantage to the distal circular penile fasciocutaneous flap is its ability to be used in the entire anterior urethra for nearly all stricture lengths. However, it does require a moderate degree of technical expertise and many surgeons may not be comfortable with the graft harvest. Some alternatives to the flap use in the penile urethra include long-segment dorsal buccal placement[10] or a different skin-based penile flap, such as the Orandi[11] or Quartey[12] flap. In some situations, a two-stage Johanson urethroplasty[13] is appropriate, especially in cases where large segments of the dorsal plate need to be removed. In the bulbar urethra, ventral or dorsal onlay of buccal mucosa can be used for strictures of up to 12 cm.[14]

CONCLUSION

The distal penile fasciocutaneous flap is a robust and reliable option for long-segment urethral stricture disease in any anterior urethral location. It has excellent long-term results with minimal morbidity, and can be combined with other tissue transfer techniques as necessary.

REFERENCES

1. McAninch JW. Reconstruction of extensive urethral strictures: circular fasciocutaneous penile flap. J Urol. 1993;149(3):488-91.
2. Breza J, Aboseif SR, Orvis BR, et al. Detailed anatomy of penile neurovascular structures: surgical significance. J Urol. 1989;141(2):437-43.
3. Buckley J, McAninch J. Distal penile circular fasciocutaneous flap for complex anterior urethral strictures. BJU Int. 2007;100(1):221-31.
4. Morey AF, McAninch JW. Ultrasound evaluation of the male urethra for assessment of urethral stricture. J Clin Ultrasound. 1996;24(8):473-9.
5. McAninch JW, Morey AF. Penile circular fasciocutaneous skin flap in 1-stage reconstruction of complex anterior urethral strictures. J Urol. 1998;159(4):1209-13.
6. Wessells H, Morey AF, McAninch JW. Single stage reconstruction of complex anterior urethral strictures: combined tissue transfer techniques. J Urol. 1997; 157(4):1271-4.
7. Erickson BA, Breyer BN, McAninch JW. Single-stage segmental urethral replacement using combined ventral onlay fasciocutaneous flap with dorsal onlay buccal grafting for long segment strictures. BJU Int. 2012;109(9): 1392-6.
8. Whitson JM, McAninch JW, Elliott SP, et al. Long-term efficacy of distal penile circular fasciocutaneous flaps for single stage reconstruction of complex anterior urethral stricture disease. J Urol. 2008;179(6):2259-64.
9. Carney KJ, McAninch JW. Penile circular fasciocutaneous flaps to reconstruct complex anterior urethral strictures. Urol Clin North Am. 2002;29(2):397-409.
10. Barbagli G, Palminteri E, Guazzoni G, et al. Bulbar urethroplasty using buccal mucosa grafts placed on the ventral, dorsal or lateral surface of the urethra: are results affected by the surgical technique? J Urol. 2005;174(3): 955-7.
11. Orandi A. One-stage urethroplasty: 4-year follow-up. J Urol. 1972;107(6):977-80.
12. Quartey JK. One-stage penile/preputial island flap urethroplasty for urethral stricture. J Urol. 1985;134(3):474-5.
13. Johanson B. The reconstruction in stenosis of the male urethra. Z Urol. 1953;46(6):361-75.
14. Wessells H. Ventral onlay graft techniques for urethroplasty. Urol Clin North Am. 2002;29(2):381-7.

10

CHAPTER

Staged Urethral Reconstruction

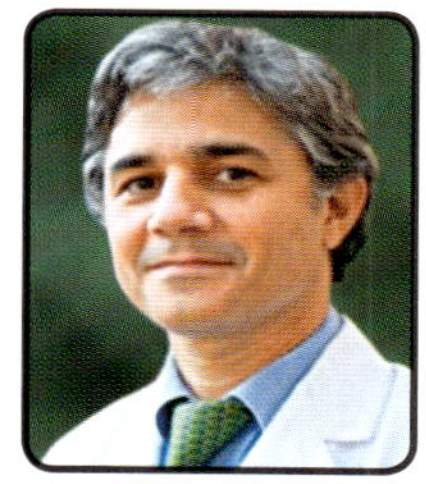

Ramón Virasoro

Ramón Virasoro, Gerald H Jordan

Chapter Outline

Abstract

Lichen sclerosis or BXO is a chronic inflammatory disease and when affecting the male genitalia can cause real bad strictures. Here we cannot use the local skin for flap urethroplasty. The way out is buccal mucosa graft. In real bad strictures especially of the anterior urethra, it is prudent to do it in a staged procedure. Professor Jordan has very explicitly described the steps in harvesting the BMG and using it for staged urethroplasty. What is important is the graft care which will decide our results of the 2nd stage neourethral tubularization. This is also a very good procedure in cases of stricture cripples and hypospadias cripples.

Keywords

Lichen sclerosis, Phimosis, Urethral stenosis, White patches, Fossa navicularis, Orotracheal tube, Stenson's duct, Epinephrine soaked packs, Graft onlay, Thiersch-Duplay strip, Urethrotomy, Proximal "V" flap, Xeroform™, Coban® bandage, Tubularization of neourethra, Tunica dartos flap.

INTRODUCTION

Lichen sclerosis (LS) is a chronic, inflammatory skin disease of unknown origin. When affecting the male genitalia and perineum, LS can progress to phimosis, urethral stenosis and eventually urethral stricture.[1] These can affect both urinary and sexual function. Medical treatment has limited indications for early and mild stages of the disease, and most patients with meatal involvement will eventually need urethral reconstruction.

The physical findings on the male genitalia in most cases are white patches that coalesce into plaques. If the glans is involved there can be a mottled appearance, and patients complain of itching and loss of sensation. With progression the skin has the pathognomonic whitish appearance, and the meatus can be almost obliterated by the scar **(Figs 10.1 and 10.2)**. Patients present with both local as well as voiding symptoms, including dysuria, urethral discharge and obstructive lower urinary tract symptoms.

There is no consensus concerning whether LS progresses into the fossa navicularis and anterior urethra, or the involvement of urethra is secondary to the initial process at the level of meatus with development of meatal stenosis. Chronic high pressure voiding will then affect the proximal urethra. The evaluation includes urethral X-rays **(Fig. 10.3)**, and when possible, urethroscopy with a small pediatric rigid scope.

This chapter describes the techniques to reconstruct the urethra in stages utilizing oral mucosa grafts.[2,3]

STAGED RECONSTRUCTION OF THE FOSSA NAVICULARIS[4,5]

In some patients, the process is limited to the meatus and fossa navicularis **(Fig. 10.2)**.[6,7]

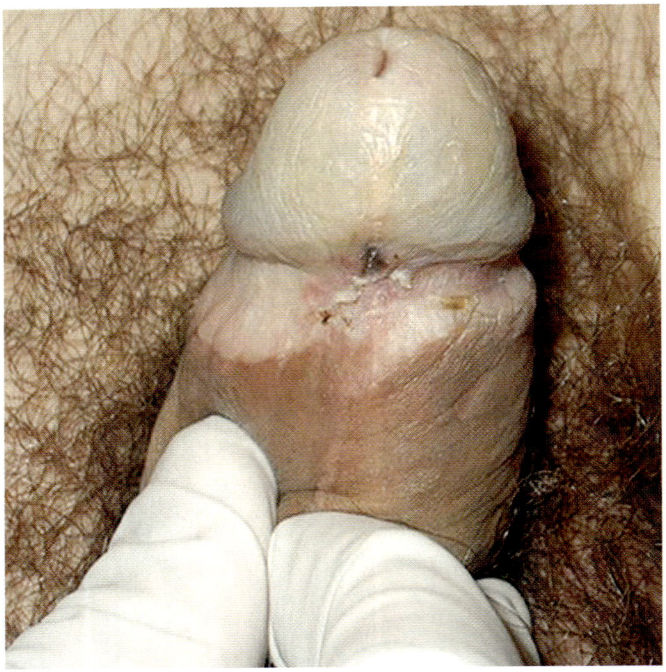

Fig. 10.1: Lichen sclerosis developed after circumcision in a 35-year-old man. Note the definite line between normal and affected skin, and meatal stenosis. LS was confirmed by histology of the circumcision specimen

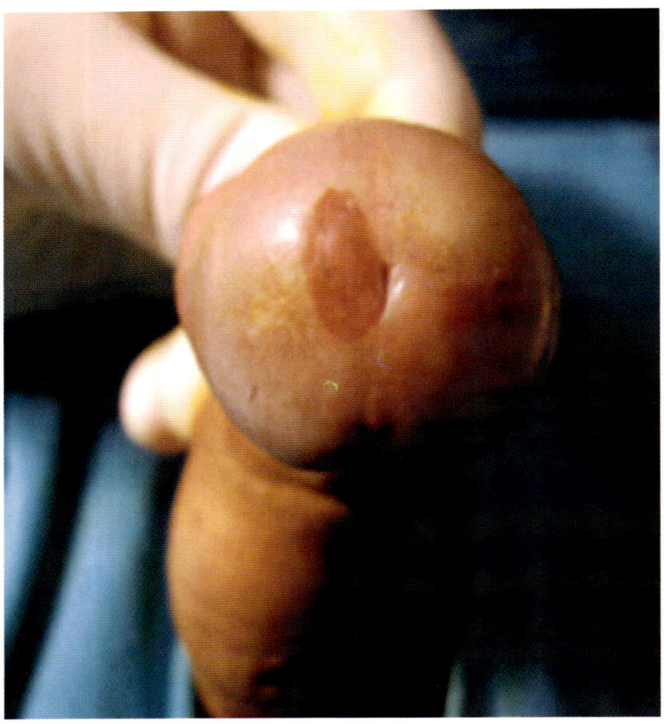

Fig. 10.2: Lichen sclerosis affecting the glans and meatus in a 23-year-old man. Glans biopsy confirmed histology

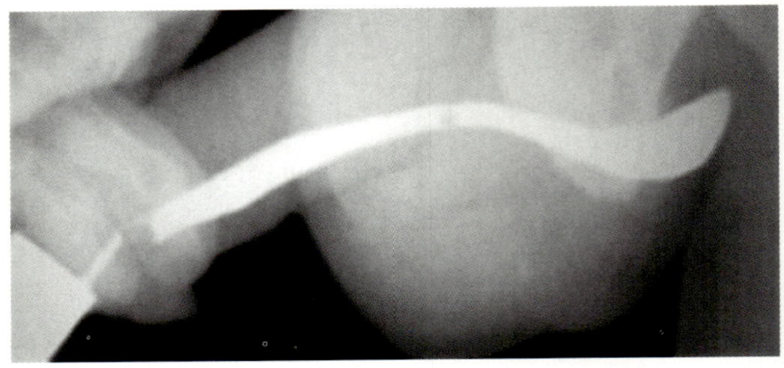

Fig. 10.3: Retrograde urethrogram of a 23-year-old man with lichen sclerosis, showing a localized fossa navicularis stricture

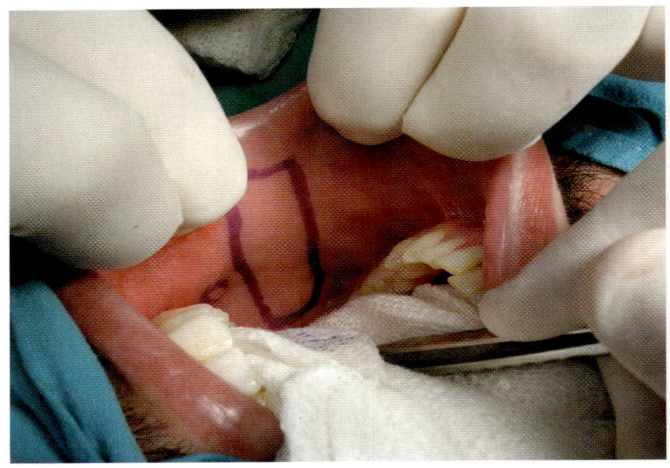

Fig. 10.4: Proper identification and marking of the Stenson's duct (marked as a circle) is essential to avoid injury further on graft harvest. A sponge is useful to displace the tongue opposite to the field

Evaluation with both retrograde and voiding urethrograms reveals the location and extent of the stricture **(Fig. 10.3)**.

First Stage: Grafting

Buccal Mucosa Graft Harvesting[8,9]

The patient is placed supine in the operating room table. The orotracheal tube is lateralized contralateral to the donor site. The face and mouth is prepared with an oral rinse containing 0.12% chlorhexidine gluconate in a near-neutral solution (pH range 5–7). The head is draped. Stay sutures are applied at both sides of the labial commissure for proper exposure. Stenson's duct is properly identified and marked, and the graft is marked **(Fig. 10.4)**. Stenson's duct is found adjacent to the second molar.

Injection of lidocaine with epinephrine helps both in dissection and hemostasis **(Fig. 10.5)**. The fluid is

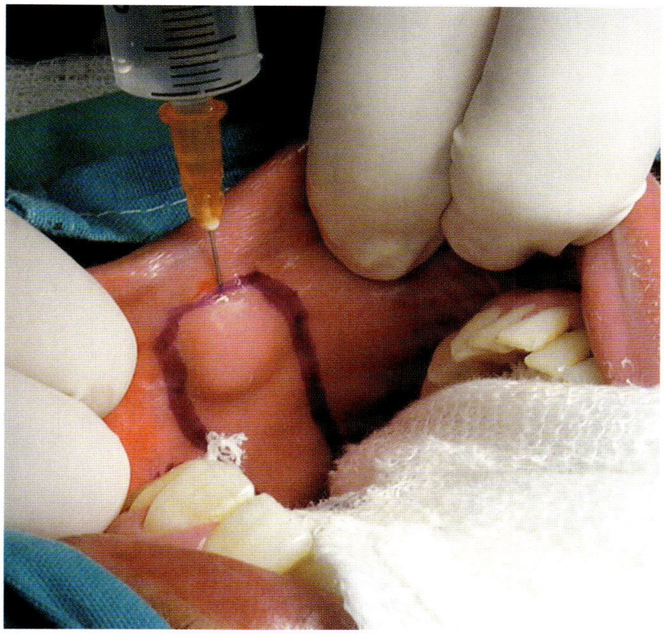

Fig. 10.5: Injection of lidocaine with epinephrine in the submucosal plane

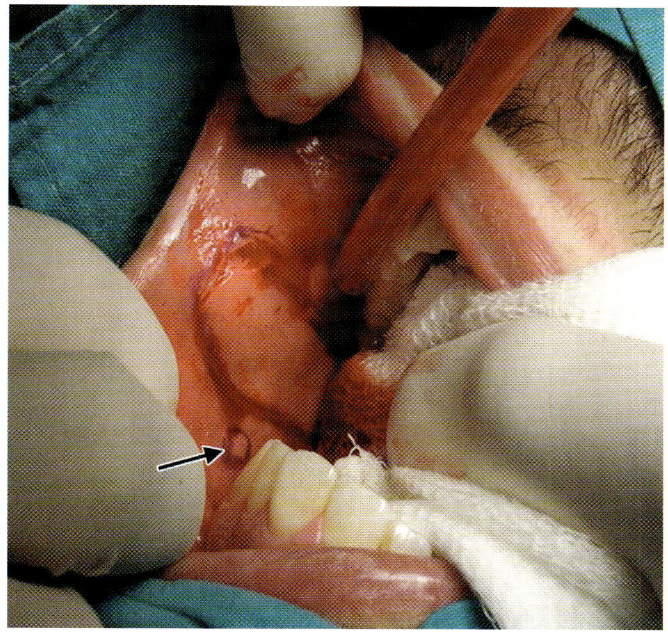

Fig. 10.6: The graft is completely incised, from the left buccal mucosa and the spared Stenson's duct is perfectly visualized (marked as a circle), shown by an arrow

delivered in the submucosal plane. If the patient is allergic to lidocaine, one can use normal saline with epinephrine.

With a no. 15 blade on a long arm scalpel, we first incise the deeper margin of the graft, followed by the margin adjacent to Stenson's duct, thus avoiding limitation in identifying the duct and avoiding injury **(Fig. 10.6)**.

The elevation of the graft is achieved with tenotomy scissors. The goal is to develop a plane at juncture of the submucosa and the muscle **(Figs 10.7 and 10.8)**.

Hemostasis of the donor defect is achieved with bipolar electrocautery **(Fig. 10.9)**.

Major bleeders are cauterized and epinephrine-soaked packs are left in the donor site; those will be checked at the end of the case, prior to extubating the patient.

The decision on whether to close completely, partially or leave the graft defect open depends on the size of the graft and on surgeon's preference.[10] Larger defects preclude closing without tension. If one decides to close the graft donor site, a 4/0 Vicryl running suture with a tapered needle is appropriate **(Figs 10.10 and 10.11)**.

We use serrated-edge scissors to clean the excess submucosa tissue **(Figs 10.12 and 10.13)**. There is no agreement as to the optimal thickness of the graft. We prefer thin grafts.

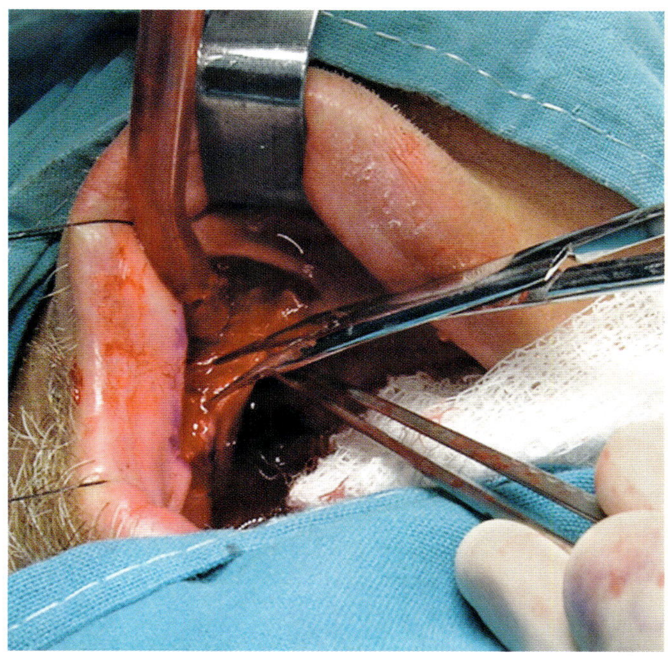

Fig. 10.7: Traction with fine forceps and opposing force with the suction device are helpful for graft elevation. Delicate scissors such as tenotomy (or Stevens) are appropriate

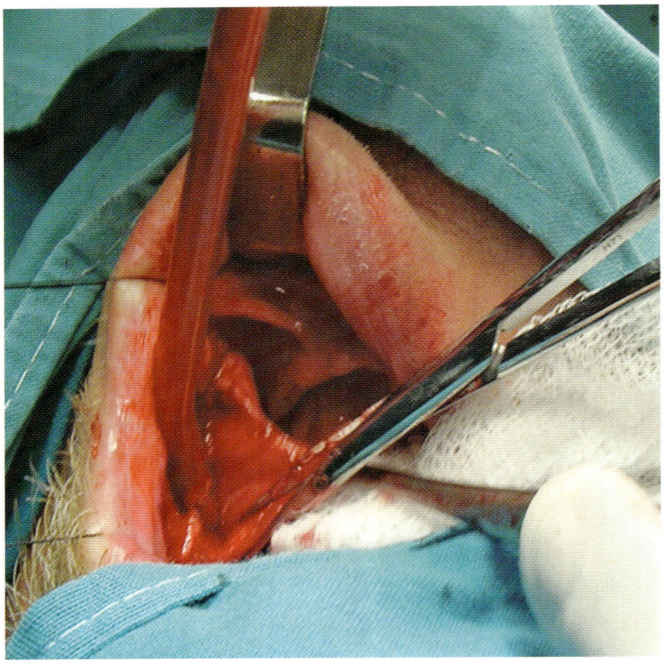

Fig. 10.8: Graft is completely detached and placed on a saline soaked sponge

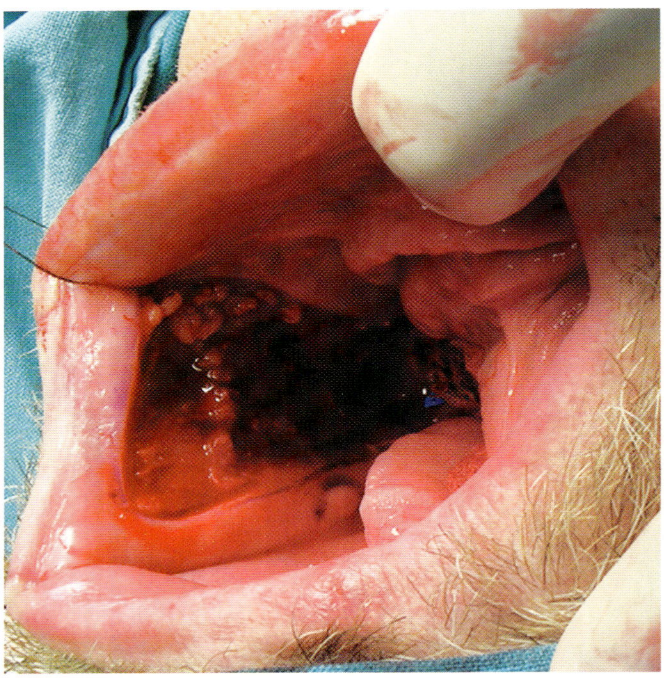

Fig. 10.9: Inspecting the site for hemostasis

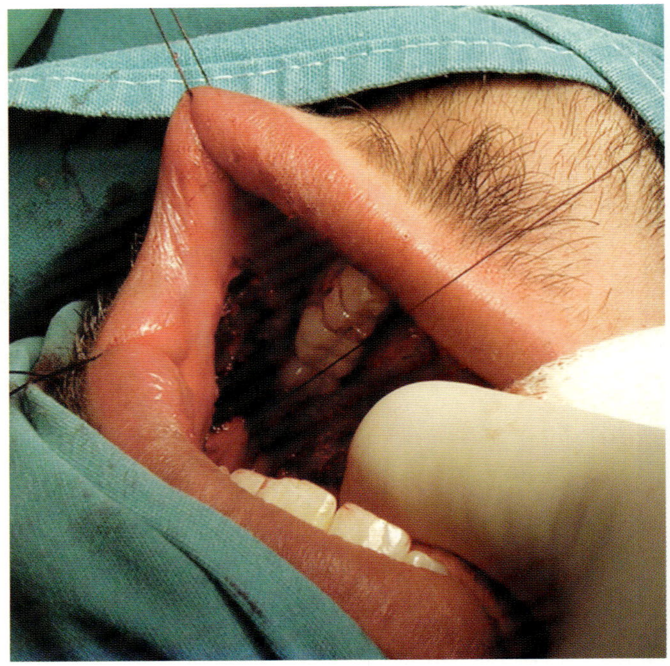

Fig. 10.10: Starting from the deepest aspect to the surface, a running 4/0 Vicryl suture on a tapered needle is carefully placed, again, sparing the Stenson's duct

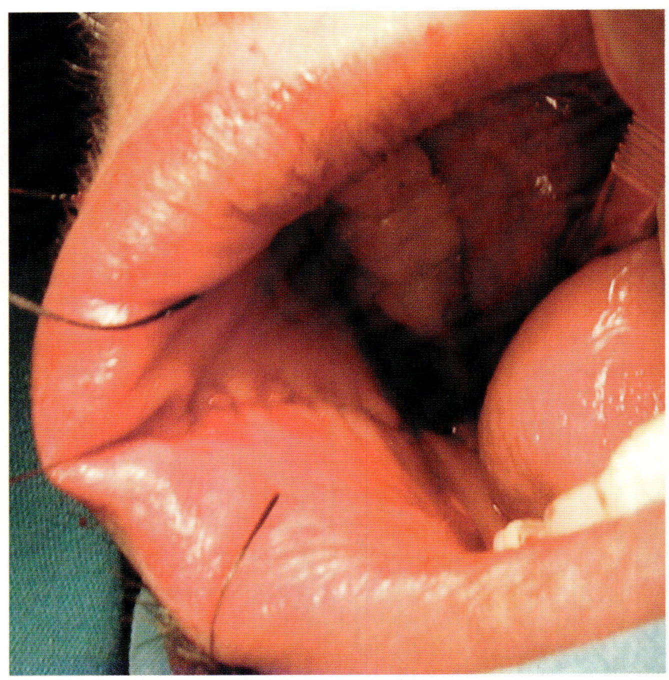

Fig. 10.11: The defect is closed without tension. Closing often helps to achieve better hemostasis

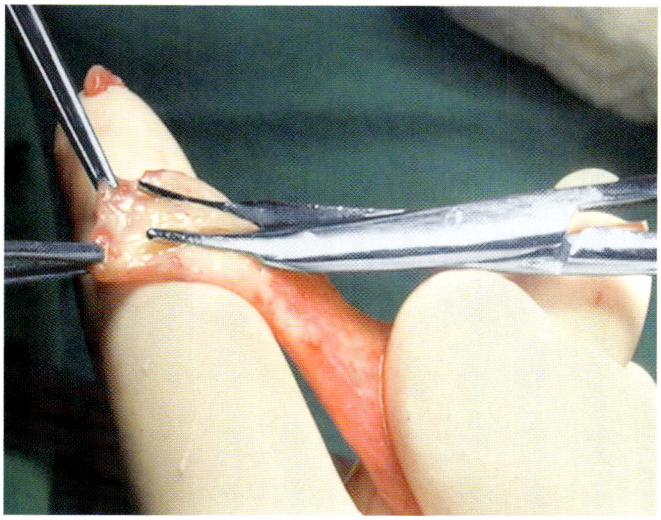

Fig. 10.12: Serrated tenotomy scissors are useful to remove the excess submucosal tissue from the graft. This removal will enhance graft take

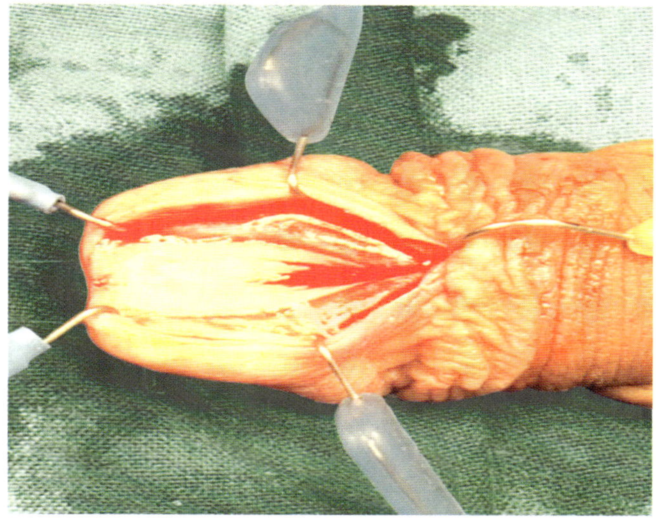

Fig. 10.14: The fossa navicularis has been exposed with the urethrotomy. A Scott's retractor with hooks can be useful to expose the field

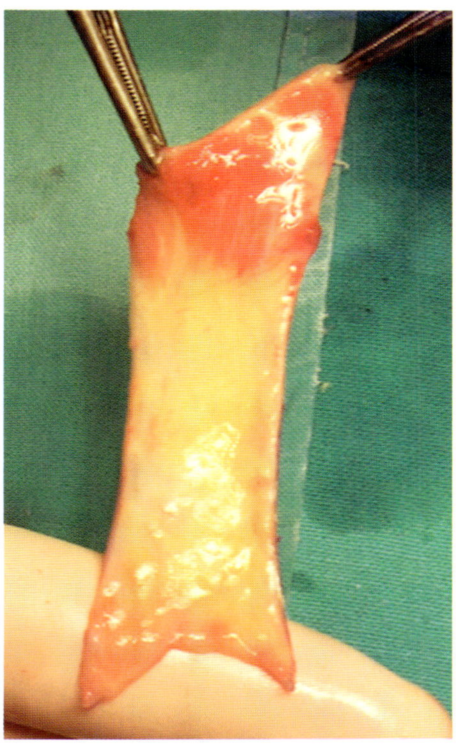

Fig. 10.13: Partial cleaning of the graft has been done. Note the submucosal tissue and muscle fibers on the superior aspect of the graft

Graft Onlay

At our centre the entire team rescrubs and instruments from the head table are not transferred to the urethral reconstruction table. The patient is repositioned into the split-leg frog-leg position. The lower abdomen, genitalia and perineum are prepped with betadine solution and draped in the usual fashion. A glans traction stitch is placed. Using a groove director, a clean urethrotomy is created on the ventrum of the penis **(Fig. 10.14)**. Once normal urethral epithelium is visualized, proximal calibration of the lumen is determined with bougies. Deep bilateral longitudinal incisions in the erectile tissue of the glans, parallel to the mucosal line on the urethrotomy, are created. The incisions should extend to the level of the tips of the corpora in order to create an adequate bed for the graft. If the epithelium is badly scarred, it is excised.

The graft is sutured and tailored into the urethrostomy defect **(Fig. 10.15)**. The goal is to achieve at least 3 cm wide graft onlay to allow eventual urethral tubularization.

The graft is sutured to the urethral margins with 4/0 Vicryl suture and mattress sutured to the bed with 6/0 Vicryl suture **(Fig. 10.16)**.

We use a mixture of 50%/50% of sterile liquid vaseline and normal saline to soak the gauze for dressing purposes **(Fig. 10.17)**.

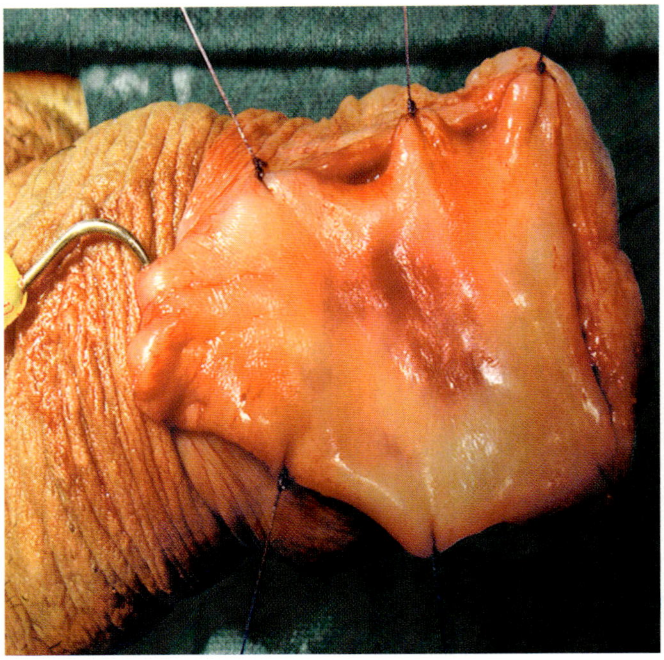

Fig. 10.15: The buccal graft has been sutured into place. The 4/0 Vicryl stay sutures are applied for further dressing purposes

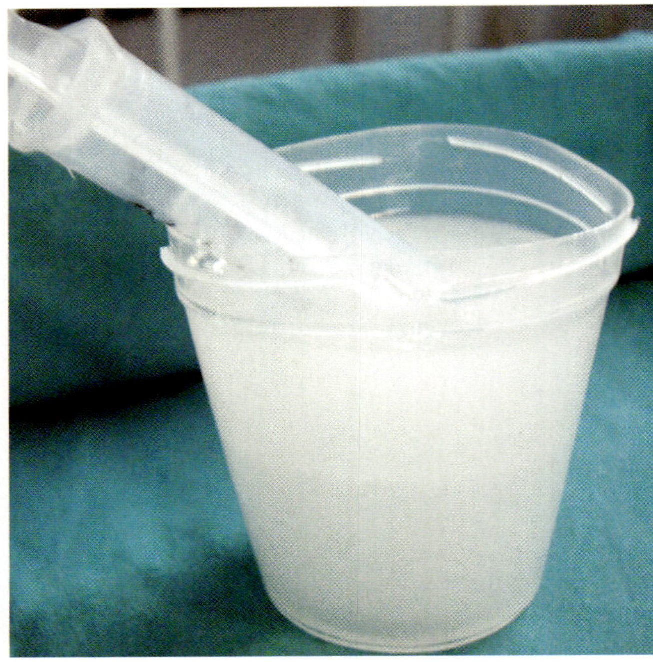

Fig. 10.17: The gauge pieces are soaked in the solution

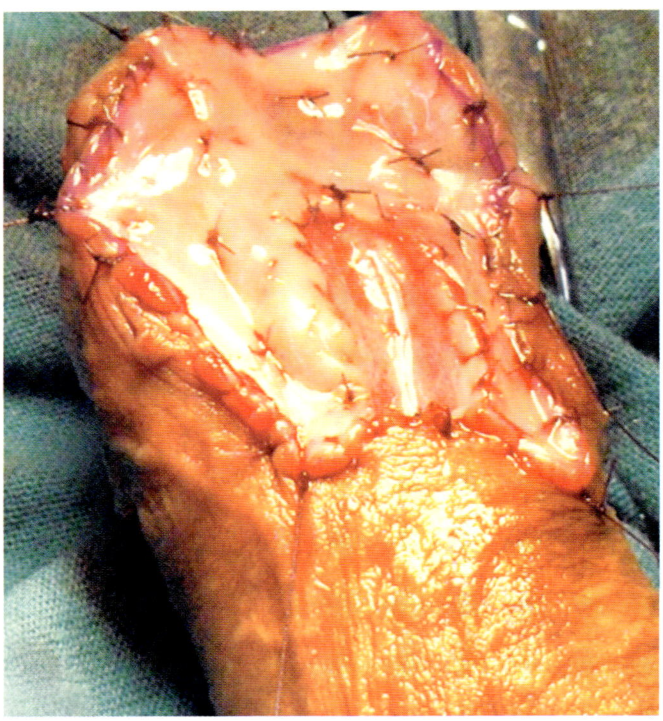

Fig. 10.16: Note the residual urethral plate in the center

The graft is covered with Xeroform™ and soaked gauzes. The dressing is held in place with the stay sutures. A mildly compressive Coban® layer is placed over the bolster. We use a 14 Fr Rüsch urethral catheter through the meatus for diversion **(Fig. 10.18)**.

The patient is hospitalized, at bed rest, for 4 days. During the initial postoperative period, they receive broad spectrum antibiotics, which are based on the preoperative urine cultures. Prior to discharge, the bolster and the diverting catheter are removed **(Fig. 10.19)**. Proper care of the graft is taken and Xeroform™ gauze is placed on the graft for a period of 4–7 days.

The patient is seen around the 7th postoperative day. Further, 3 months and 6 months follow-up visits are encouraged. Regarding the graft donor site care, the patient's diet is as tolerated. We encourage saline gargles early after the surgery **(Fig. 10.20)**.

The second stage is planned for around 6 months, depending on the neomeatal calibration and proximal urethroscopy **(Fig. 10.21)**.

Second Stage: Neourethral Tubularization

The patient is positioned flat on the table, slightly frog-legged supine. A glans traction stitch is placed **(Fig. 10.22)**.

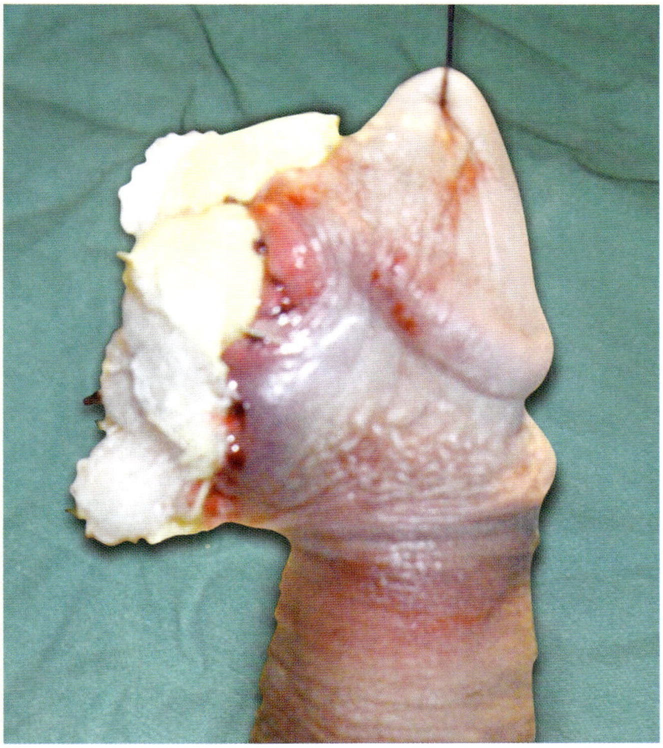

Fig. 10.18: The dressing of Xeroform and soaked gauge pieces held in place by long stay sutures all-round the graft area

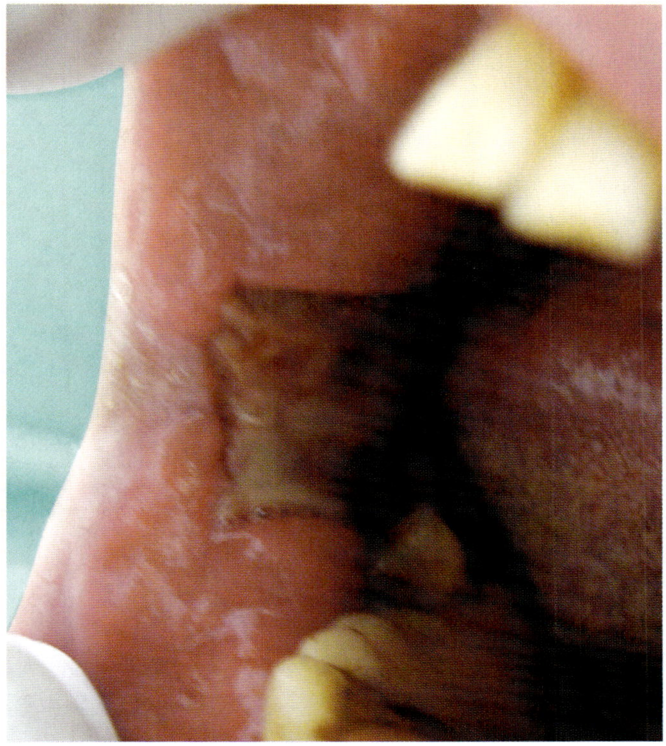

Fig. 10.20: The appearance of the graft donor site at 1 week, when left opened

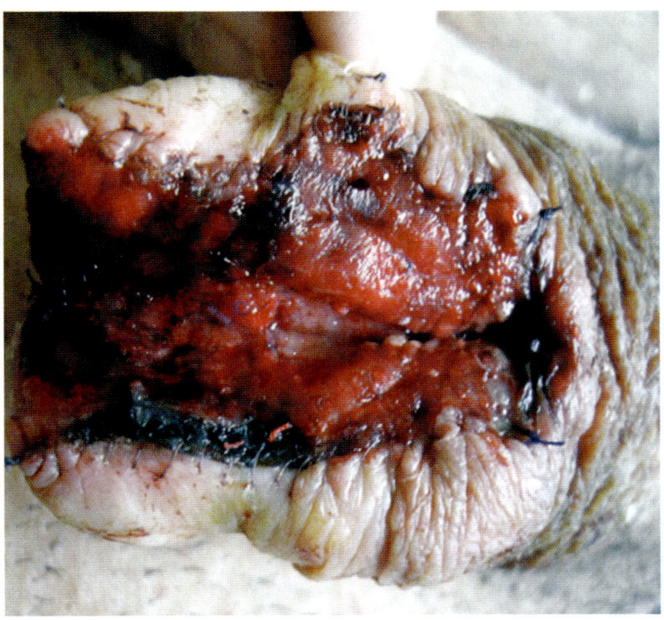

Fig. 10.19: The appearance of the graft after removing the bolster at 4–5 postoperative days

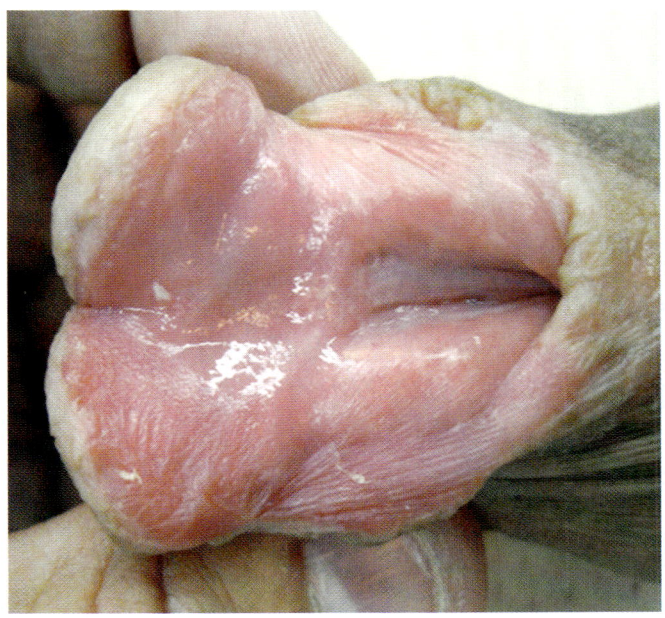

Fig. 10.21: The appearance of the graft at about 6 months after the first stage

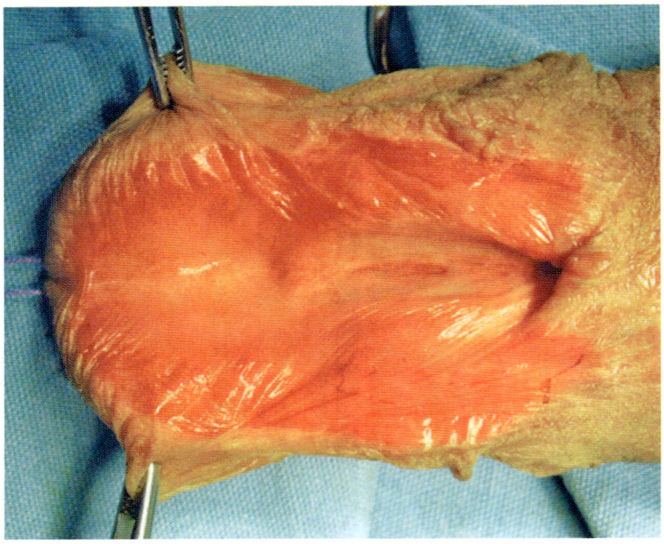

Fig. 10.22: A glans traction stitch being taken

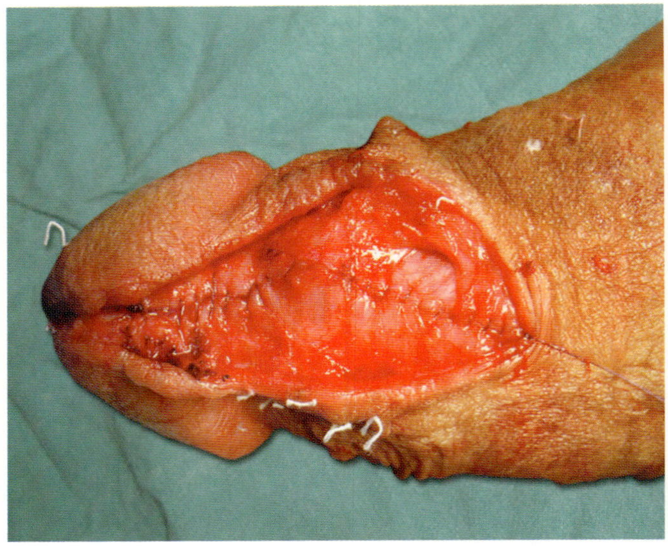

Fig. 10.24: The appearance of the tubularized neourethra. The adjacent dartos fascia is closed, providing a second layer closure

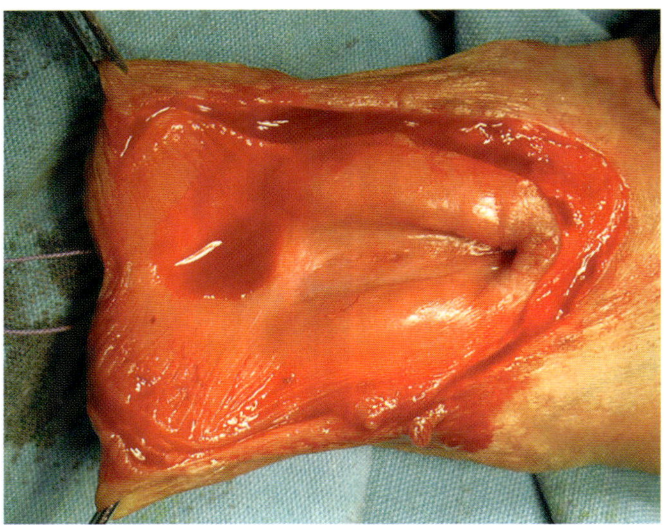

Fig. 10.23: The appearance of urethral strip after incisions, which are created to allow elevation of the adjacent tissue

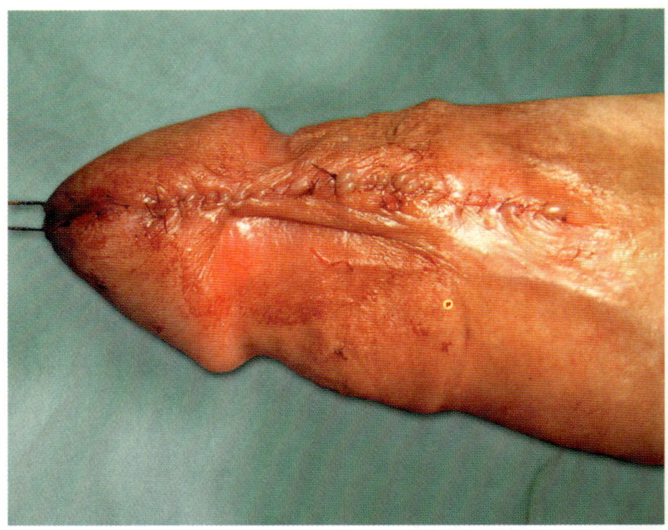

Fig. 10.25: The appearance of ventrum of the penis after closure

A Thiersch-Duplay strip measuring 3 cm wide from the meatus to the spatulated area at the proximal urethrostomy is marked **(Fig. 10.23)**.

The tissues adjacent to the urethral strips are elevated; the urethral strip is minimally elevated, only enough to allow tubularization. The urethra is tubularized with a watertight 4/0 Vicryl extraepithelial suture. Glans wings are then elevated and the meatus is created **(Fig. 10.24)**. The dartos fascia is interposed between the urethral and skin suture lines.

The skin is closed with 5/0 Vicryl suture **(Fig. 10.25)** and a 14 Fr Foley catheter is placed. The patient is hospitalized for 23 hours. A voiding trial with contrast is done at 2–3 weeks depending on the condition of the wounds.

ANTERIOR PANURETHRAL STAGED BUCCAL MUCOSA GRAFT RECONSTRUCTION

First Stage

For patients with urethral strictures associated with LS, sparing of the proximal urethra is characteristic. However, a more aggressive approach is needed. Preoperative evaluation has already been discussed **(Figs 10.26 and 10.27)**.

For more extensive reconstructions, a larger amount of oral graft is required. Usually bilateral harvest of buccal grafts is sufficient, although lingual or bladder epithelial grafts can be used to augment the repair. It is imperative to use bladder mucosa only if oral donor sites have been considered. A bladder epithelial graft cannot be used for staged reconstruction. When harvesting large grafts from the cheeks, it is recommended to leave the donor site open or partially closed, leaving the proximal area open to avoid contracture **(Figs 10.28 and 10.29)**. If bilateral grafting is planned, nasal intubation can be helpful.

Urethrotomy is created to normal appearing urethral epithelium and corpus spongiosum as confirmed by appearance and bouginage **(Figs 10.30 to 10.32)**.

Once a normal urethra is achieved, calibration is done **(Fig. 10.32)**, and proximal urethroscopy will rule out proximal urethral lesions.

A small V-flap is developed in the scrotum and sutured to the most proximal area of urethral spatulation **(Figs 10.33 and 10.34)**.

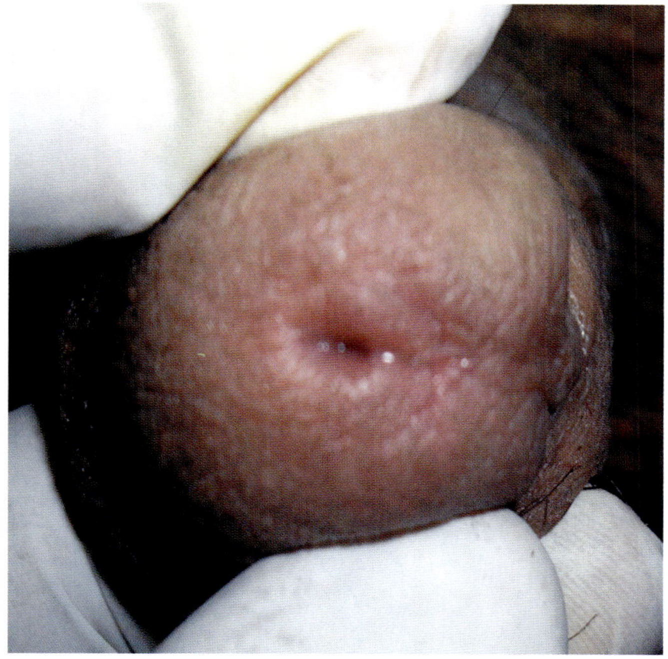

Fig. 10.27: Pinpoint meatus in the patient with more aggressive urethral involvement

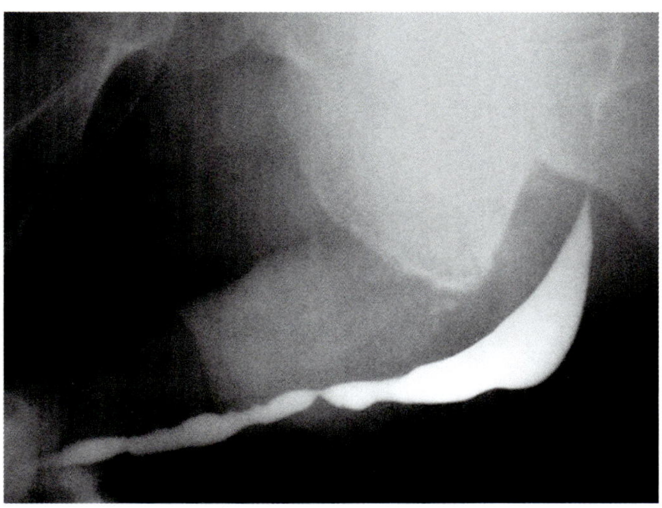

Fig. 10.26: The retrograde urethrogram of a 58-year-old lichen sclerosus patient shows a beaded appearance of the urethra extending from the meatus to the distal bulb. Sparing of the proximal urethra is characteristic

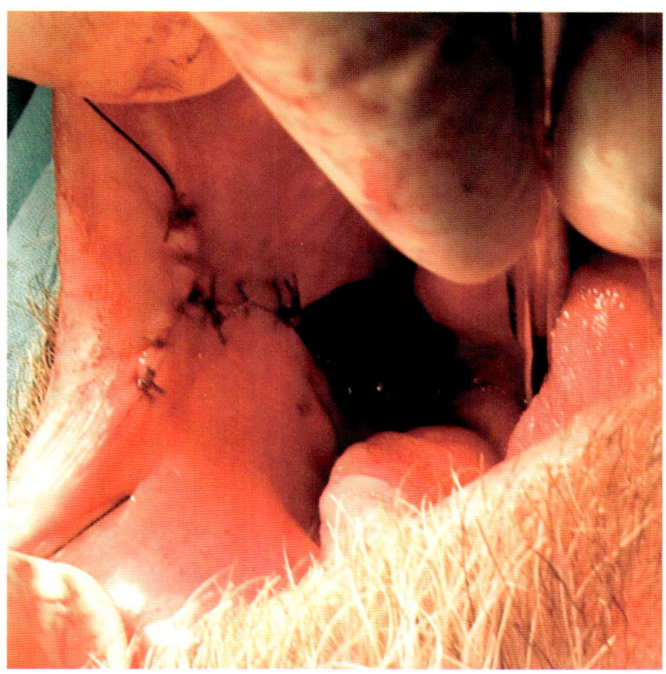

Fig. 10.28: Left cheek is partially closed. The distal area is triangulated

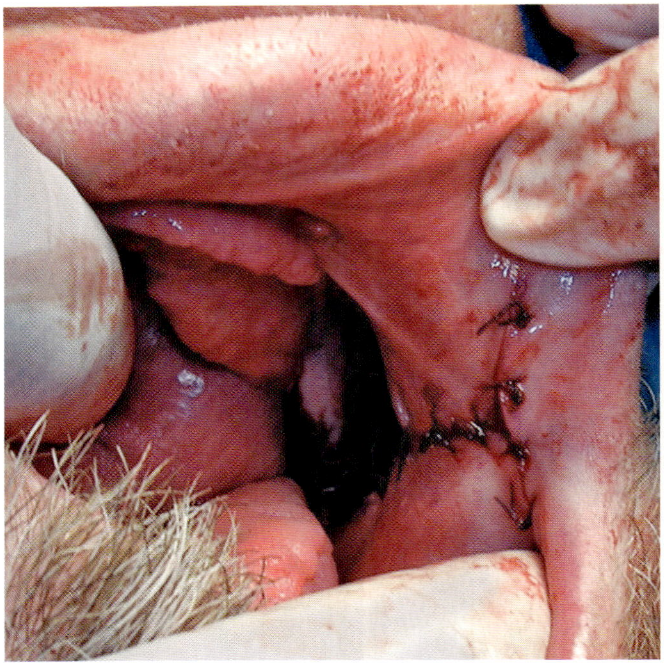

Fig. 10.29: Right cheek is partially closed. Both proximal areas are left open

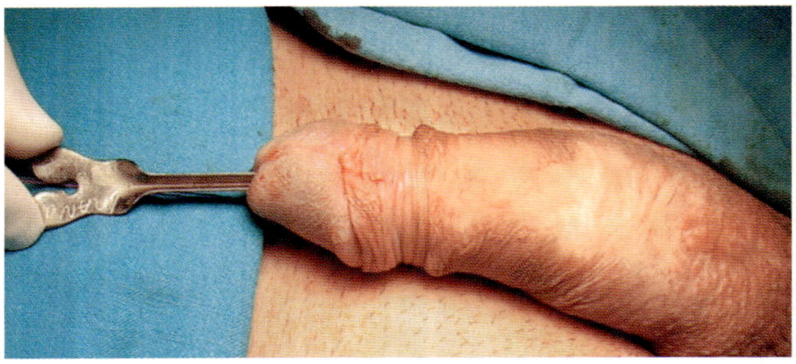

Fig. 10.30: A groove sound is useful to guide the urethrotomy

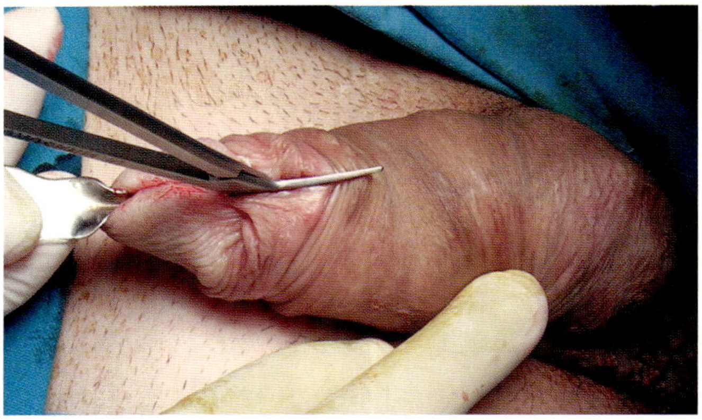

Fig. 10.31: External urethrotomy starts at the meatus

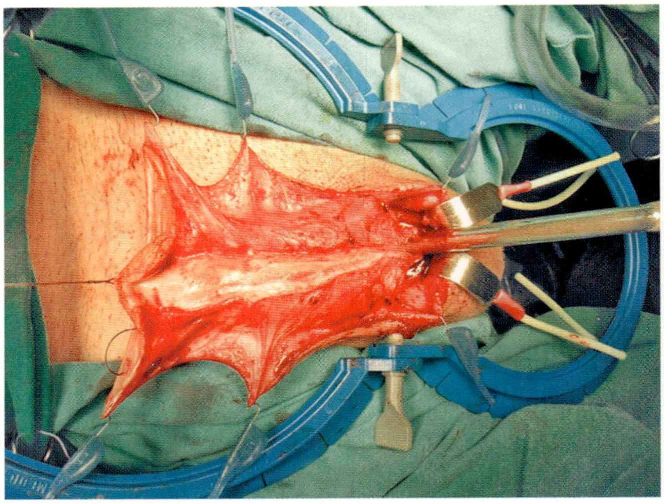

Fig. 10.32: The urethrotomy is completed; the normal appearance of the urethral epithelium is noted and the urethral caliber is confirmed by bouginage. Elevation of the glans flaps has been accomplished

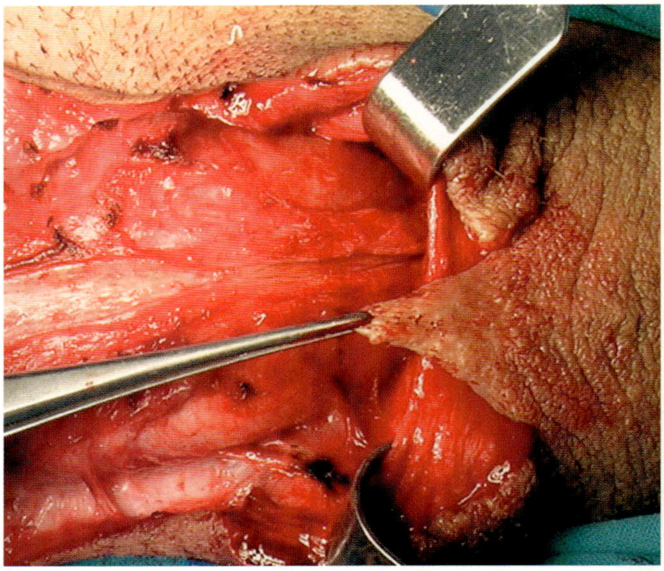

Fig. 10.33: A proximal V-flap is advanced into the proximal urethral spatulation

The defect is measured **(Fig. 10.35)**. If there is a need for additional graft material, one should strongly consider harvest from the tongue.[11]

In this particular case, bilateral buccal grafts measuring 4 × 7 cm are harvested **(Figs 10.36 and 10.37)**.

The 4/0 chromic tie-over sutures are positioned, and the grafts are tailored, pie-crusted and quilted in place **(Figs 10.38 and 10.39)**.

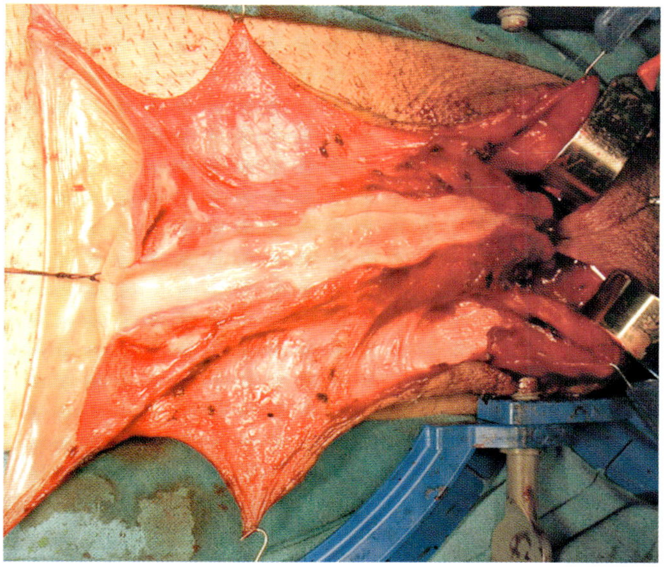

Fig. 10.34: The appearance of stenotic portion of the urethra is noted and prepared for the graft onlay

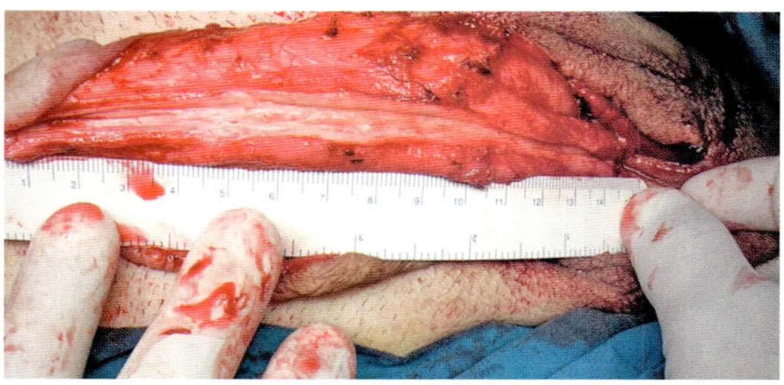

Fig. 10.35: The urethral defect measures 15 cm

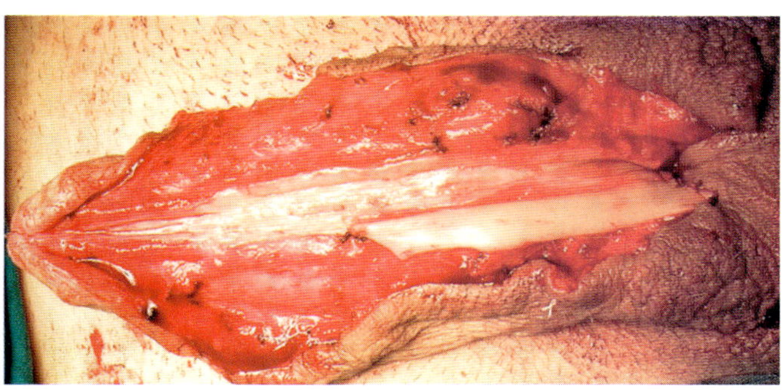

Fig. 10.36: Harvested grafts are divided and sutured to the preserved urethral strip and to the adjacent tissues

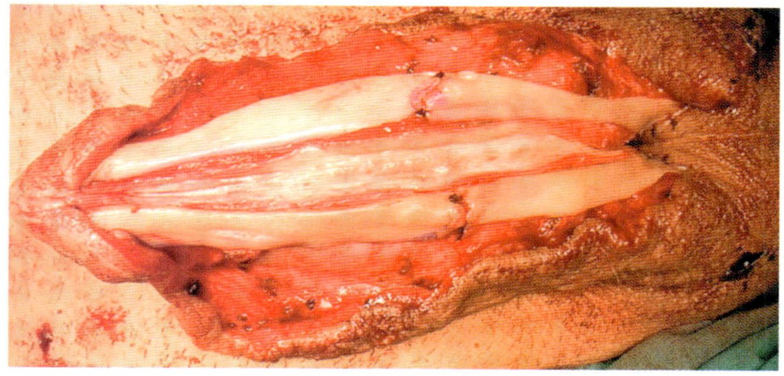

Fig. 10.37: The graft material has been sutured adjacent to the urethral strip

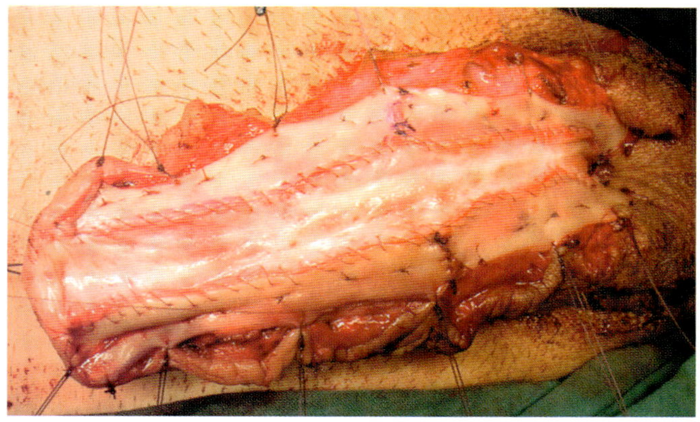

Fig. 10.38: The 4/0 chromic tacking sutures are applied alongside the lateral margins

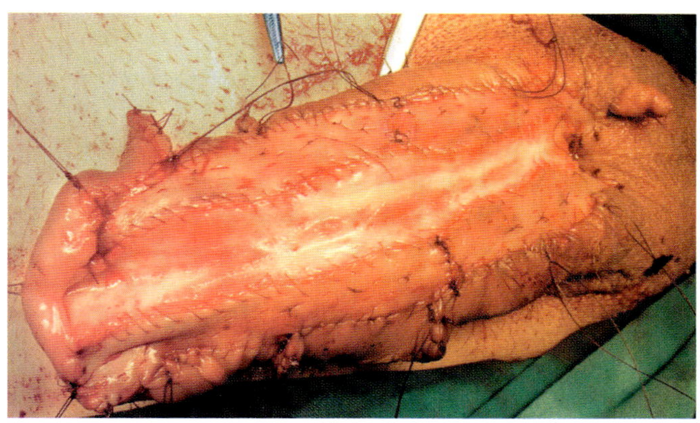

Fig. 10.39: The grafts are completely inset quilted and pie-crusted

Xeroform™ is placed as the deep layer of the bolster and covered with vaseline embedded gauzes **(Fig. 10.40)**.

A Coban® bandage covers the gauze, and a 14 Fr Rüsch urethral diverting catheter is placed **(Fig. 10.41)**.

The patient is at bed rest initially, and initial postoperative care has already been described. The bolster and the urethral catheter are removed around 5th postoperative day **(Fig. 10.42)**.

Second Stage

It can be accomplished at 6–12 months, depending on the graft appearance, urethrostomy bouginage and the patient's desire **(Fig. 10.43)**.

Prior to scheduling the second stage, proximal urethroscopy is essential to rule out other stenotic process.

Patient is placed in frog leg supine position. A glans traction suture is applied. A neourethral strip is measured and incised, measuring 3 cm across **(Fig. 10.44)**.

The urethral strip edges are then minimally elevated and tubularized in Thiersch-Duplay fashion. The tubularization is accomplished with 4/0 Vicryl subepithelial suture **(Figs 10.45 and 10.46)**.

The left hemiscrotum is dissected and a tunica dartos flap is elevated and transposed to the ventral aspect of the shaft. This interpose a robust second layer over the entire urethral closure **(Figs 10.47 and 10.48)**.

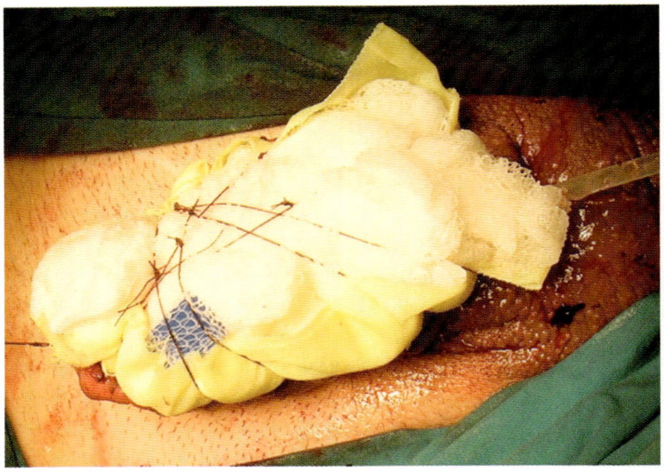

Fig. 10.40: The bolster is tied against the graft with the 4/0 chromic tacking sutures

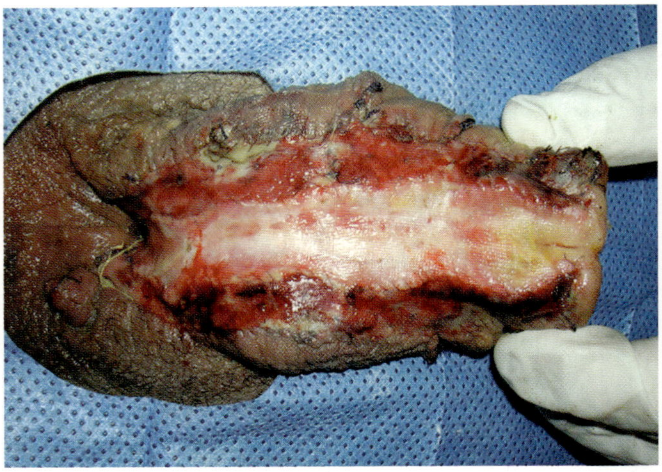

Fig. 10.42: The characteristic appearance of the grafts on 5th postoperative day

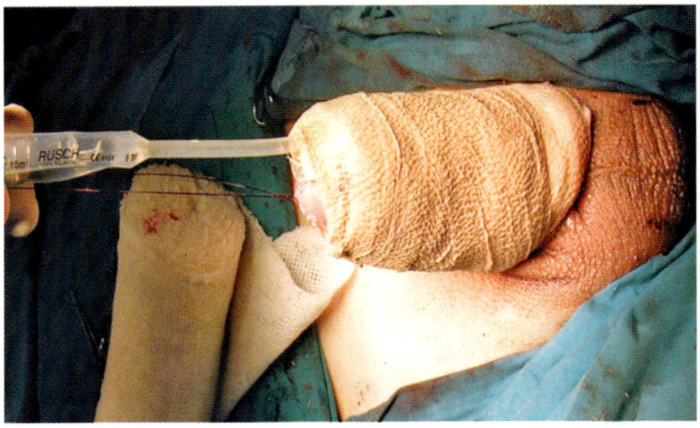

Fig. 10.41: The bolster is held in place with a moderately compressive Coban® bandage

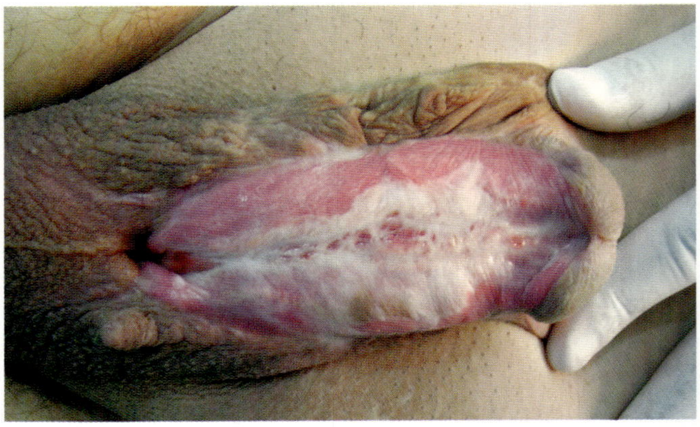

Fig. 10.43: Nine months after first stage, the grafts have a smooth and pink surface. The neourethra is 3 cm wide

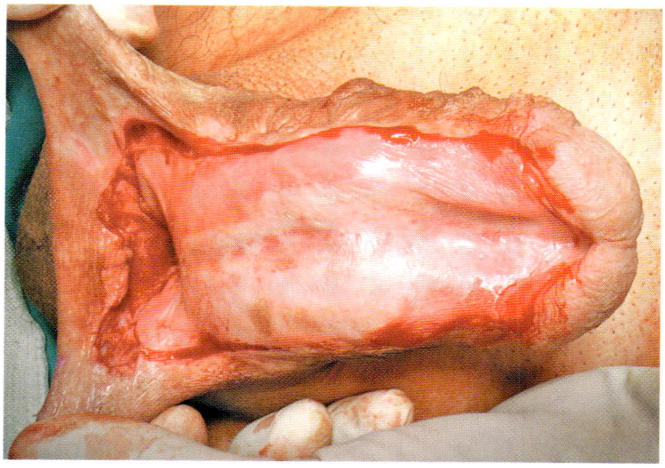

Fig. 10.44: Incisions to develop the Thiersch's strip are noted and the proximally advanced V-flap is re-elevated

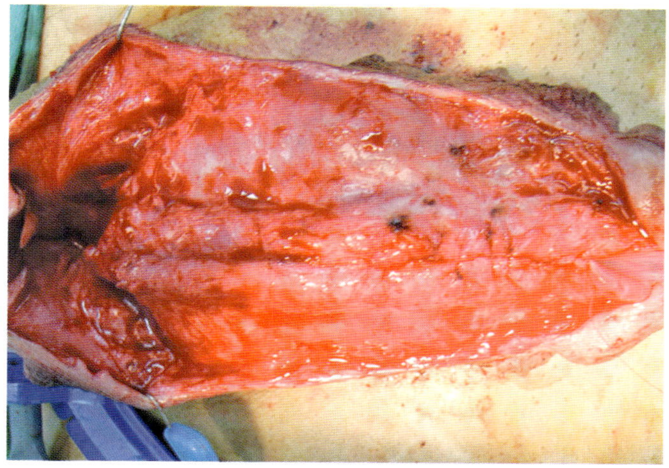

Fig. 10.46: The appearance of the tubularized urethral strip

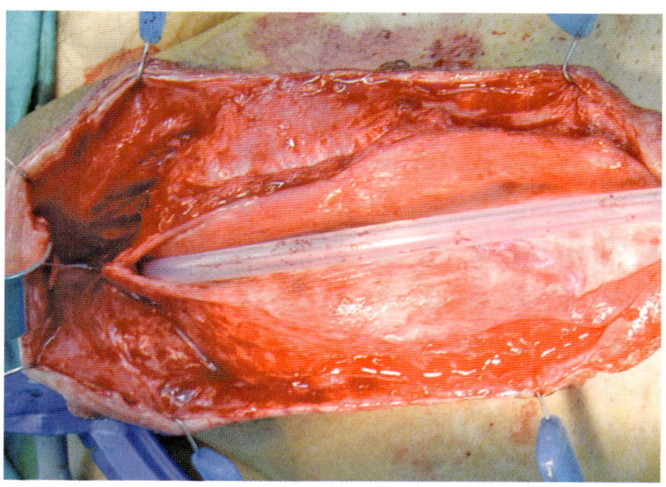

Fig. 10.45: Tubularization of the neourethra with 6/0 subcuticular running Vicryl suture over a 14 Fr Rüsch catheter

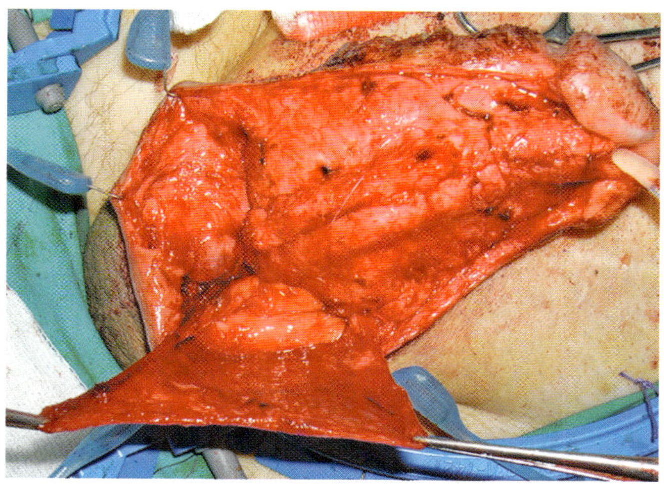

Fig. 10.47: The appearance of the tunica dartos flap

The glans and the penis are closed using 5/0 interrupted Vicryl sutures. The urethral catheter is fixed to the glans to avoid ventral traction against the suture lines **(Figs 10.49 and 10.50)**.

A voiding trial with contrast is done at 2–3 weeks depending on the condition of the wounds. Follow-up is encouraged at 6 months and 12 months after the surgery and yearly thereafter.[12]

COMPLICATIONS

Oral Mucosa Graft Harvesting

When placing the tacking sutures on the angles of lip, if there is bleeding on the needle tract, pressure is recommended to avoid hematomas **(Fig. 10.51)**.

The main concern during the elevation of the graft is sparing the Stenson's duct. The best way to avoid it is by

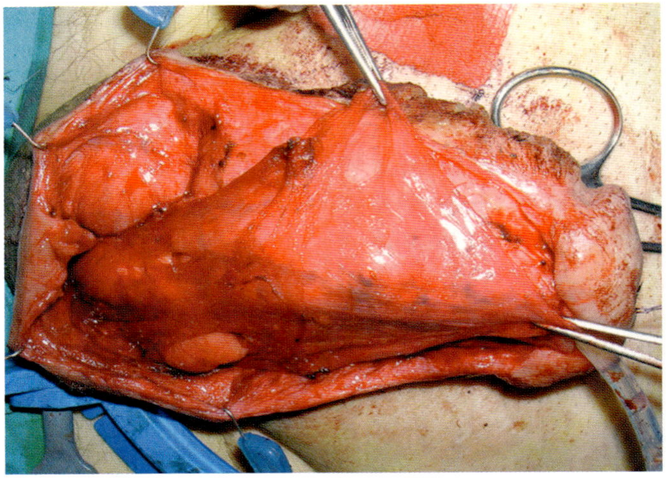

Fig. 10.48: The tunica dartos flap is fixed to the coronal sulcus, covering the entire ventral surface of the urethra

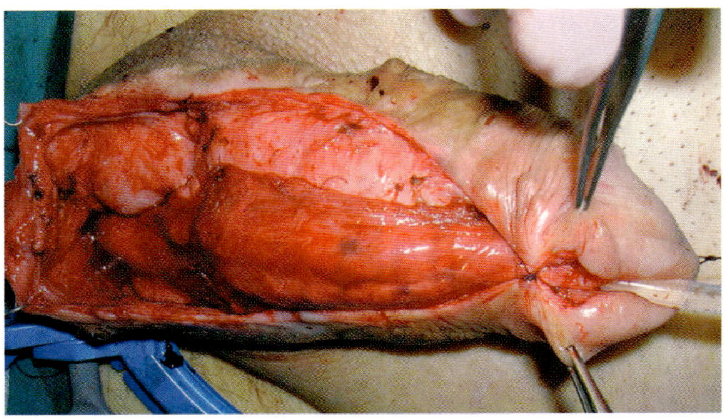

Fig. 10.49: Skin closure. A slit-shaped meatus, when possible, is created

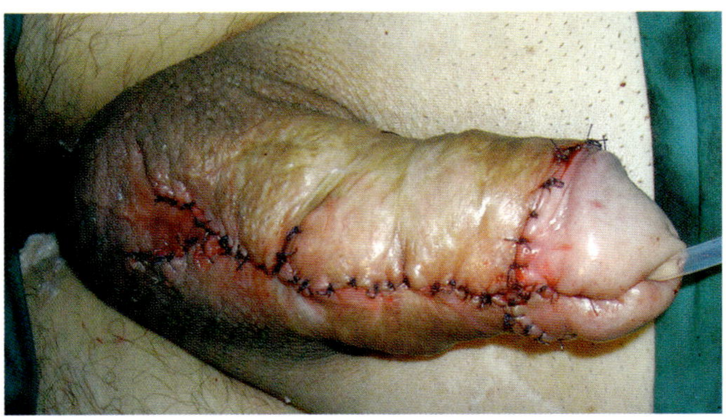

Fig. 10.50: Final appearance of the penis

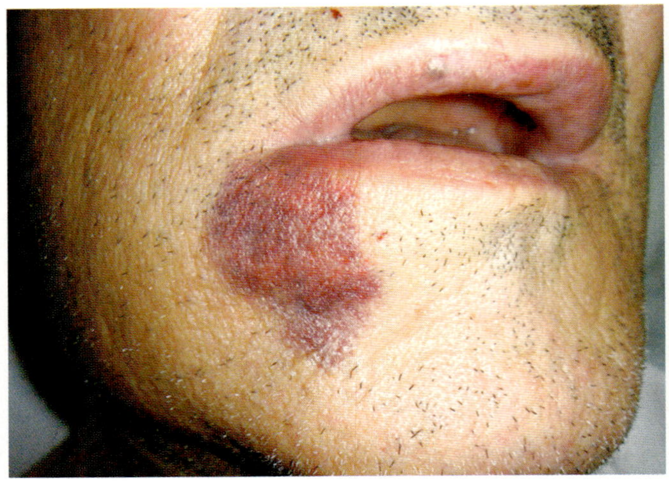

Fig. 10.51: Facial hematoma resulting from the traction sutures

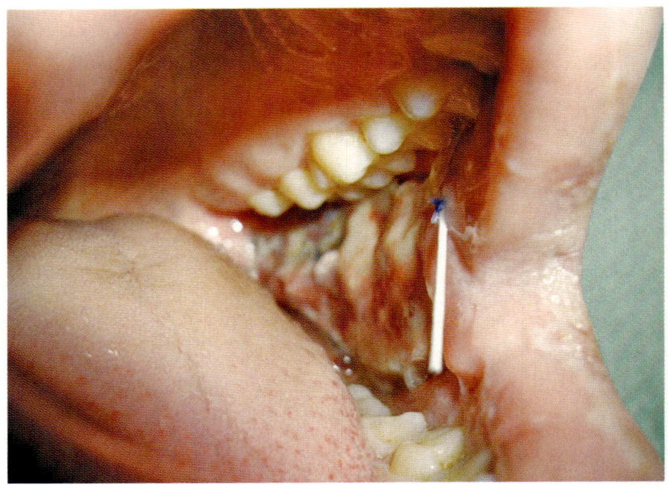

Fig. 10.52: In this case, Stenson's duct has been injured during the graft harvest. The opening of the duct is identified and stented with a small caliber feeding tube for 1 week. The defect is left open

marking it prior to injecting the lidocaine/epinephrine solution, for that would modify the anatomy and can obscure the opening of the duct. If the duct is injured, then identification and proper stenting is essential, and the defect must be left open to close by second intention **(Fig. 10.52)**.

Careful hemostasis is recommended by using the bipolar electrocautery in the mucosal defect to avoid nerve damaging.

Second Stage: Neourethral Tubularization

Fistulae, along the suture line are the most common complication. The tunica dartos flap used to cover the suture line, goes a long way in reducing this complication. Also one should not place too tight a Foley's catheter. It should not be snuggly fitting the neourethra. A loose catheter allows for free drainage of the urethral secretions, lest they do not get inspissated along the suture line and predispose to infection and suture line disruption.

CONCLUSION

Conservative methods to manage urethral strictures, such as internal urethrotomy and frequent dilations, have been ineffective for urethral strictures associated with LS.

Meatal dilation can certainly buy time, but the trauma of repeated dilations cannot be underestimated.

Meatotomy is seldom a long-term fix. Whether it is the Koebner phenomenon that dooms meatotomy to failure or just the fact that LS is a "skin disease" is not clear.[13]

When there is meatal or perimeatal compromise, more aggressive therapy is required. Patients with meatal and perimeatal involvement frequently have developed panurethral stricture disease, probably the result of a combination of disease progression and high pressure voiding against meatal stenosis. Additionally, many patients have had many "minimally invasive" procedures almost certainly damaging the proximal urethra.[14]

Several meatoplasty techniques have been proposed in the past, with variable functional and cosmetic results.

More aggressive reconstruction techniques with genital and/or extragenital skin grafts and flaps have been proposed, but considering the pathophysiology of the disease, they are not supported by the literature.

In a review of our series of strictures of the meatus and fossa navicularis, corrected with the ventral transverse skin island elevated on a dartos fascial flap, 12 patients (34%) had LS. Lichen sclerosis recurred at the fossa or meatus in 6 patients (50%), with a mean follow-up of 8.9 years and a median of 8.3 years.

Early on, authors applied this technique to every patient with a fossa stricture; in fact, they believed that it was the solution for those patients with a meatal stricture secondary to LS. With better understanding of the physiopathology of LS, they know that the process will recur in the flap. Since then, they have treated LS fossa navicularis strictures with primary or staged oral mucosa graft onlay, and did so in over 50% of their patients in the follow-up period analyzed. For primary reconstruction, they used the Asopa technique for dorsal buccal mucosal graft onlay. The graft was 20% larger than the defect to allow shrinkage during the graft taking; by doing this, they have not had graft necrosis/loss due to shrinkage. They have also not encountered graft loss secondary to dryness in their series in cases of staged buccal graft.

EDITORIAL COMMENTS

Dr Rajesh Gulia

Staged procedures have never failed. In the quest for single stage, various single stage pedicled flap procedures have been tried, but not with an overall good success rate. In LS, since it is a skin disease, we definitely should not use local skin even if adequately available. In another case, which we call stricture cripples, or hypospadias cripples, the local vascularity is questionable. It is always better to do a staged procedure in these cases. Further these patients have had multiple reconstructive procedures, repeated endoscopic urethrotomies or blind dilatations. They are both financially and emotionally drained with a very poor quality of life, to the extent of going into depression and having suicidal tendencies. We have to offer one last solution that works. If enough expertise is not available, a good perineal urethrostomy is also a good solution.

REFERENCES

1. Akporiaye LE, Jordan GH, Devine CJ Jr. Balanitis xerotica obliterans (BXO). AUA Updates Series. 1997;16:162.
2. Depasquale I, Park AJ, Bracka A. The treatment of balanitis xerotica obliterans. BJU Int. 2000;86:459-65.
3. Venn SN, Mundy AR. Urethroplasty for balanitis xerotica obliterans. Br J Urol. 1998;81:735.
4. Jordan GH. Reconstruction of the fossa navicularis. J Urol. 1997;138:102.
5. Nahas BW, Hart AJ. Letter to the editor. Re: Reconstruction of resistant strictures of the fossa navicularis and meatus. J Urol. 1999;161:924.
6. Armenakas NA, Morey AF, McAninch JW. Reconstruction of resistant strictures of the fossa navicularis and meatus. J Urol. 1998;160:359.
7. Bracka A. Re: Reconstruction of resistant strictures of the fossa navicularis and meatus. J Urol. 1999;162:1389.
8. Bürger RA, Müller SC, el-Damanhoury H. The buccal mucosal graft for urethral reconstruction: a preliminary report. J Urol. 1992;147(3):662-4.
9. Dubey D, Sehgal A, Srivastava A, et al. Buccal mucosal urethroplasty for balanitis xerotica obliterans related urethral strictures: the outcome of 1 and 2-stage techniques. J Urol. 2005;173(2):463-6.

10. Morey AF, Lin HC, DeRosa CA. Fossa navicularis reconstruction: impact of stricture length on outcomes and assessment of extended meatotomy (first stage Johanson) maneuver. Urologia Internationalis. 2007;79(1): 8-12.
11. Simonato A, Gregori A, Lissiani A, et al. The tongue as an alternative donor site for graft urethroplasty: a pilot study. J Urol. 2006;175:589-92.
12. Virasoro R, Eltahawy EA, Jordan GH. Long-term follow-up for reconstruction of strictures of the fossa navicularis with a single technique. BJU International. 2007;100(5):1143-5.
13. Malone P. A new technique for meatal stenosis in patients with lichen sclerosus. J Urol. 2004;172:949-52.
14. Kulkarni S, Barbagli G, Kirpekar D, et al. Lichen sclerosus of the male genitalia and urethra: surgical options and results in a multicenter international experience with 215 patients. Eur Urol. 2009;55:945-56.

11

CHAPTER

Perineal Urethrostomy

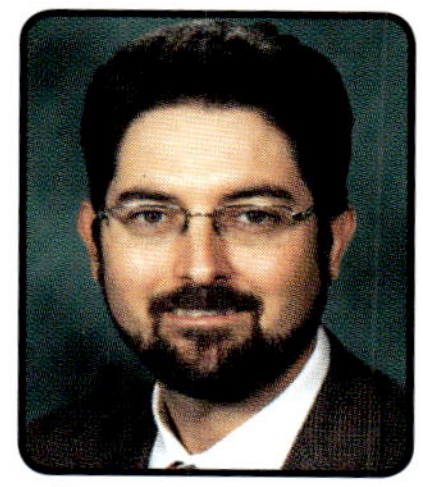

Jeremy B Myers

Jeremy B Myers, William O Brant

Chapter Outline

- Indications and Contraindications
  - Indications
  - Relative Contraindications
- Surgery
  - Recommended Equipment
  - Patient Preparation
  - Positioning
  - Surgical Steps
  - Postoperative Care
- Outcomes
- Surgical Pearls
- Editorial Comments

Abstract

Perineal urethrostomy is an essential procedure for any surgeon that treats lower urinary tract pathology involving the urethra or penis. Patients who are stricture cripples, can be motivated for only one last surgery that gives results. Here, a well done perineal urethrostomy provides the answer. The key to success is take the "skin to the bulbar urethra," rather than the "bulbar urethra to the skin." Patients are so satisfied with a well done perineal urethrostomy that they do not want to come back for the 2nd stage procedure if planned. A well done perineal urethrostomy with a thin perineal flap does not require regular dilatations of the urethrostomy. In the video compilations along with this atlas, the procedure of perineal urethrostomy shown has been done by Professor Barbagli.

Keywords

Perineal urethrostomy, Diversion of urine, Partial penectomy, Fournier's gangrene, Periurethritis, Suprapubic cystostomy, Inverted "U" advancement, Ventral urethrotomy, Dorsal urethral plate, Avascular necrosis of the flap.

INTRODUCTION

Perineal urethrostomy is an essential procedure for any surgeon that treats lower urinary tract pathology involving the urethra or penis. A perineal urethrostomy is placed, in the bulbar urethra, just distal to the external sphincter and it allows for diversion of urine proximal to the majority of the anterior urethra.[1] It is most commonly employed for patients with difficult to treat urethral strictures, but is indispensable for treating several other pathologic conditions of the penis and urethra.

There are several conditions that make urethroplasty challenging and may decrease its ultimate success; in these cases perineal urethrostomy may be a good alternative to urethral reconstruction. One example of unfavorable urethral disease is lengthy strictures involving the entire anterior urethra **(Fig. 11.1)**. These "pan" urethral strictures can arise from a variety of causes, but are notorious in the setting of lichen sclerosis. Panurethral strictures that arise from lichen sclerosis are very prone to urethroplasty failure and for this reason many surgeons advocate for perineal urethrostomy as a first line therapy.[2] There are several other conditions, which can also decrease the success of urethroplasty, for example, those patients with multiple failed urethroplasties in the past,[3,4] patients with a history of hypospadias repair[5] and those with prior pelvic radiation therapy.[6] *Although these cases need to be carefully considered individually, sometimes the best functional outcomes may be from abandoning the idea of further urethral reconstruction and instead creating a permanent perineal urethrostomy.*

In addition to difficult to treat strictures, perineal urethrostomy is an essential technique as an adjunct to the treatment of men with urethral and penile carcinoma. Even when some of the penis can be spared, as in a partial

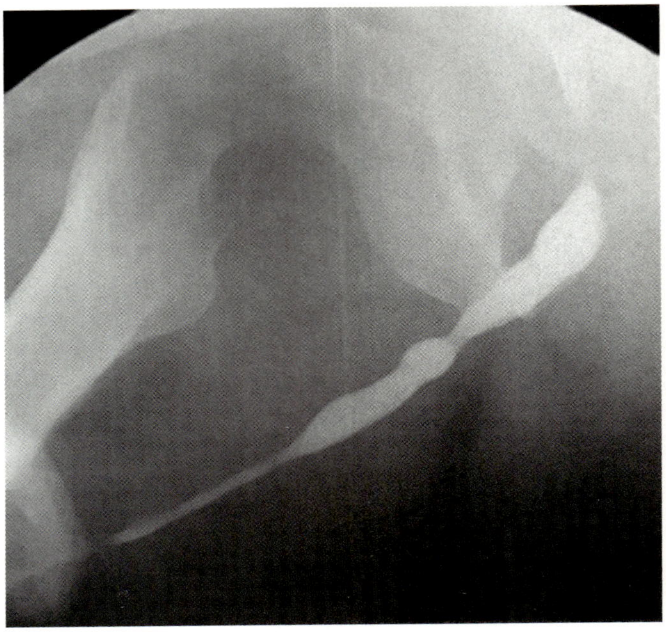

Fig. 11.1: A retrograde urethrogram that shows panurethral stricture arising from the lichen sclerosis

penectomy for penile cancer, men do not urinate well from a urethrotomy at the penoscrotal junction or further into the scrotum, and consideration should be given to creation of a proximal perineal urethrostomy to ensure a good urinary outcome.

Another condition in which perineal urethrostomy is useful is in men with Fournier's gangrene. This condition classically arises from periurethritis from a catheter or urethral stricture disease. Often, due to the necrotizing infection, the penile skin has to be removed and if there is underlying stricture disease through the penis or urethral loss from urethritis, the options are very limited for subsequent urethral repair once the penis has been skin grafted **(Fig. 11.2)**. Usually these men are temporized with a suprapubic cystostomy until they have healed completely and then consideration can be given to elective creation of a perineal urethrostomy.

The final scenario in which, perineal urethrostomy is very helpful is elderly men with urethral stricture disease. The incidence of stricture disease increases with age[7] and although many elderly men can be managed conservatively some will require surgical intervention beyond dilation or internal urethrotomy. Elderly men are often not bothered by needing to sit to void after surgery and are happy to forgo urethroplasty, especially for complicated strictures, that may have less success than a permanent perineal urethrostomy.

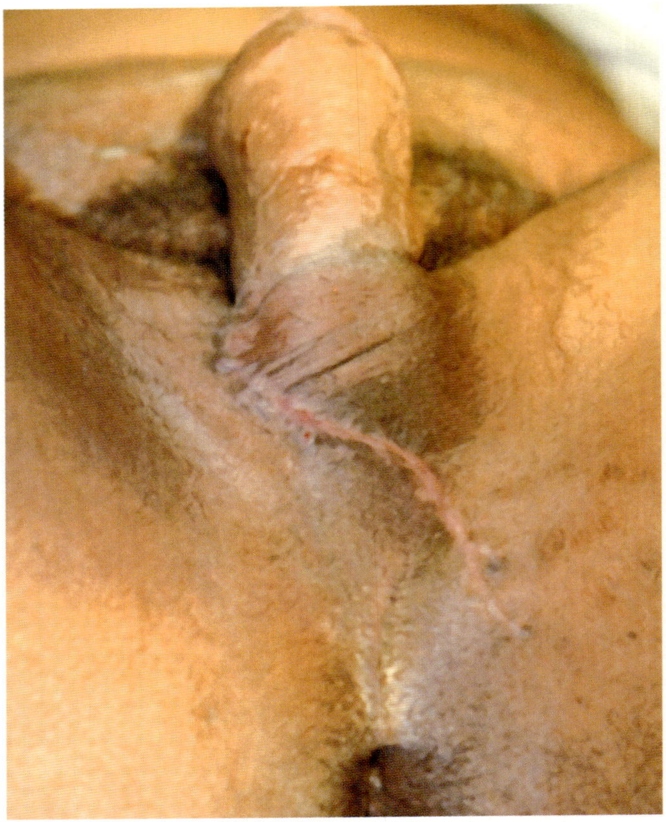

Fig. 11.2: A difficult case of Fournier's gangrene with penile skin grafting, primary perineal closure and relocation of the testes in thigh pouches. This patient had diffused bulbar and pendulous urethral stricture disease

BACKGROUND

Perineal urethrostomy has a reputation of being prone to stenosis at the level of the perineum. This reputation may arise from creation of the perineal urethrostomy by transection of bulbar urethra and bringing the urethra up to the skin surface. This technique creates a small opening at the level of the perineum and also decreases the blood supply through the urethra by cutting the bulbar arteries as they course longitudinally through the urethra. Recent series, reporting perineal urethrostomy outcomes, generally describe an alternative technique where the urethra is opened ventrally, rather than transected, and the dorsal plate and longitudinal blood supply of the urethra is preserved.[2,8–10]

The concept of this surgical approach is not new and it was probably first described by Johanson. He described opening the urethra along the ventrum and sewing it to the perineal and scrotal skin, in order to subsequently perform a second stage tubularization of this repair with adjacent skin that had healed to the urethra.[11] Blandy described a similar concept for approach to proximal strictures with an inverted "U" advancement flap as is described in this chapter and eventual tubularization of this repair similarly to Johanson's repair.[1] The idea of the inverted "U" was to decrease tension on the skin where it was sewn to the urethra.

While these surgeries were described with the purpose of ultimate definitive repair and retubularization of the urethra, in creation of a perineal urethrostomy the steps are identical, but the patient never undergoes subsequent closure. In fact, it is the experience of many surgeons that patients who undergo first stage urethroplasty for complex bulbar strictures often do not choose to subsequently undergo closure as the urinary outcome is so satisfactory to them without closure.[2,8]

INDICATIONS AND CONTRAINDICATIONS

Patients who choose to undergo perineal urethrostomy either have unfavorable urethral pathology for reconstruction or do not desire extensive urethral reconstructive surgery. Patients with contraindications to perineal urethrostomy are those with extensive disease proximal to the bulbomembranous junction such as prostatic urethral stenosis or bladder neck contracture. In addition, poor external sphincteric function, especially combined with a history of prostate resection or ablative procedures, is a relative contraindication unless a bladder neck artificial urinary sphincter is feasible. In addition, those patients who have had complete loss of their perineal soft tissue and skin from Fournier's gangrene may not be good candidates for a perineal urethrostomy, as the creation of advancement flaps may not be possible.

Indications

- Intractable anterior urethral strictures (especially, in cases of panurethral lichen sclerosis)
- Penile or urethral carcinoma requiring penectomy
- Cases of Fournier's gangrene with urethral involvement
- Older patients not desiring extensive urethral reconstruction.

Relative Contraindications

- Urethral disease involving or proximal to the external sphincter
- Incontinence and need for an artificial urinary sphincter
- Skin grafted perineum.

SURGERY

Recommended Equipment

- Perineal retractor (e.g. perineal Bookwalter, Lone Star retractor)
- Sacral elevation (folded bean bag or blankets)
- Atraumatic forceps
- Fine serrated dissecting scissors.

Patient Preparation

A preoperative urine culture is done to assure sterile urine in patients undergoing perineal urethrostomy. Patients are given preoperative broad-spectrum antibiotics prior to making an incision. Sequential compression devices are used during the operation.

Positioning

After undergoing general endotracheal anesthesia, patients are placed into a high lithotomy position, using "candy cane" stirrups. Sacral elevation (authors use a bean bag covered by a gel pad) is used to support and rotate the pelvis so that the perineum and proximal urethra are easily accessible to the surgeon **(Fig. 11.3)**. Care is taken to make sure that all pressure points are adequately padded. Complications in this position are rare[12] and generally should not occur if the duration of the operation is less than 5 hours.[1,13] In addition to establishing an optimal position for access to the proximal urethra, the high lithotomy position allows two standing surgeons to operate side by side with ease.

Surgical Steps

After patients are positioned into the high lithotomy position an inverted "U" shape incision is made **(Figs 11.4A and B)**. The apex of the inverted "U" is located in the upper portion of the perineum where it meets the scrotum; this incision acts to relax the perineum and facilitates a tension-free anastomosis between the skin and urethra. This relaxing incision is especially important when patients are obese or have had previous perineal surgery. An important component to the inverted "U" incision and flap is the mobilization of a full thickness fat pad underneath it, directly off of the underlying bulbospongiosus muscle. This maneuver helps assure a good vascular supply to the apex of the flap. Usually a midline incision extending cephalad from the apex of the inverted "U" is made into the lower scrotum, because the opening in the skin of the perineum is not large enough for

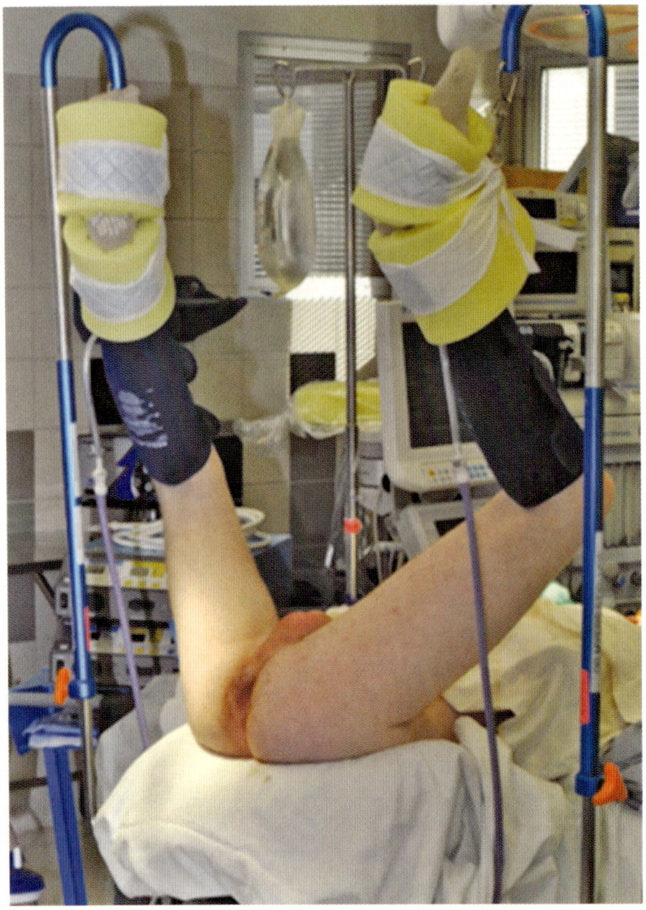

Fig. 11.3: Positioning of the patient for perineal urethrostomy. Candy cane stirrups are used along with a bean bag covered by a gel pad that is bulked under the buttocks to rotate the perineum to a more parallel position

the corresponding urethrotomy. One critical component for success is to make the inverted "U" flap long enough. A common error is to underestimate the length needed and to have tension where the flap meets the proximal urethra. The inverted "U" flap can always be shortened if there is redundant flap by trimming the apex of the "U" after it is created.

Once the inverted "U" flap is developed, the bulbospongiosus muscle is separated, exposing the bulbar urethra. The urethra is then grasped with two pairs of forceps above and below the area of planned incision. A knife is then used to make a longitudinal incision ventrally into the urethra measuring approximately 4–6 cm **(Figs 11.5A and B)**. Stay sutures are placed and the urethra is calibrated with a bougie à boule toward the bladder to make sure there is no stricture proximal to the urethrotomy. If strictured urethra is identified proximally, then the ventral urethral incision is extended toward the membranous urethra until an uninvolved area is found. Cystourethroscopy is performed in order to evaluate the distance to the external sphincter as well as to identify potential issues such as obstructive prostatic disease or bladder calculi. Typically the ventral urethrotomy abuts or is within 1 cm of the starting of the external sphincter.

The skin of the perineum is then sutured to the open urethrotomy preserving the dorsal urethral plate. This starts with bringing the apex of the inverted "U" incision to the proximal margin of the urethrotomy. During placement of stitches, care is taken to incorporate three important layers: the urethral mucosal edge, the adventitial edge of the corpus spongiosum, and lastly the skin edge **(Figs 11.6A and B)**. This method preserves blood supply within the corpus spongiosum, in contrast to the effect of a full thickness stitch through the corpus spongiosum. In order to help reduce any tension on the inverted "U" flap, several sutures are placed in the subdermal tissue of the body of the flap and secured to the dense tissue surrounding the bulbar urethra. Interrupted absorbable suture, consisting of 2-0 or 3-0 polyglactin (Vicryl, Ethicon Inc.), is used to mature the perineal urethrostomy. As the perineal urethrostomy is created, the greatest tension is usually between the lateral portion of skin of the inverted "U" and the perineal skin. Often the addition of a bolster suture over a Kittner sponge or a vertical mattress suture can aid in taking tension off of this area.

Once the skin is brought down to the urethra around entire urethrotomy, two openings exist between the urethra and the skin **(Figs 11.7A and B)**. The proximal opening of the urethra leads toward bladder and the distal urethral opening leads out toward penis. The dorsal urethral plate remains intact, as well as the longitudinal blood flow within the corpus spongiosum. A Foley catheter is placed through the proximal portion of the urethrotomy into the bladder and patients are admitted to the surgical ward for recovery.

Postoperative Care

Patients during the postoperative period are treated with antibiotics until the catheter is removed. Usually the catheter is left in place for 14 days. If there is any concern about local tissue healing at the inverted "U" advancement flap, then the catheter can be left for a longer period so that urine in the area does not complicate wound healing further. If breakdown of the incision occurs, then patients are asked to perform sitz bath twice daily.

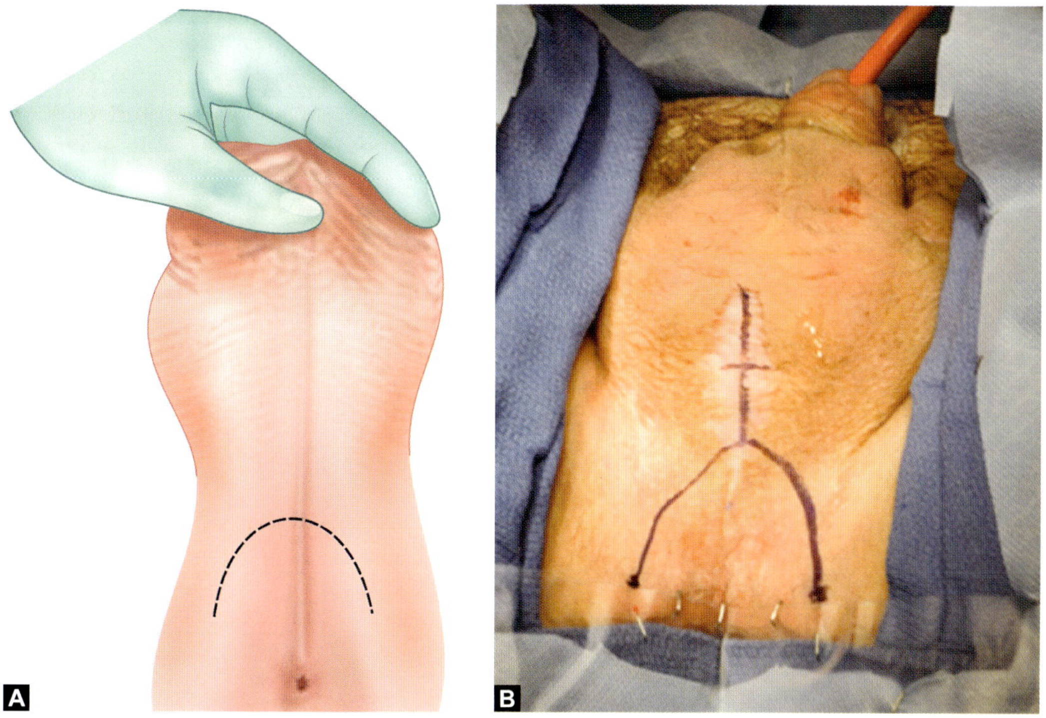

Figs 11.4A and B: The planned advancement flap. The pictures demonstrate the flap abutting the lower scrotum with a cephalad extension that is commonly needed to accommodate the urethrotomy

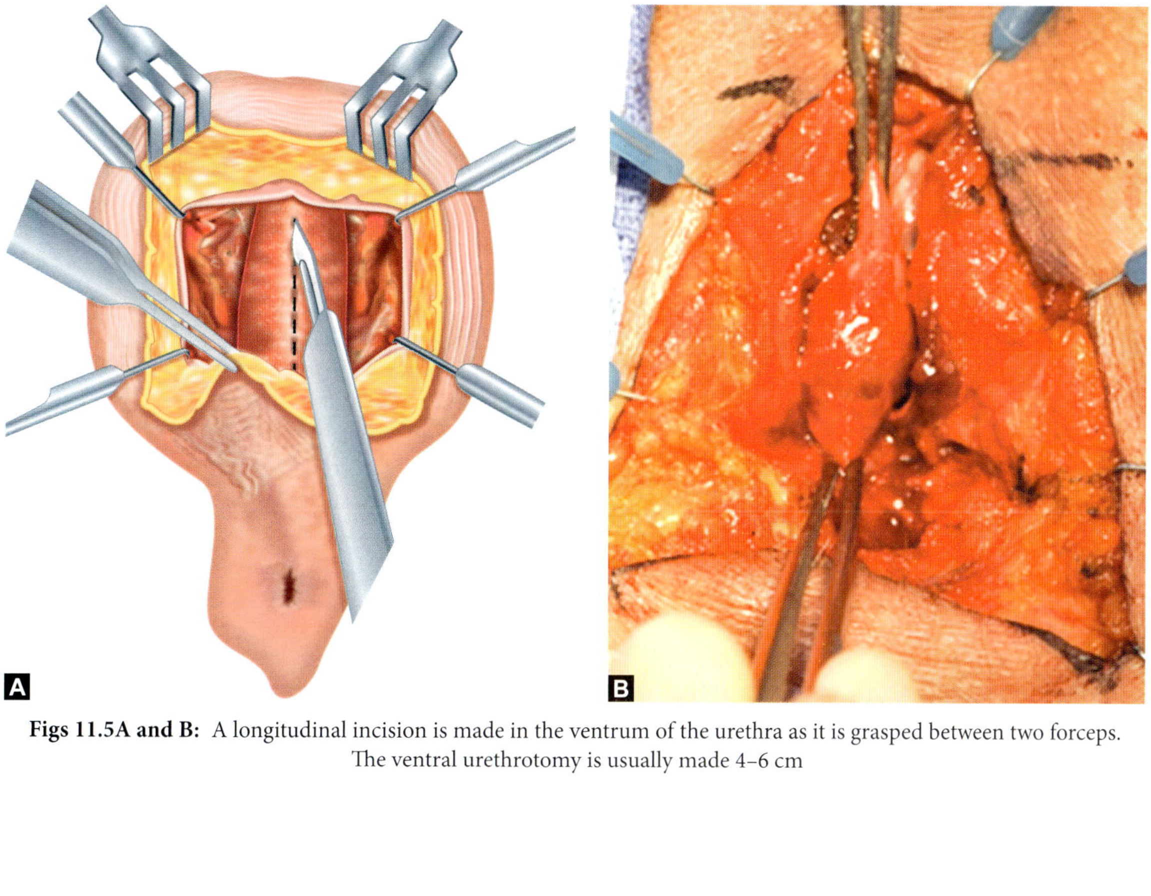

Figs 11.5A and B: A longitudinal incision is made in the ventrum of the urethra as it is grasped between two forceps. The ventral urethrotomy is usually made 4–6 cm

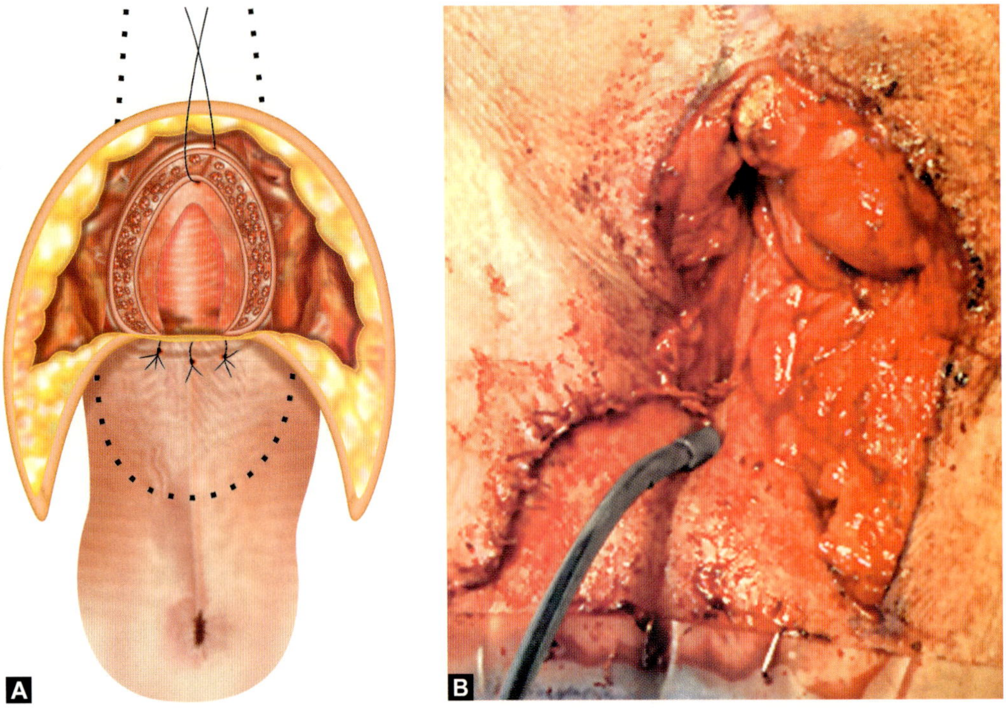

Figs 11.6A and B: Three layers, the urethral mucosa, the adventitial of the corpora spongiosus and skin, are incorporated in absorbable stitches and the urethrotomy is gradually matured. Note that left margin of the flap has been sutured and the tip of the suction cannula is at the urethrostomy opening

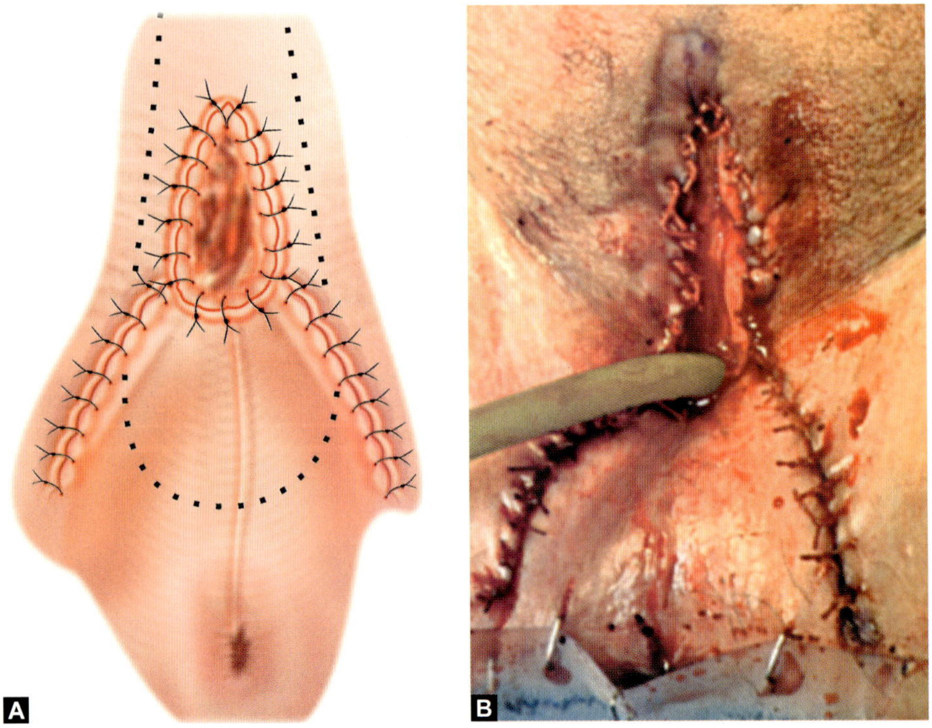

Figs 11.7A and B: The final situation: the catheter is left in for about 2 weeks or longer, if there is any wound breakdown

Patients are followed at regular intervals. Cystourethroscopy is performed at 3 months and 12 months or if there is any concern of stenosis, based upon symptoms, urinary tract infection, a low urinary flow rate, or an increase in postvoid residual urine. Patients, after 1 year, can be followed, at the surgeon's discretion, by symptoms, urinary flow rate, measurement of residual urine, all in conjunction with periodic urethral calibration or cystoscopy.

OUTCOMES

There have been three large case series within the last decade that have reported the outcomes of perineal urethrostomy.[2,8-10] Perineal urethrostomy failure in these studies was defined as a need for instrumentation such as dilation or the need for revision of the perineal urethrostomy. The overall success defined by these criteria was 78% (206/265) between the three series **(Table 11.1)**. *The only factor that predicted perineal urethrostomy failure was a history of radiotherapy for prostate cancer.*[10]

DISCUSSION AND CONCLUSION

Perineal urethrostomy is a valuable technique for treatment of men with intractable stricture disease, penile and urethral carcinoma, urethral complications from Fournier's gangrene and elderly patients who do not want urethral reconstructive surgery. Alternatives to perineal urethrostomy are the various techniques for addressing panurethral stricture, suprapubic cystotomy drainage or urinary diversion. The outcomes of perineal urethrostomy are excellent, when the longitudinal urethral blood supply and dorsal urethral plate are preserved.

Table 11.1: Patients undergoing perineal urethrostomy and the etiology of their urethral disease

	N
Idiopathic stricture disease	9 (20%)
Lichen sclerosis	9 (20%)
Severe infections	7 (16%)
XRT	6 (13%)
Prior hypospadias surgery	5 (11%)
Endoscopic or catheter trauma	5 (11%)
SCC or condyloma	4 (9%)
Total	**45**

Abbreviations: N: Number of patients; XRT: Radiation therapy for prostate cancer; SCC: Squamous cell carcinoma.

SURGICAL PEARLS

- One technical aspect of the operation that can help is the high lithotomy position. This position allows the best access to the proximal urethra and allows creation of the perineal urethrostomy up to the level of the external sphincter as necessary.
- An additional "surgical pearl" is to outline the inverted "U" flap so that it extends up to the junction of the scrotum. Once this inverted "U" flap is released off of the bulbocavernosus muscle it contracts substantially and an adequate length is crucial to prevent tension where it is sewn into the proximal urethrotomy.
- The most common intraoperative problem is stricture that extends from the area of the bulbar urethra toward the external sphincter. Usually this problem can be dealt with by extending the ventral urethrotomy up to the level of the external sphincter.
- On occasion the dorsal plate of the urethra is very diseased and not suitable for creation of the perineal urethrostomy. In these circumstances, it is worthwhile to add a dorsal buccal mucosal graft to recreate a dorsal plate for the length of the perineal urethrostomy, so that the area does not contract with wound healing and time.

Perineal urethrostomy is reliable and represents a good alternative to urethral reconstruction in men with a variety of lower urinary tract surgical issues. Surgeons, who are familiar with perineal anatomy and its proper surgical exposure, can easily learn this technique and apply it to appropriate patients.

EDITORIAL COMMENTS

Dr Rajesh Gulia

The author has very aptly said that the perineal urethrostomies were notorious for getting stenosed. He has also mentioned the reason for it. The important point (apart from preserving the blood supply) is to take the skin down and inside the urethra rather than bringing the urethra up to the skin surface. He has also stressed that "important component of the inverted "U" incision and flap is the mobilization of a full thickness fat pad underneath it, directly off of the underlying bulbospongiosus muscle. This maneuver helps assure a good vascular supply to the apex of the flap." It is an anatomical fact that the blood supply to this inverted "U" shaped flap is from the perineal artery, which is a superficial terminal branch of the internal pudendal artery. Its various branches form a subdermal arterial plexus, which arborizes with the branches of the opposite side. So rich is this plexus that avascular necrosis of this flap is rarely seen and hardly reported. It is not all that essential to take the full thickness fat pad underneath it. Doing so makes it bulky and difficult to take it to the urethral opening without tension. Keeping it without the fat, makes it supple, flexible and easy to take as deep inside the urethral opening without tension. It is very important to anastomose the skin to the healthy portion of the proximal bulbar/membranous urethra and that too without tension. In the quest for healthy mucosa we have gone so proximally so as to be able to have a peek at the verumontanum. One technical difficulty that may arise is in taking sutures so deep inside. What helps is preplacing three sutures with a double armed needle in the proximal healthy urethra. Then with the other needle of the double armed suture, they are placed at the corresponding three points on the apex of the flap, and holding the three sutures taut the flap is slid/telescoped into the depth to approximate to the healthy edges of the proximal urethra. A well done perineal urethrostomy is so satisfying to these so called stricture cripples that they never come back for any further definitive reconstruction.

REFERENCES

1. Blandy JP, Singh M, Tresidder GC. Urethroplasty by scrotal flap for long urethral strictures. Br J Urol. 1968;40(3):261-7.
2. Peterson AC, Palminteri E, Lazzeri M, et al. Heroic measures may not always be justified in extensive urethral stricture due to lichen sclerosus (balanitis xerotica obliterans). Urology. 2004;64(3):565-8.
3. Breyer BN, McAninch JW, Whitson JM, et al. Multivariate analysis for risk factors for long-term urethroplasty outcome. J Urol. 2010;183(2):613-7.
4. Barbagli G, Selli C, Tosto A. Reoperative surgery for recurrent strictures of the penile and bulbous urethra. J Urol. 1996;156(1):76-7.
5. Barbagli G, De Angelis M, Palminteri E, et al. Failed hypospadias repair presenting in adults. Eur Urol. 2006;49(5):887-94; discussion 895.
6. Elliott SP, McAninch JW, Chi T, et al. Management of severe urethral complications of prostate cancer therapy. J Urol. 2006;176(6):2508-13.
7. Santucci RA, Joyce GF, Wise M. Male urethral stricture disease. J Urol. 2007;177(5):1667-74.
8. Barbagli G, De Angelis M, Romano G, et al. Clinical outcome and quality of life assessment in patients treated with perineal urethrostomy for anterior urethral stricture disease. J Urol. 2009;182(2):549-57.
9. Kulkarni S, Barbagli G, Kirpekar D, et al. Lichen sclerosus of the male genitalia and urethra: surgical options and results in a multicenter international experience with 215 patients. Eur Urol. 2009;55:945-56.
10. Myers JB, Porten SP, McAninch JW. The outcomes of perineal urethrostomy with preservation of the dorsal urethral plate and urethral blood supply. Urology. 2011;77(5): 1223-7.
11. Johanson B. Reconstruction of the male urethra in strictures. Acta Chir Scand. 1953;176:3-89.
12. Angermeier KW, Jordan GH. Complications of the exaggerated lithotomy position: a review of 177 cases. J Urol. 1994;151(4):866-8.
13. Anema JG, Morey AF, McAninch JW, et al. Complications related to the high lithotomy position during urethral reconstruction. J Urol. 2000;164(2):360-3.

CHAPTER 12

Female Urethroplasty

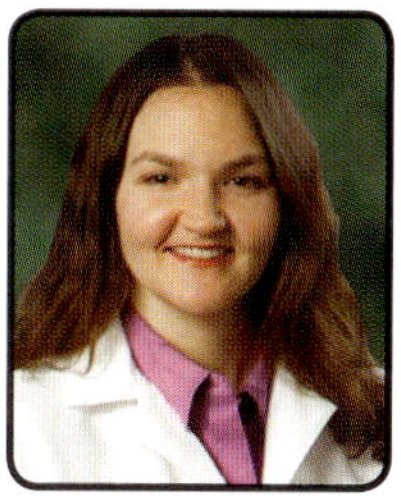

Anne Pelletier-Cameron

Allen McNeil Haraway, Anne Pelletier-Cameron

Chapter Outline

Abstract

Keeping in view the rarity of urethral stricture disease in women, this chapter very succinctly explains the etiopathogenesis of urethral stricture disease in women. It also clearly stresses that urethral dilation should not be performed on female patients with lower urinary tract symptoms and no evidence of a urethral stricture since this can actually cause urethral strictures. Female urethroplasty has been very nicely diagrammatically explained stepwise. Both vaginal flap urethroplasty and buccal mucosa graft urethroplasty have been detailed. Also if the patient develops stress urinary incontinence later on, one should use an autologous pubovaginal sling at the bladder neck rather than a synthetic midurethral sling.

Keywords

Female urethral stricture, Urethral dilation, Self-obturation, Vaginal inlay flap, Vaginal advancement flap, Weighted vaginal speculum, Vestibular flap, Pubocervical fascia, Martius flap, Suprameatal inverted "U," Clitoral bodies, Vaginal pack, Urethrovaginal fistula, Stress incontinence, Autologous pubovaginal sling.

INTRODUCTION

Bladder outlet obstruction in females is a rare entity, and urethral stricture makes up only a small component of this diagnosis. The incidence of true urethral stricture in women has been estimated to be 0.1–1%[1] of the population. Female urethral stricture is typically iatrogenic from inappropriate urethral dilations or traumatic catheterization, urethral surgeries, pelvic radiation, trauma (pelvic fracture) or chronic urethritis/cystitis leading to fibrosis. Since true urethral stricture disease is rare, little has been written about the etiology, diagnosis or treatment.

The diagnosis of urethral stricture in women is made when there are irritative and/or obstructive voiding symptoms and an inability to pass even a small catheter due to stenosis in the distal urethra.[2] Urodynamics will typically reveal high pressure with a low flow. The combination of urodynamics with fluoroscopic imaging during voiding can provide additional information about stricture location and length.[3-5] *Failure of the bladder neck and proximal urethra to open upon initiation of detrusor contraction suggests proximal bladder outlet obstruction, not a urethral stricture.* When video urodynamics or voiding cystourethrogram is nondiagnostic, cystoscopy is usually done for confirmation.[1] Cystoscopy combined with bougie à boule can help in determining the caliber of the urethra. Characteristics of strictures are apparent at cystoscopy as circumferential scars, similar to urethral strictures in men.

FEMALE URETHRAL ANATOMY

For a successful outcome, it is important to understand the female urethral anatomy. The urethra is a thin fibromuscular tube, 2–5 cm in length and is responsible for both drainage and continence. The female urethra comprises several tissue layers. The proximal two-thirds of the female urethra is lined by transitional cells that are a continuation from the urothelial lining of the bladder. In the distal urethra, the urothelial lining transitions into stratified squamous epithelial cells. The mucosa is redundant with multiple folds, which contribute to continence by acting as a seal. The musculature of the female urethra is comprised of an inner smooth layer and a striated external layer. The inner smooth layer runs longitudinally along the entire urethra. The proximal third of the external sphincter completely encircles the urethra. The middle of the external urethral sphincter covers the ventral surface of the urethra in a horse-shoe shape. The relative lack of musculature in the distal third of the female urethra allows it to act as a nozzle to direct the flow of urine.

URETHRAL DILATION AND URETHROTOMY

Urethral dilation has been used in the past to treat a variety of disorders in females with one of those being urethral strictures. This was first reported by Massey and Abrams.[6] In this study, urodynamics tests were not done on these patients and the subset of patients with true urethral stricture disease is unclear. In a more recent study, Smith et al.[7] reported on seven patients managed by initial urethral dilation to 30 F who were maintained on clean intermittent catheterization (CIC) with an 18–20 F catheter daily for 6 months. Patients reported a mean improvement in the American Urological Association (AUA) symptom score of 10.7 points. A prospective, randomized trial of 49 patients compared urethral dilation with female urethral sounds to simple CIC for the management of recurrent urethral strictures.[8] Patients who did CIC alone had better objective urinary flow rates and better subjective quality-of-life scores. This study also noted an increased frequency of urinary tract infections in patients treated with dilation alone compared to those patients doing CIC. There is no definitive clinical evidence to suggest that this procedure has any benefit in this disease. It is reasonable in selected patients with mild complaints and evidence of urethral strictures. If dilation is performed, then these patients should be maintained on self-obturation. It is unknown what the risk of stricture recurrence is after dilation. Authors feel that it is reasonable to offer someone with a true urethral stricture the option of urethral dilation. **Figure 12.1** is an example of a female with a urethral stricture, whose uroflow improved after dilation **(Fig. 12.2)**. Authors would not recommend multiple urethral dilations.

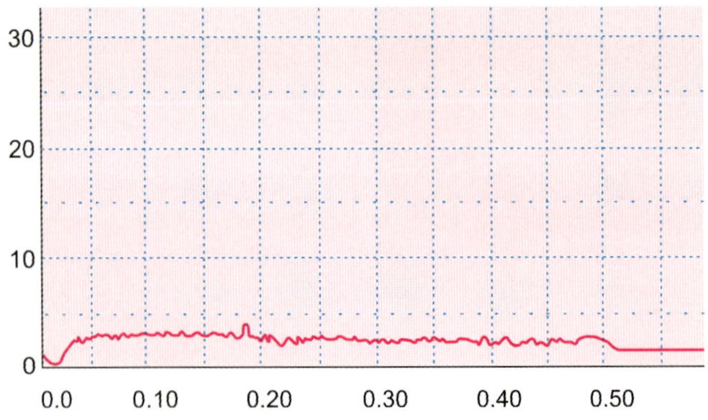

Fig. 12.1: Uroflow of a female with a urethral stricture

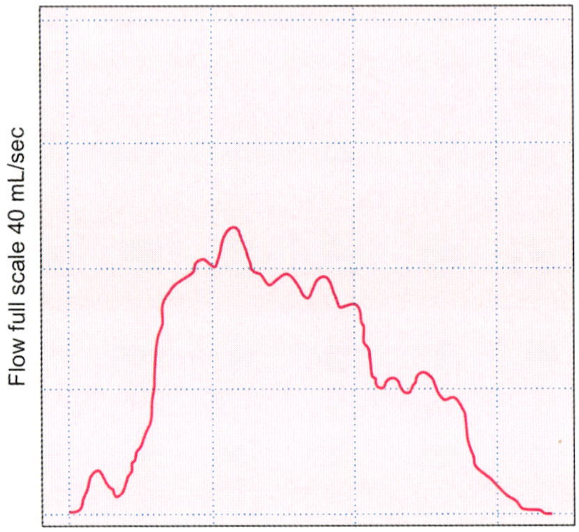

Fig. 12.2: This is the uroflow of the same patient after urethral dilation

Urethral dilation should not be performed on female patients with lower urinary tract symptoms and no evidence of a urethral stricture since this can actually cause urethral strictures. Santucci et al.[9] showed that dilating the unstrictured female urethra is still a common practice despite the unproven efficacy. The persistence of this practice is probably due to a lack of clinical guidelines and the financial reimbursement of this simple office procedure.

FEMALE URETHROPLASTY TECHNIQUES

There are no good guidelines for the management of female urethral stricture disease as there are in male stricture disease. We can extrapolate from the male data, and it is reasonable to offer open surgery to women who have failed one or more simple dilations. Women with long, fibrotic strictures would also be candidates for an open urethroplasty. Those who are unable to do intermittent self-catheterization may do better with an open repair since this may not put them at higher risk of recurrence.

The Vaginal Inlay Flap

This method was originally described, but never reported by Blandy. It has since been reported by Gormley and McGuire[10] and later updated by Gormley.[11] Twelve symptomatic women with a history of urethral stricture underwent a vaginal flap urethroplasty. Follow-up was from 3 months to 9 years. All patients had subjective relief of their symptoms and were able to catheterize with a 14 Fr catheter. No patients had stress urinary incontinence. Irritative symptoms, particularly urgency, persisted in some patients postoperatively despite having a technically good repair.

The advantage of this method is that there is no graft or flap to harvest, it is technically easy to perform and there is a lower risk of fistula formation. The largest published case series also supports this technique. The disadvantage is hypospadiac appearing meatus as a result of this repair.

The surgery is performed with the patient in the dorsal lithotomy position. A weighted vaginal speculum is placed in the vagina and a U-shaped vaginal flap is outlined with the apex at the urethral meatus. Sharp dissection is used to develop a plane between the vaginal mucosal flap and the periurethral fascia. This vaginal flap is dissected 2–3 cm proximally **(Fig. 12.3)**.

Once this is complete, a nasal speculum is inserted into the urethral meatus to visualize the stricture, and the urethra is incised from the strictured area posteriorly at the 6 o'clock position. The nasal speculum is advanced into the urethra as the incision is made to ensure that the most proximal portion of the stricture is incised. Once the stricture is finally incised, the urethra often "springs" open. Any severe scar tissue can be excised **(Fig. 12.4)**. The stricture is usually distal to the external sphincter. Due to the small risk of malignancy in any stricture, all excised tissue is typically sent to pathology **(Figs 12.3 and 12.4)**.

After the incision of the urethral stricture is completed, the flap of mobilized vaginal tissue is advanced into the defect and sutured into place. The apex of the U-shaped vaginal flap is approximated to the apex of the incision in the urethral mucosa **(Fig. 12.5)** and the edges of the vaginal flap are approximated to the urethral mucosal edges using an interrupted absorbable suture.

A 22 Fr cystoscope is passed and the urethra and bladder are inspected at the conclusion of the procedure. A 16 Fr Foley's catheter is placed **(Fig. 12.6)**.

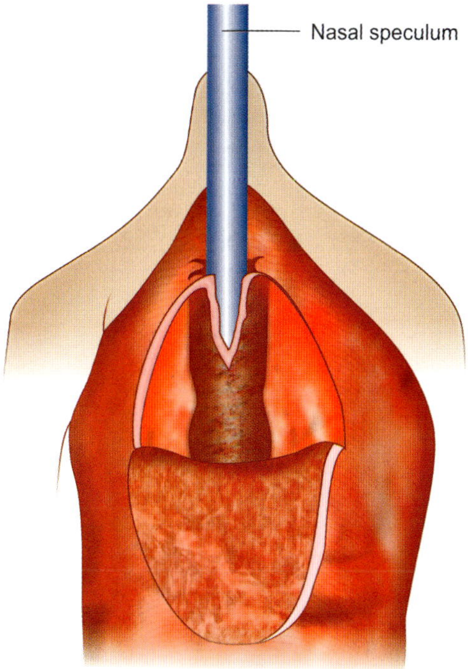

Fig. 12.3: The vaginal flap is outlined

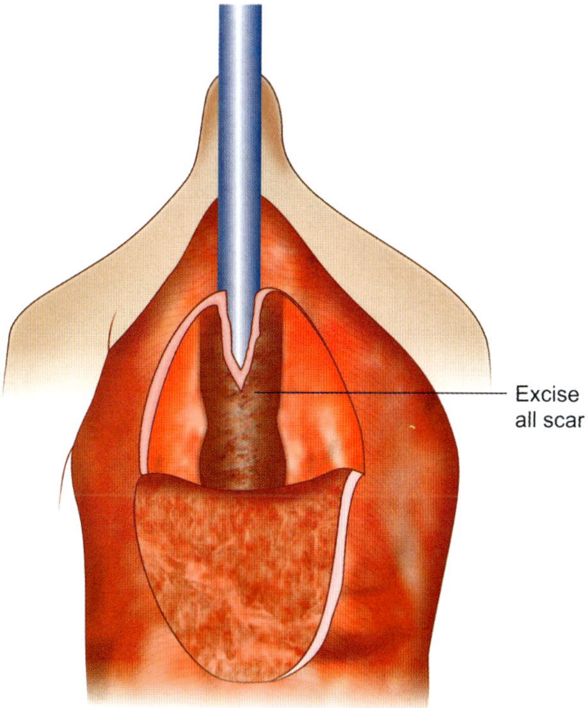

Fig. 12.4: All the scar tissue is excised

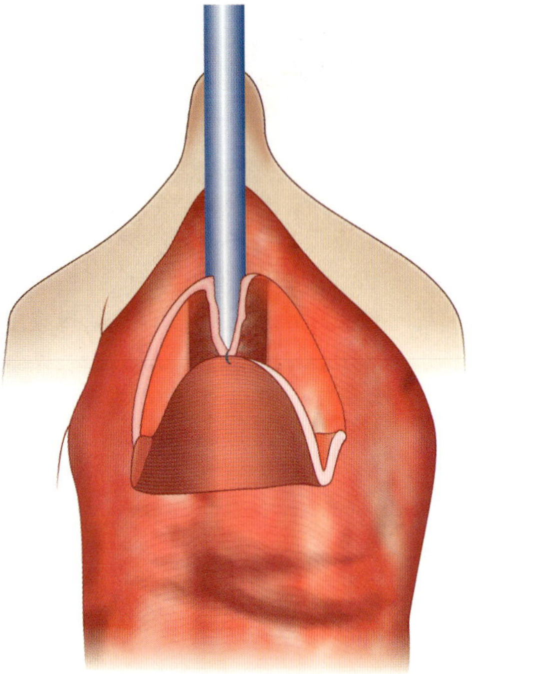

Fig. 12.5: The apex of the flap is approximated to the apex of the healthy urethra

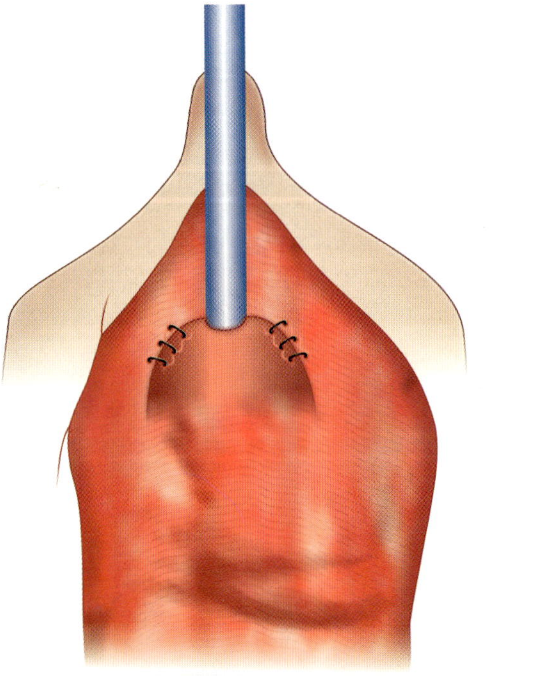

Fig. 12.6: A 16 Fr Foley's catheter is placed

There are other flap-based urethroplasty techniques described in the literature. Tanello et al.[12] described the use of a pedicle flap from the labia minora as a treatment for distal urethral strictures in two patients. This was a ventral approach, and both patients had reportedly excellent outcomes with normal micturition and resolution of the stricture on cystourethrography at 2 years. A dorsal approach using a vestibular flap with underlying muscular tissue has also been described.[13] The distal tip of the flap is anastomosed to the proximal urethral margin with the epithelial surface facing the urethral lumen. Flow rates and AUA symptom index scores improved. Two of the seventeen patients complained of persistent obstructive voiding symptoms despite an improvement in urethral caliber.

Female Urethroplasty with Buccal Mucosa

The advantages of this technique are a more normal appearance of the urethral meatus and more scar can be excised. The disadvantage is the increased risk of fistula formation and the paucity of literature supporting this technique. It is important to cover the repair with another layer of tissue.

The patient is placed in a dorsal lithotomy position. A weighted vaginal speculum is placed. The vaginal epithelium is injected with 1% lidocaine with epinephrine to assist with hydrodissection.

An inverted "U" incision is made with the apex at the external urethral meatus **(Fig. 12.7)**. Using tenotomy scissors, the plane between the vaginal epithelium and pubocervical fascia is identified. Once this is started, Metzenbaum scissors are used to complete the dissection of the vaginal flap. A nasal speculum and cystoscopy are used to identify the urethral stricture. The urethra is entered at the 6 o'clock position using a no. 15 blade **(Fig. 12.8)**.

The pubocervical fascia is dissected free from the urethra to be used later as a pedicle-based flap to cover the repair. The scar tissue is completely excised **(Fig. 12.9)**. Cystoscopy is performed to ensure that the stricture has been incised and to inspect the bladder for any other pathology. A 16 Fr Foley's catheter is placed, if this has not already been done. The buccal graft is prepared for placement. The buccal mucosal graft is 5–6 cm in length and 2–3 cm wide and then this is tailored to accommodate the urethral defect. Two 5-0 polydioxanone sutures are placed at the apex of the urethral incision in an interrupted fashion to secure the graft **(Fig. 12.10)**. A 5-0 Monocryl is used in a running fashion on either side to the distal apex.

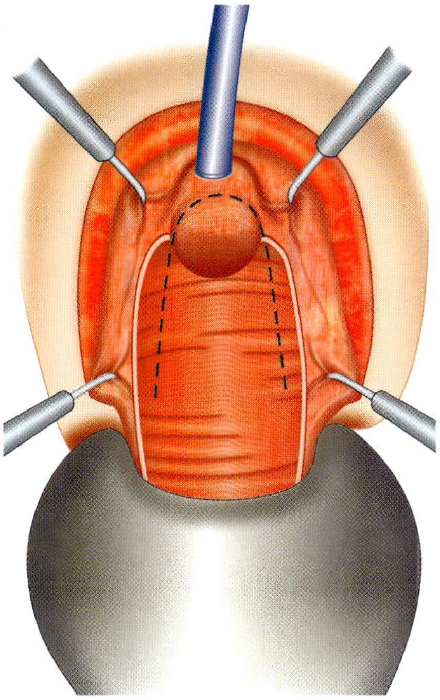

Fig. 12.7: An inverted "U" incision

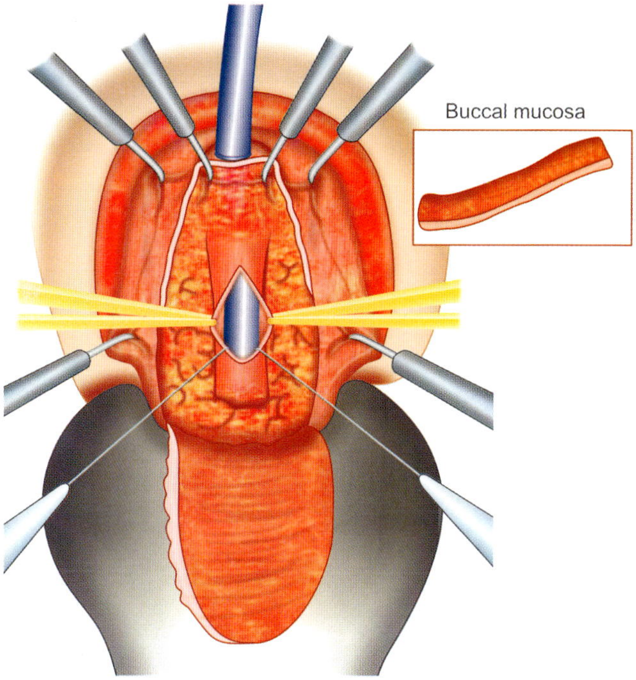

Fig. 12.9: After complete excision of the scar tissue, two stay sutures are taken

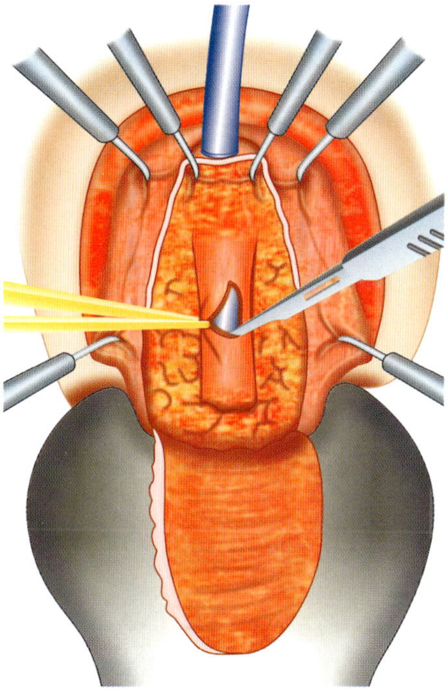

Fig. 12.8: The strictured portion of the urethra being cut by no. 15 blade

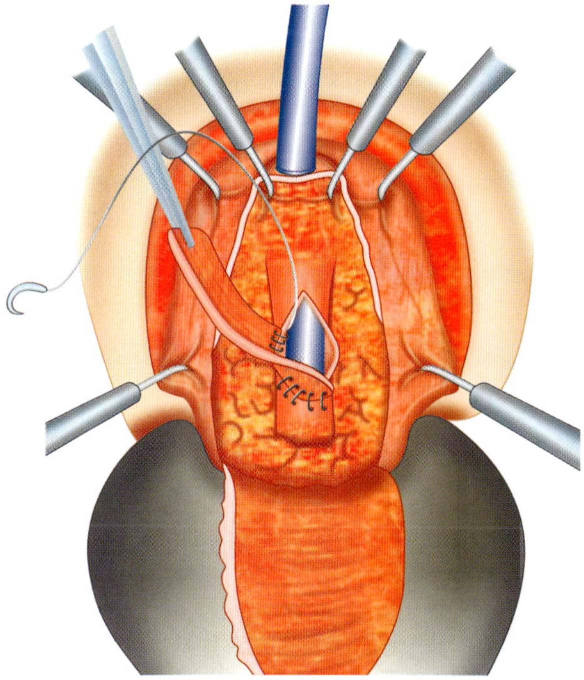

Fig. 12.10: The buccal graft being positioned at one of the apex of the urethral incision

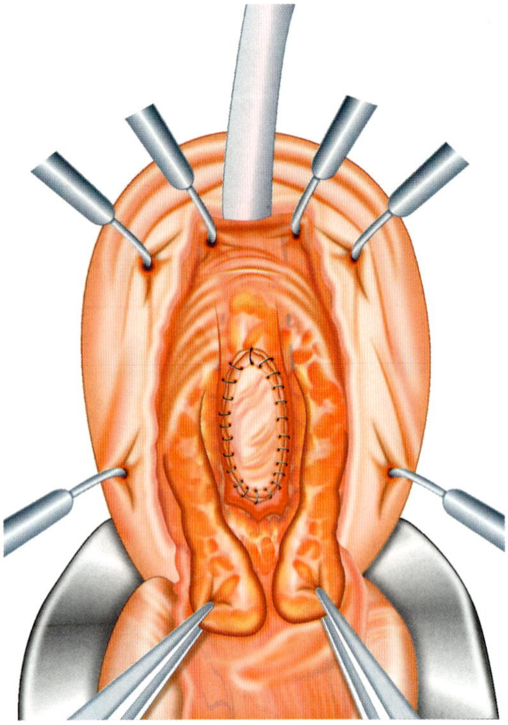

Fig. 12.11: The surrounding pubocervical fascia is identified and lifted

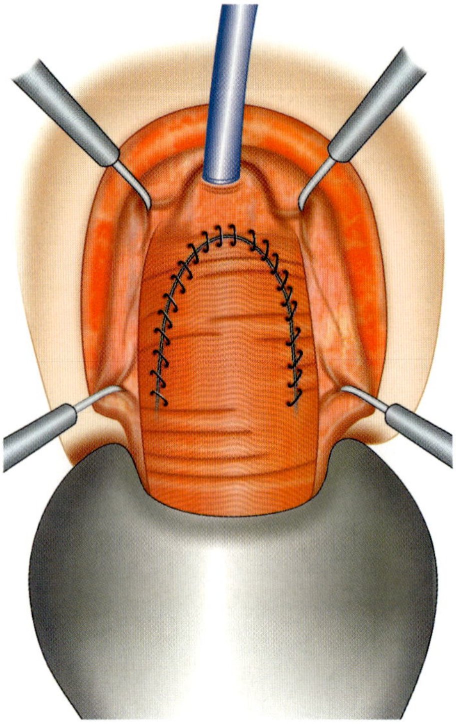

Fig. 12.12: Closure of vaginal epithelium

The pubocervical fascia is closed in a "vest-over-pants" fashion with a 4-0 Vicryl suture to give two additional layers of coverage **(Fig. 12.11)**. The vaginal epithelium is then closed in a running fashion **(Fig. 12.12)**.

Berglund et al.[14] described two patients managed with a ventral buccal mucosal graft urethroplasty. This was performed in a similar fashion to the technique described above. The urethra was exposed through a midline anterior vaginal incision. A Martius flap was used for additional coverage. One patient had complete resolution of symptoms, while the other developed a meatal stenosis distal to the graft requiring dilation.

Urethroplasty Using a Dorsal Buccal Graft

This procedure has been used to treat three patients with urethral strictures.[15] A suprameatal inverted "U" incision is made from the 3 o'clock to the 9 o'clock position. The urethra is mobilized inferiorly, developing a plane dorsally between the urethra and the overlying clitoral bodies. Following incision of the stricture, a 5 cm by 3 cm buccal graft is sutured in place to the defect and quilted to the clitoral bodies to provide structural and vascular support. The surrounding tissues are reapproximated over a catheter. In 2 years of follow-up, all three patients obtained a nonobstructive pattern on urodynamics. No significant complications occurred.

POSTOPERATIVE CARE

Instructions for the vaginal advancement flap are as follows:

After 7–10 days of catheter drainage, the catheter is removed and the patient is advised to start once daily CIC with a 14 Fr catheter. It is possible that catheterization may not be necessary, but that daily catheterization will allow the patient to know sooner, if and when the urethra begins to stricture to a caliber of less than 14 Fr. There is no data to know if less frequent catheterization would be enough, but anecdotally patients who catheterize daily seem to have fewer difficulties with it as it quickly becomes a habit. Over 3 months catheterization, interval can be lengthened and eventually discontinued.

For all urethroplasties, a vaginal pack is left in overnight, and can be removed on the morning of 1st postoperative day and the patient can be discharged for home. A voiding cystourethrogram is performed at 2–3 weeks (7–10 days for vaginal advancement flap). If this shows no extravasation and the patient can void to completion, then the Foley's catheter is removed. Antibiotics should be given around the time of catheter removal.

COMPLICATIONS

Urinary tract infections can be avoided with a negative preoperative urine culture, appropriate preoperative antibiotics and antibiotics given around the time of catheter removal. A vaginal pack overnight along with meticulous surgical dissection will help to prevent any postoperative bleeding. Urethrovaginal fistulas are rare with the vaginal advancement flap due to the fact that there are few suture lines. To prevent urethrovaginal fistulas forming in the buccal mucosal graft procedures, authors recommend nonoverlapping suture lines and a multiple-layered closure over the repair. The patient should understand that CIC may be needed in the future, if the stricture happens to recur. Stress incontinence, surprisingly, is uncommon after such extensive surgery, but it can be treated with an autologous pubovaginal sling placed at the bladder neck. Placing a synthetic, midurethral sling over the buccal graft is ill-advised and with the vaginal advancement flap, there is no anatomical midurethra. *Again, if stress urinary incontinence is to be treated in this situation, authors would recommend avoiding a synthetic midurethral sling.*

CONCLUSION

There is currently no consensus on the best female urethroplasty technique. The method chosen depends on stricture characteristics and individual surgeon's comfort with each approach. With stricture recurrence after dilation or in patients with severe stricture disease, proceeding to a urethroplasty is recommended. The techniques described in this chapter are what authors have used in the past with success. They recommend that dilation or urethrotomy can be used judiciously in women with a true urethral stricture.

EDITORIAL COMMENTS

Dr Rajesh Gulia

My teacher, the late Professor HS Bhat, used to say "the surgeons stop looking below the symphysis and gynecologist looks well below the female urethral region. Hence, it is for the urologists to look at this region and understand regarding it". His second often repeated statement regarding female urethra used to be "it is an outlet for many a problem in the ladies, so ensure that it is patent, lest you face the fallbacks of a blocked drain. The problem here is the numbers. No large numbers to evaluate and compare the outcomes of various procedures". All said and done, a subset of patients who have a urethral stricture will benefit from urethroplasty. A well done vaginal flap inlay has excellent outcomes. This is a locally available tissue and must be used to its full advantage. Also, it has no additional morbidity of harvesting a flap/graft and lower risk of fistula formation.

REFERENCES

1. Ackerman AL, Blaivas J, Anger JT. Female urethral reconstruction. Curr Bladder Dysfunct Rep. 2010;5(4):225-32.
2. Gormley EA. Vaginal flap urethroplasty for female urethral stricture disease. Neurourol Urodyn. 2010;29 (Suppl 1): S42-5.
3. Nitti VW, Tu LM, Gitlin J. Diagnosing bladder outlet obstruction in women. J Urol. 1999;161 (5):1535-40.
4. Kuo HC. Videourodynamic characteristics and lower urinary tract symptoms of female bladder outlet obstruction. Urology. 2005;66(5):1005-9.
5. Groutz A, Blaivas JG, Chaikin DC. Bladder outlet obstruction in women: definition and characteristics. Neurourol Urodyn. 2000;19(3):213-20.
6. Massey JA, Abrams PH. Obstructed voiding in the female. Br J Urol. 1988;61(1):36-9.
7. Smith AL, Ferlise VJ, Rovner ES. Female urethral strictures: successful management with long-term clean intermittent catheterization after urethral dilatation. BJU Int. 2006;98(1):96-9.
8. Ngugi PM, Kassim A. Clean intermittent catheterization in the management of urethral strictures. East Afr Med J. 2007;84(11):522-4.
9. Santucci RA, Payne CK, Anger JT, et al. Office dilation of the female urethra: a quality of care problem in the field of urology. J Urol. 2008;180(5):2068-75.
10. Schwender CE, Ng L, McGuire E, et al. Technique and results of urethroplasty for female stricture disease. J Urol. 2006;175(3):976-80.
11. Gormley EA. Vaginal flap urethroplasty for female urethral stricture disease. Neurourol Urodyn. 2010;29 (Suppl 1): S42-5.
12. Tanello M, Frego E, Simeone C, et al. Use of pedicle flap from the labia minora for the repair of female urethral strictures. Urol Int. 2002;69(2):95-8.
13. Montorsi F, Salonia A, Centemero A, et al. Vestibular flap urethroplasty for strictures of the female urethra. Impact on symptoms and flow patterns. Urol Int. 2002;69(1):12-6.
14. Berglund RK, Vasavada S, Angermeier K, et al. Buccal mucosa graft urethroplasty for recurrent stricture of female urethra. Urology. 2006;67(5):1069-71.
15. Migliari R, Leone P, Berdondini E, et al. Dorsal buccal mucosa graft urethroplasty for female urethral strictures. J Urol. 2006;176(4):1473-6.

13

CHAPTER

Stricture after Transurethral Resection of the Prostate, Radical Retropubic Prostatectomy and Radiation Therapy

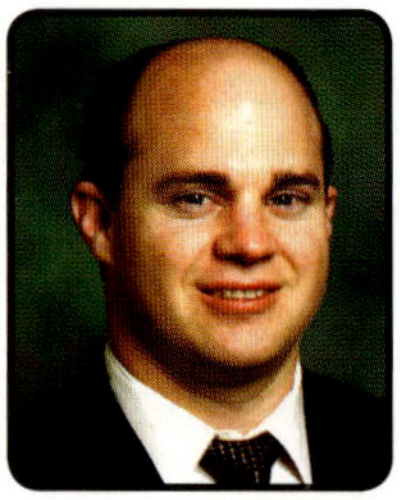

Daniel D Dugi III

Daniel D Dugi III, Allen F Morey

Chapter Outline

Abstract

With increasing use multimodality treatment for prostate carcinoma and newer techniques and modalities, such as intensity modulated radiation therapy (IMRT) and proton beam therapy, continue to be introduced with an overall trend towards increasing dose rates over the past decades, the incidence of stricture urethra in these patients seems to be on the rise. The treatment is much akin to that of pelvic fracture urethral distraction defect (PFUDD), but the results may be poorer. The reason being the naked eye cannot see the ischemia caused by obliteration of microvasculature caused by radiation therapy (RT), unlike the gross fibrosis which is both visible and palpable following PFUDD. The other bad prognostic feature is that these strictures are quite proximal involving the bulbomembranous urethra and have a significant risk of postsurgery urinary incontinence as high as 40% in one series and patients must be counseled accordingly. Strictures following RRP are more difficult to treat. These require extensive mobilization and superior pubectomy.

Keywords

External beam radiation therapy, Brachytherapy, IMRT, Proton beam therapy, Disordered collagen deposition, Dysfunctional fibroblasts, Microvascular obliteration, Postsurgery urinary incontinence, Urethral rest, Capped suprapubic catheter, Moderate lithotomy position, Spongiofibrosis, Radioactive seed, Type I, II, and III strictures, Bladder neck contracture, Reconstructive ladder, Anterior bladder flap, Superior pubectomy, Vesicourethroplasty, Omental flap.

INTRODUCTION

Urethral strictures that develop after treatment of prostate disease are a heterogeneous group of problems. The prostate may be present or absent, and the stricture may result from postsurgical scarring or radiation damage. These strictures are difficult to treat due to their typical location deep in the pelvis near the membranous urethra, and treatment involves the risk of urinary incontinence. In contrast to strictures of the anterior urethra or postpelvic fracture urethral injuries, endoscopic procedures play a prominent role in treatment of urethral stenosis after prostate therapy.

STRICTURE AFTER RADIATION THERAPY FOR PROSTATE CANCER

Radiation therapy for prostate cancer may be administered as external beam radiation therapy, brachytherapy or a combination of both. Newer techniques and modalities,

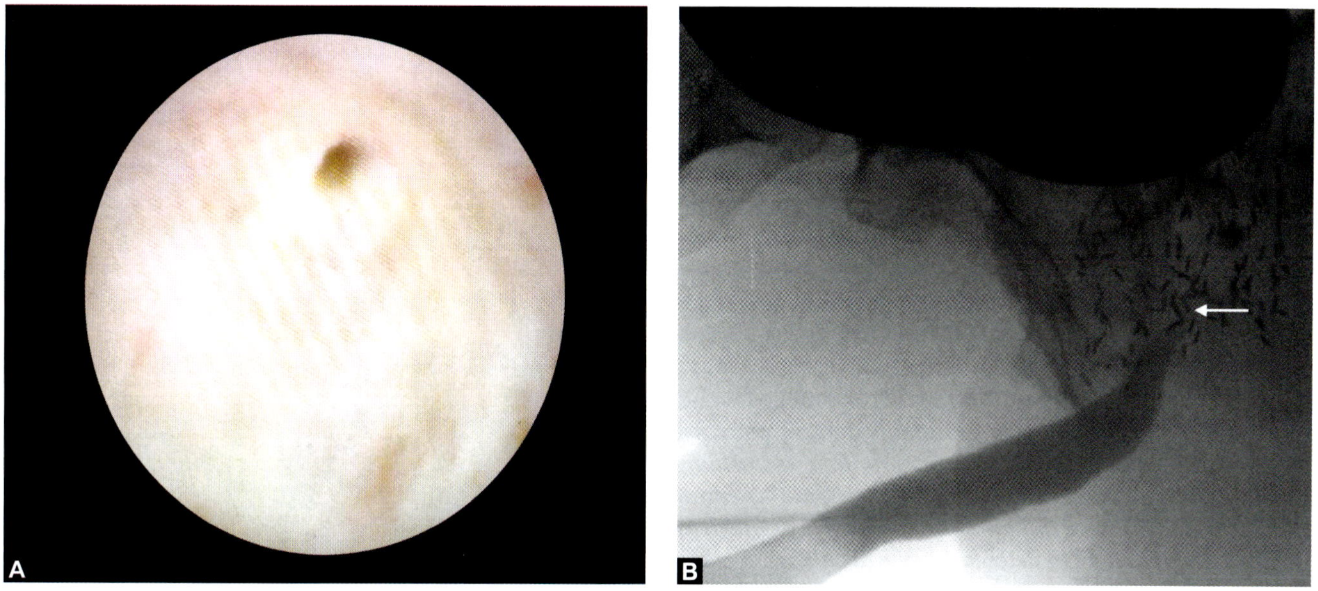

Figs 13.1A and B: Bulbomembranous urethral stricture after brachytherapy. (A) Endoscopic view of the stricture. Note blanched appearance of irradiated tissue; (B) Retrograde urethrogram. Brachytherapy seeds extend distal to the membranous urethra (arrow)

such as intensity modulated radiation therapy (IMRT) and proton beam therapy, continue to be introduced with an overall trend toward increasing dose rates over the past decades. Large database studies have found a stricture rate of less than 2% for external beam or brachytherapy as monotherapy and approximately 5% for combined therapy.[1] Studies of high dose radiation therapy suggest a much higher 10–12% stricture rate for combined therapy.[2,3] At this time, modalities such as cryotherapy and high-frequency focused ultrasound have not been reported in sufficient numbers to confidently assess their stricture rate.

Strictures occur most frequently in the bulbomembranous urethra **(Figs 13.1A and B)**, with strictures of the bladder neck or within the prostatic urethra being less common.[2] Independent risk factors for stricture formation include prior transurethral resection of prostate, higher dose rate administration and a higher calculated dose to the membranous urethra.[2,3] While the precise mechanisms leading to urethral stricture are not fully known, they may include injury to urethral epithelium inciting an inflammatory response, disordered collagen deposition by dysfunctional fibroblasts[4] and microvascular obliteration with tissue ischemia leading to fibrosis.[5]

Urethroplasty for radiation-induced strictures has a lower reported success rate than nonradiation strictures.[6] This is most likely because the area of tissue damage includes all the tissue proximal to the stricture, and radiation damage has diminished the tissue's potential for healing after surgery. Much like strictures of the anterior urethra and postpelvic fracture urethral disruption, stricture dilation or internal urethrotomy are palliative measures for those patients who are unable or unwilling to undergo urethroplasty.

Treatment of strictures involving the bulbomembranous urethra have a significant risk of postsurgery urinary incontinence, 40% in one series,[6] and patients must be told to expect this risk before surgery. Surgery to address urinary incontinence after urethroplasty, e.g. artificial urinary sphincter (AUS) placement, must be staged several months later to allow tissue revascularization.

URETHROPLASTY FOR RADIATION-INDUCED STRICTURES OF THE BULBOMEMBRANOUS URETHRA

Urethroplasty for radiation-induced strictures requires consideration of the effects of radiation on surrounding tissue. The membranous urethra and surrounding tissue have poor vascularity and reduced healing capacity due to the radiation injury. Excision and anastomotic urethroplasty should be the primary goal as it removes avascular, scarred urethra and brings in viable, better vascularized distal urethra to the anastomosis. Genital skin flaps are generally not necessary. Free grafts of skin or buccal mucosa may have decreased success due to poor

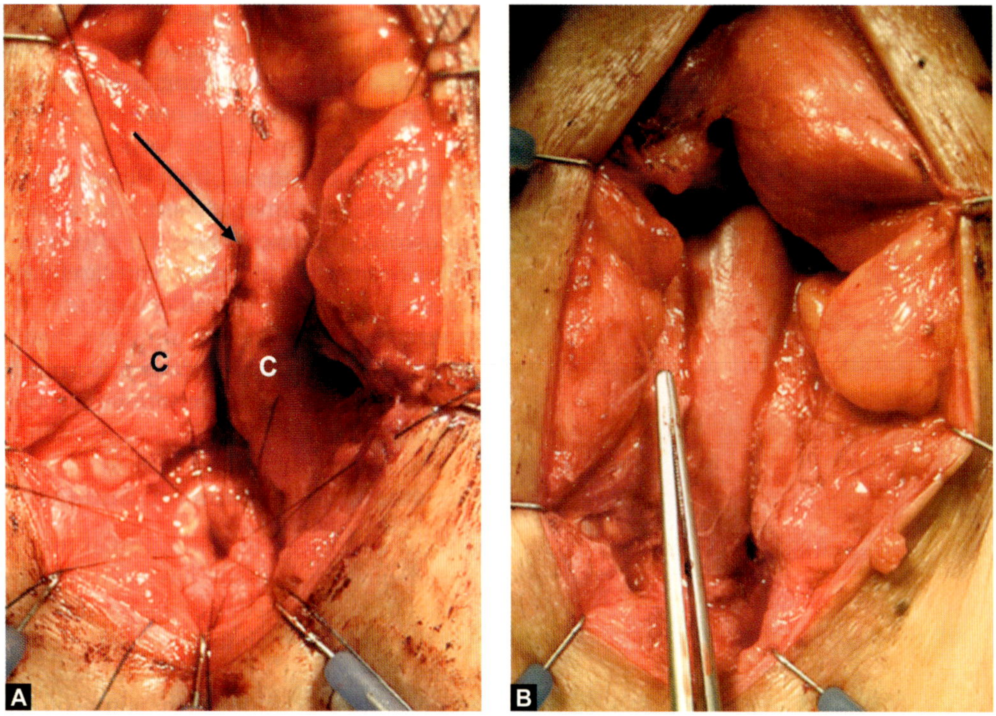

Figs 13.5A and B: (A) Anastomotic sutures are preplaced in the proximal urethral margin, clamped and numbered according to their position as if on the face of a clock. Note that the corporal bodies "C" have been separated to the level of the arrow in order to shorten the distance to the anastomosis; (B) Bulbospongiosum after completion of anastomosis. Forceps demonstrates position of corpora after corporal splitting. The two corporal bodies are split in midline and distal urethra is seen to pass between them

proximal urethra once the proximal 6 o'clock suture has been placed. Placing the catheter, after more sutures have been placed, increase the risk of tangling the catheter in the sutures.

After all anastomotic sutures are placed, begin tying down the sutures, beginning at the 12 o'clock position and moving either clockwise or counterclockwise. The assistant should use forceps to hold the distal urethra down to the anastomosis while the first sutures are being tied to take tension off the sutures and insure mucosa-mucosal approximation.

Closure

Close the wound in layers with absorbable suture. Authors have not found drains to be necessary. They retain the capped suprapubic tube for 5 weeks and it is removed 1 week after Foley's catheter removal after normal voiding is assured.

Follow-up

Authors prefer to leave the catheter anchored to the abdomen securely for 4 weeks as healing potential of radiated tissue is diminished. A voiding cystourethrogram is performed at the time of catheter removal to insure that there is no extravasation of urine. Follow-up is done at 3 months after the catheter is removed. Measurement of uroflow and postvoid residual urine volume may help in follow-up of urethral patency.

Continence

If the patient is incontinent of urine after urethroplasty, placement of an AUS may be considered. Artificial urinary sphincter placement should be delayed at least 6 months to allow for collateral circulation to develop, and transcorporal placement of the AUS cuff may be prudent.[10]

STRICTURE AFTER TREATMENT FOR BENIGN PROSTATIC DISEASE

Surgical treatment for prostatic obstruction of the bladder outlet removes the obstructing prostatic tissue. Endoscopic treatment is most common and uses an energy source, such as monopolar or bipolar electric current or laser energy, to resect or ablate prostatic tissue. This may result in a circumferential or near-circumferential surgical wound within the prostate fossa and bladder neck. The natural healing process leads to wound contraction, and in some cases, this may cause clinically significant stenosis of the urethral lumen.

Strictures of the prostate have been categorized as Types I–III by location and inciting insult.[11] Type I strictures are frequently referred to as bladder neck contractures as they involve circumferential contraction of hypertrophic circular fibers at the bladder neck as it joins the prostate. Bladder neck contractures have been reported in up to 9.7% of patients undergoing transurethral resection of the prostate, *with higher rates among patients who had prostate adenoma weights less than 30 g*,[12] while it has been reported after laser prostate enucleation in 6% at long-term follow-up.[13] Types II and III strictures involve the midprostate fossa or entire prostatic urethra, respectively, and typically result from complications of simple prostatectomy.

Treatment for strictures following surgery for benign prostate disease is first focused on endoscopic therapy. The principle of a "reconstructive ladder" is often used, beginning with less invasive therapies and progressing into more invasive treatments if initial treatments fail. This may begin with simple stricture dilation, followed by transurethral incision or resection of the stricture. Up to 58% of patients may respond to the initial treatment.[14] In strictures after benign prostate treatment also, surgeons have attempted to manipulate the healing process by injecting steroids or other medications into the stricture at the time of incision.[2,3]

The hope of any treatment to incise a stricture is to disrupt the circumferential scar tissue and allow for healing with less contraction. Although, transurethral incision of anterior urethral strictures is rarely successful,[15] the surrounding tissue at the bladder neck is much more robust, allowing aggressive incision through the scar down to healthy tissue in more than one location. Also, the morbidity of open surgery for these types of strictures is much greater than urethroplasty for anterior urethral strictures, so a higher chance of failure of endoscopic management is acceptable. Yet some men will not have a durable response to endoscopic treatment. Open surgical management is a good option for those men who have not had radiation tissue damage and have otherwise healthy lower urinary tracts.

OPEN SURGERY FOR BLADDER NECK CONTRACTURE: ANTERIOR BLADDER FLAP

Due to the morbidity of open surgery, the patient considering this approach has typically failed multiple endoscopic attempts at treatment. Since the stricture most oftenly involves the bladder neck and not the membranous urethra, the risk of incontinence as a result of reconstructive surgery is low. Authors use a rotational random bladder flap to span the stenotic area. They prefer to use this as an anterior onlay with the anterior bladder neck and prostate divided to allow flap insertion. This is a highly variable problem requiring flexibility and creativity from the surgeon.

Patient Positioning

The patient is placed in the supine position with the umbilicus at the break in the table, which is gently flexed. Hair is removed from the lower abdomen and genitals, and the penis is prepped into the field. Patients typically have a suprapubic catheter, so remove this prior to skin preparation and replace the catheter on the field.

Exposure

A midline incision is made from inferior to the umbilicus to the pubic symphysis. The abdominal fascia is incised and the space of Retzius exposed and developed bilaterally. A self-retaining retractor (i.e. Bookwalter) is placed. Fat is swept away from the prostate and anterior bladder for better visualization. There may be extensive inflammation near the bladder neck from prior aggressive endoscopic incisions. If greater exposure is needed, a superior pubectomy may be performed (see under "Vesicourethroplasty after Radical Prostatectomy" for description).

Bladder Flap Development

Fill the bladder with antibiotic irrigation via the suprapubic catheter or a small urethral catheter. Flexible urethroscopy is performed to place a wire and then an open-ended catheter across the bladder neck contracture to aid in identifying the urethral lumen. Mobilize the bladder from surrounding anterior attachments, which is necessary to advance the bladder flap across the stenotic bladder neck and close the bladder incisions.

An anterior bladder incision is made down through the bladder neck, completely incising the anterior prostate into the stenotic urethral lumen, until a normal caliber lumen is encountered. This allows direct visualization of the ureteral orifices and location of the bladder neck. A small wedge of fibrotic tissue may be removed anteriorly if necessary. Complete the incision of the bladder flap. Inspect the tip and excise any fibrotic tissue resulting from prior endoscopic therapies.

Mark the planned incision for the laterally-based bladder flap, with its tip at the bladder neck (**Figs 13.6A to C**). We use a flap 3 cm wide to allow for partial tubularization.

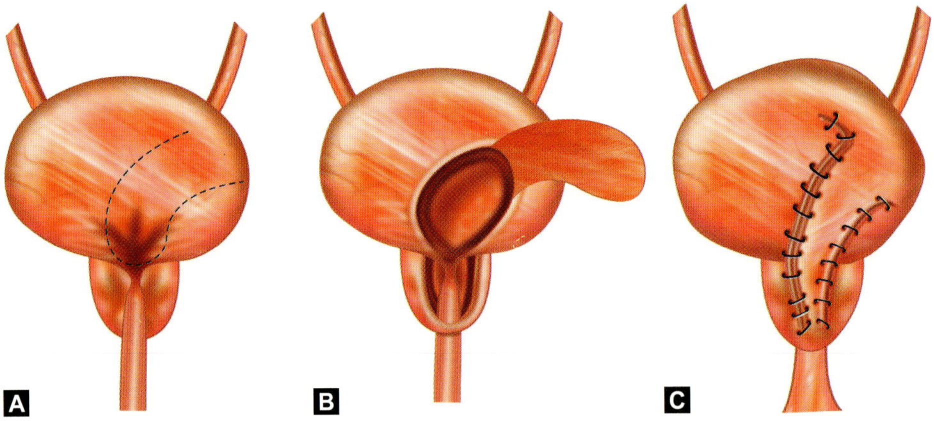

Figs 13.6A to C: (A) Outline of urethral lumen seen below the bladder neck. Dashed line shows markings for the laterally-based bladder flap. The tip is based at the bladder neck; (B) Bladder flap has been developed and an incision carried through the stenosis and distally through the prostate into normal caliber urethral lumen; (C) The bladder flap is advanced and sewn across the bladder neck

The length-to-width ratio of the flap should not exceed 3:1, which is the maximal ratio for adequate blood supply to a random flap. Stay sutures along the lines of the flap may help in later dissection.

Inset of Flap and Closure

Mobilization of the bladder should allow the flap to easily be advanced across the bladder neck. Preplacing traction sutures through the surrounding tissues of the bladder neck is helpful in a tight working space. The bladder flap is rotated distally and sewn into position anteriorly using 3-0 or 4-0 absorbable suture. Place knots outside the lumen.

Place an 18 F catheter across the anastomosis, but wait to inflate the balloon until the bladder has been closed to avoid damaging the balloon. Once the distal flap has been inset with a few interrupted sutures, it is usually easy to close the rest of the bladder with running suture. Test the anastomosis for leakage by filling the bladder with saline. Leave a 19 F round (Blake) drain in the retropubic space away from the anastomosis and close the wound.

Follow-up

We leave both a urethral catheter and suprapubic catheter for at least 4 weeks. We perform a voiding cystourethrogram to assure no extravasation **(Fig. 13.7)**. After the patient voids well for the next 2 weeks, the suprapubic catheter is removed.

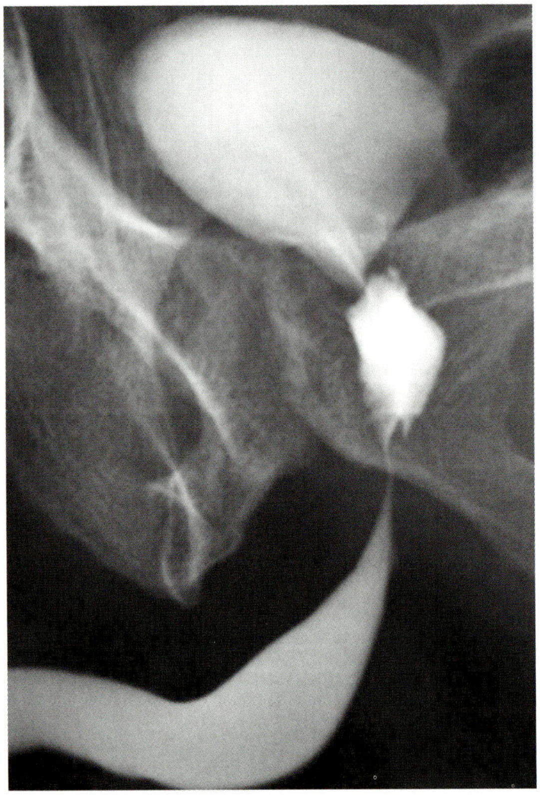

Fig. 13.7: Urethrogram after superior pubectomy and anterior bladder flap to treat resistant bladder neck contracture after simple prostatectomy. Note the wide open bladder neck

STRICTURE AFTER RADICAL PROSTATECTOMY

Anastomotic strictures after radical prostatectomy are reported in 0.5–17.5% of men after open prostatectomy and 0–3% after laparoscopic or robotic prostatectomy;[16] *these are also referred to as bladder neck contractures.* These strictures are distinctly different from the rare cases of stenosis after anastomotic disruptions **(Fig. 13.8)**, which are conceptually similar to pelvic fracture urethral disruption injuries.

Multiple factors may predispose a patient toward developing a bladder neck contracture, including an overly-narrowed bladder neck reconstruction at the time of prostatectomy, postoperative bleeding, cigarette smoking and radiation therapy.[14,17,18] Ischemia may play a role as well, as there is diminished blood flow to the membranous urethra after prostatectomy even in patients without strictures.[19]

As discussed above in strictures after treatment for benign disease, initial therapy for bladder neck contractures is focused on endoscopic therapy. This often begins with simple dilation and then progresses into endoscopic incision or resection. Treatment of recalcitrant recurrent stenosis by permanent urethral stent placement (i.e. urolume) has been advocated as an acceptable option in refractory cases,[20] although authors have found that urolume placement frequently complicates management due to tissue ingrowth and collateral damage to normal surrounding urethra.

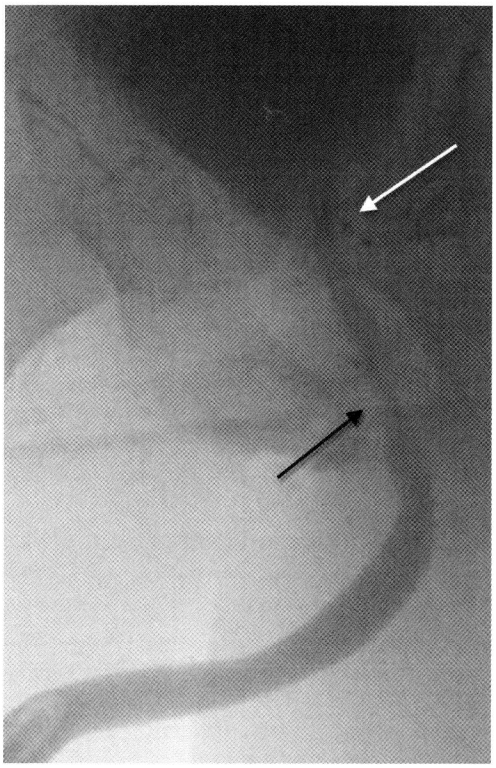

Fig. 13.8: Defect in urethral continuity due to disruption of vesicourethral anastomosis after radical prostatectomy. This patient was managed by indwelling catheter for 2 years prior to referral for reconstruction. Note distraction defect between bladder neck (white arrow) and membranous urethra (black arrow)

Open surgery should be reserved for patients who have failed multiple endoscopic treatments. Vesicourethroplasty is one of the several options to consider, with one series reports primary success of 60% with almost all patients with recurrent stenosis successfully managed endoscopically.[21] Because of the proximity of the stricture to the membranous urethra or its involvement with the stricture, patients must expect urinary incontinence after open reconstruction. This can be treated in a staged fashion several months later by AUS placement. Erectile function is usually already compromised in these patients, but remaining erectile function will likely to be lost after this extensive surgery. *Vesicourethroplasty must, therefore, be reserved for the well-counseled and highly motivated patient. For some men, a better option may be a continent catheterizable channel with or without bladder augmentation or another form of urinary diversion.*

Several factors make open surgery for vesicourethral anastomotic strictures both technically difficult and morbid surgery. Surgical access to the stricture is one of the greatest challenge. The bladder neck and membranous urethra are perhaps the hardest structures to access from an abdominal approach as they are at the pelvic outlet and behind the pubic symphysis. After prostatectomy, all the anterior tissues and the posterior bladder neck have been mobilized and can be expected to be densely adherent to surrounding tissue. In order to excise the scarred tissue and making a tension-free anastomosis, both the bladder base and urethra must be mobilized, suggesting an abdominoperineal approach with partial or complete resection of the pubic symphysis. From the perineum, the target area is also quite deep with the pelvic inlet limiting access to the bladder neck, although some advocate a strictly perineal approach.[22]

The pubic symphysis is important in rotational stability of the pelvis, especially with ambulation. Additionally, the pubis is the site of attachment of the rectus abdominis muscle as well as several muscles from the lower extremity **(Fig. 13.9)**. Complete pubectomy has been used in difficult urethroplasty for many years;[23] however, this leads to increased stress on the sacroiliac joint and may cause late posterior pelvic instability and pain.[24] *Authors*

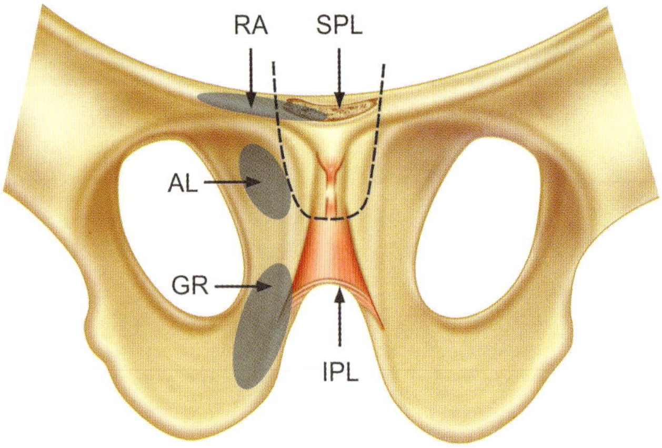

Fig. 13.9: Ligaments and muscular attachments are pertinent to the superior pubectomy. Dotted line indicates area of resection of pubis (RA: Rectus abdominis; AL: Adductor longus; GR: Gracilis; SPL: Superior pubic ligament; IPL: Inferior pubic ligament)

prefer superior pulpectomy when possible as this leaves the important inferior pubic ligament to maintain anterior pelvic stability.[25]

VESICOURETHROPLASTY AFTER RADICAL PROSTATECTOMY

Coordination and Patient Positioning

Authors prefer an abdominoperineal approach with a two team approach to expedite the surgery. One team works with the abdominal approach, while simultaneously, another team performs the perineal dissection and urethral mobilization. The patient is placed in a moderate lithotomy position with adjustable stirrups so that the legs can be repositioned throughout the case.

Abdominal Approach

A midline incision is made from inferior to umbilicus to base of the penis to expose the superior pubic symphysis. The rectus fascia is divided in the midline. A self-retaining retractor should be placed. An Omni-Flex retractor **(Fig. 13.10)** with its point of fixation over the upper abdomen and the open end toward the feet will minimize interference with the perineal field. The bladder will likely to be adherent to surrounding structures as the space of Retzius will have already been dissected during the initial prostatectomy. Carefully mobilize the bladder into the pelvis. Sometimes, the best plan for dissection will leave the anterior pelvic periosteum on the bladder. Sharply dissect the bladder neck as far distally as possible until the urethra has been mobilized from the perineal approach. This dissection is painstaking and difficult due to postsurgical fibrosis. It is critical to conduct the dissection in close proximity to the pubis to prevent soft tissue injury.

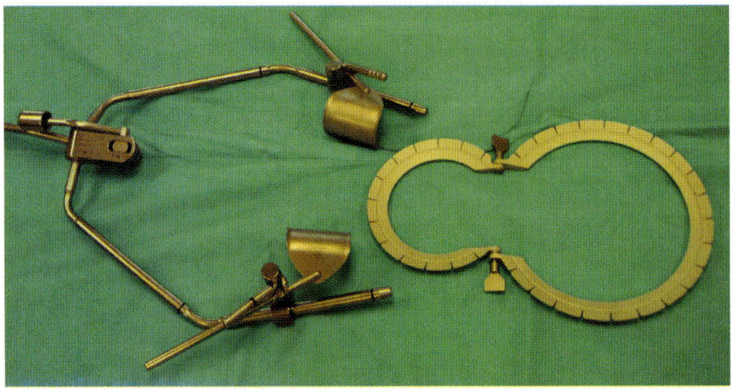

Fig. 13.10: Omni-Flex retractor (left) is open at the bottom, which allows for minimal conflict with the perineal Lone star retractor (right)

Perineal Approach

A midline incision is made in the perineum for standard urethral exposure. The bulbar urethra is mobilized to the level of stenosis at the membranous urethra. The urethra is transected as close to the level of stenosis as possible, ideally within the stenosis. The distal segment of the stricture is resected until healthy urethra is reached, which should easily accept a 28 F probe.

Superior Pubectomy

Extend the midline incision to allow exposure of the pubic symphysis. Detach the medial attachments of the rectus abdominis from the symphysis as far laterally as necessary to allow resection of a 2–3 cm section of superior portion of the pubic symphysis **(Fig. 13.11)**. The bone segment to be removed should first be free from all surrounding tissue. An osteotome and mallet is the simplest method for bone excision, although an oscillating saw is faster. Hemostasis should be obtained with electrocautery or absorbable hemostatic agents; bone wax is useful but may cause a foreign body reaction.[26]

Continue to dissect under lower edge of the symphysis, hugging the bone during sharp dissection, until the perineal space is encountered. Spreading scissors forcefully under the symphysis will drop the periurethral tissues down and allow passage of the amputated bulbar urethra up to the retropubic area, where the anastomosis can then be easily performed under direct vision. Additional bone may be resected, if necessary, to facilitate creating the anastomosis.

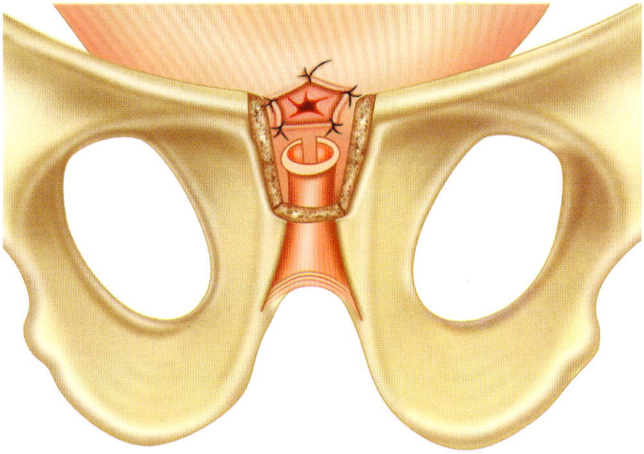

Fig. 13.11: Pubis after superior symphysectomy showing bladder mucosa eversion prior to urethral anastomosis

Urethral Anastomosis

The anastomosis between the distal urethra and bladder is done under direct vision. Authors prefer 4-0 synthetic absorbable suture (i.e. PDS) in interrupted sutures. Sutures may be placed through both the proximal side and distal side, then clamped to be tied once all sutures have been placed.

Closure

If available, an omental flap may be used to cover anastomosis and close the dead space left by the partial pubectomy. A 19 F round (Blake) drain is left in the perivesical space. The abdominal and perineal wounds are closed in routine fashion.

Follow-up

The catheter is left in place for 4–6 weeks, and a voiding cystourethrogram is performed upon catheter removal to rule out urine extravasation. The patient should return to check for urethral patency at 3 months and 6 months by cystoscopy. If the urethra remains patent at 6 months, the patient may proceed to placement of an AUS;[22] again, a transcorporal approach should be considered due to the increased risk of urethral erosion after urethroplasty.[10]

REFERENCES

1. Damico CF, Mebust WK, Valk WL, et al. Triamcinolone: adjuvant therapy for vesical neck contractures. J Urol. 1973;110(2):203-4.
2. Vanni AJ, Zinman LN, Buckley JC. Radial urethrotomy and intralesional mitomycin C for the management of recurrent bladder neck contractures. J Urol. 2011;186(1):156-60.
3. Eltahawy E, Gur U, Virasoro R, et al. Management of recurrent anastomotic stenosis following radical prostatectomy using holmium laser and steroid injection. BJU Int. 2008;102(7):796-8.
4. Dormand EL, Banwell PE, Goodacre TE. Radiotherapy and wound healing. Int Wound J. 2005;2(2):112-27.
5. Yarnold J, Brotons MC. Pathogenetic mechanisms in radiation fibrosis. Radiother Oncol. 2010;97(1):149-61.
6. Meeks JJ, Brandes SB, Morey AF, et al. Urethroplasty for radiotherapy induced bulbomembranous strictures: a multi-institutional experience. J Urol. 2011;185(5):1761-5.
7. Hussain M, Lal M, Askari SH, et al. Holmium laser urethrotomy for treatment of traumatic stricture urethra: a review of 78 patients. J Pak Med Assoc. 2010;60(10):829-32.
8. Jin T, Li H, Jiang LH, et al. Safety and efficacy of laser and cold knife urethrotomy for urethral stricture. Chin Med J (Engl). 2010;123(12):1589-95.
9. Terlecki RP, Steele MC, Valadez C, et al. Urethral rest: role and rationale in preparation for anterior urethroplasty. Urology. 2011;77(6):1477-81.
10. Aaronson DS, Elliott SP, McAninch JW. Transcorporal artificial urinary sphincter placement for incontinence in high-risk patients after treatment of prostate cancer. Urology. 2008;72(4):825-7.
11. Pansadoro V, Emiliozzi P. Iatrogenic prostatic urethral strictures: classification and endoscopic treatment. Urology. 1999;53(4):784-9.
12. Lee YH, Chiu AW, Huang JK. Comprehensive study of bladder neck contracture after transurethral resection of prostate. Urology. 2005;65(3):498-503.
13. Krambeck AE, Handa SE, Lingeman JE. Experience with more than 1,000 holmium laser prostate enucleations for benign prostatic hyperplasia. J Urol. 2010;183(3):1105-9.
14. Borboroglu PG, Sands JP, Roberts JL, et al. Risk factors for vesicourethral anastomotic stricture after radical prostatectomy. Urology. 2000;56(1):96-100.
15. Santucci R, Eisenberg L. Urethrotomy has a much lower success rate than previously reported. J Urol. 2010;183(5):1859-62.
16. Breyer BN, Davis CB, Cowan JE, et al. Incidence of bladder neck contracture after robot-assisted laparoscopic and open radical prostatectomy. BJU Int. 2010;106(11):1734-8.
17. Gotto GT, Yunis LH, Vora K, et al. Impact of prior prostate radiation on complications after radical prostatectomy. J Urol. 2010;184(1):136-42.
18. Huang G, Lepor H. Factors predisposing to the development of anastomotic strictures in a single-surgeon series of radical retropubic prostatectomies. BJU Int. 2006;97(2):255-8.
19. John H, Suter S, Hauri D. Effect of radical prostatectomy on urethral blood flow. Urology. 2002;59(4):566-9.

20. Elliott DS, Boone TB. Combined stent and artificial urinary sphincter for management of severe recurrent bladder neck contracture and stress incontinence after prostatectomy: a long-term evaluation. J Urol. 2001;165(2):413-5.
21. Pfalzgraf D, Beuke M, Isbarn H, et al. Open retropubic reanastomosis for highly recurrent and complex bladder neck stenosis. J Urol. 2011;186(5):1944-7.
22. Simonato A, Gregori A, Lissiani A, et al. Two-stage transperineal management of posterior urethral strictures or bladder neck contractures associated with urinary incontinence after prostate surgery and endoscopic treatment failures. Eur Urol. 2007;52(5):1499-504.
23. Pierce JM Jr. Exposure of the membranous and posterior urethra by total pubectomy. J Urol. 1962;88:256-8.
24. Moore RS Jr, Stover MD, Matta JM. Late posterior instability of the pelvis after resection of the symphysis pubis for the treatment of osteitis pubis. A report of two cases. J Bone Joint Surg Am. 1998;80(7):1043-8.
25. Grace JN, Sim FH, Shives TC, et al. Wedge resection of the symphysis pubis for the treatment of osteitis pubis. J Bone Joint Surg Am. 1989;71(3):358-64.
26. Sudmann B, Bang G, Sudmann E. Histologically verified bone wax (beeswax) granuloma after median sternotomy in 17 of 18 autopsy cases. Pathology. 2006;38(2):138-41.

CHAPTER 14

Tissue Engineering in the Management of Urethral Strictures

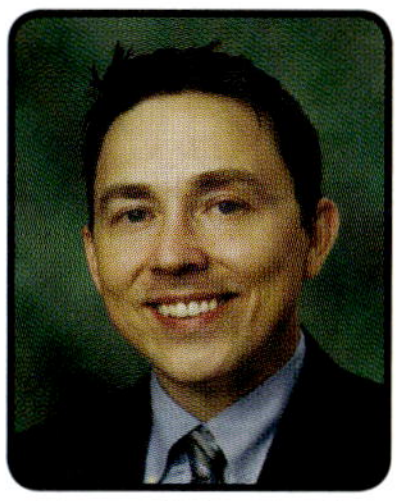

Ryan P Terlecki

Ryan P Terlecki, Anthony Atala

Chapter Outline

- Biomaterials and Wound Healing
- Choosing a Biomaterial
- Classes of Biomaterials
  - Acellular Tissue Matrices
  - Synthetic Polymers
  - Comparison of Biological and Synthetic Materials
- Synthetic Biomaterials in Urethral Reconstruction
- Natural Biomaterials in Urethral Reconstruction
  - Unseeded Matrices
  - Seeded Matrices
- Future Directions
  - Alternative Cell Sources for Scaffold Seeding
  - Cell-seeded Synthetic Materials

Abstract

This is a beautifully written chapter. A complex topic made easy. It gives an insight into what all has been tried and being tried in this field of tissue engineering. Avoiding a stricture is a race between regenerative response and inflammatory response. In urethra the additional factor to accommodate is the biomechanical stress of erection. Various biomaterials have been tried and tested. The outcomes are promising and encouraging. This chapter definitely encourages young fertile minds to go into this side of urethral research.

Keywords

Regenerative response, Inflammatory response, Collagen deposition, Fibrosis, Cell suspensions, Cell adhesion substrate, Extracellular matrix, Biomaterial, Acellular tissue matrices, Synthetic polymers, PGA, PLA, PLGA, Urine derived stem cells (USCs).

INTRODUCTION

Urethral strictures can present in a multitude of fashions, and the management strategies employed by the reconstructive urologist may be equally diverse. Research has shown that internal urethrotomy and dilation procedures rarely provide lasting success.[1] Choosing a surgical approach for definitive correction involves assessment of etiology, length, location and prior interventions. The level of experience and surgeon's preference are also critical in this process. While excision and primary anastomosis provide excellent results for strictures within the proximal bulbar urethra, many strictures may require substitution urethroplasty using flaps or grafts.[2] This is especially true in the setting of lengthy strictures associated with lichen sclerosus et atrophicus. Graft selections for complex urethroplasties have included skin as well as buccal, lingual, bladder and colonic mucosa. Regardless of the source, graft harvest undoubtedly contributes to longer operating times as well as increased morbidity. Additionally, graft materials require competent vascularity in the recipient bed as tubularized grafts have had an unacceptably high failure rate.[3,4] Recognizing these limitations, tissue engineering represents a promising strategy to advance the field of urethral reconstruction.

BIOMATERIALS AND WOUND HEALING

Following tissue injury, the body can initiate cell ingrowth from the wound edges in order to cover the defect. The cells from the edges of native tissue are able to traverse short distances without any detrimental effects, and thus smaller wounds can heal well. However, if the wound is large (more than a few millimeters in distance or depth), the body's regenerative response to injury can be overwhelmed, and an inflammatory response can take over in order to seal the wound. When this occurs, increased collagen deposition, fibrosis and scar formation ensue. In the urethra, these processes ultimately manifest as a stricture.

Various strategies have been employed to promote the healing process while impeding scarring. Direct injection of cell suspensions has been attempted in order to regenerate various tissues, but the majority of mammalian-cell types are anchorage-dependent and will die, if not provided with a cell-adhesion substrate.[5,6] Thus, injections of cell suspensions are limited as a viable strategy for improving wound healing.

Attempts to mimic the body's own tissue scaffold, the extracellular matrix (ECM), to assist with the regenerative process have proved much more successful. The ECM consists mostly of collagen, but also contains elastin, proteoglycans and glycosaminoglycans (GAGs). It functions by bringing cells together into tissue, controlling the tissue structure and regulating the cell phenotype.[7] By serving as ECM surrogates, biomaterials can elicit similar biological and mechanical functions when used in tissue engineering strategies, including localization and delivery of cells and/or bioactive factors (e.g. cell adhesion peptides, growth factors) to desired sites in the body, definition of a three-dimensional (3D) space for the formation of new tissues with appropriate structure and guidance of the development of new tissues with appropriate function.[8] Furthermore, biomaterial-based matrices implanted in wound beds can greatly increase the distances that cells can traverse without initiating an adverse fibrotic response.

CHOOSING A BIOMATERIAL

The design and selection of an appropriate biomaterial is critical in the development of engineered tissues. Generally, the biomaterial should be biocompatible, promote cellular interaction and tissue development, and possess the proper mechanical and physical properties. In addition, the material should be biodegradable and bioresorbable to support the reconstruction of a completely normal tissue without inflammation, thereby avoiding the risk of inflammatory or foreign-body responses. It is important to consider that in the urethra, as well as other areas of the urinary tract, implanted structures will be exposed to urine and may serve as a nidus for calcification.

The biomaterial should also provide temporary mechanical support, which is sufficient to withstand the various *in vivo* forces exerted by the surrounding tissue. The male urethra is unique in this respect, as it must accommodate the biomechanical stress of erection. The physical support of the biomaterial should be maintained until the engineered tissue has sufficient mechanical integrity to support itself.[9]

CLASSES OF BIOMATERIALS

Generally, two classes of biomaterials have been used for engineering of urethral tissues. The first, *acellular tissue matrices*, have been created from tissues such as bladder submucosa, small intestine submucosa (SIS), corpus spongiosum, amnion, aorta and dermis.[10-16] The second class of biomaterials used in urethral tissue engineering are the *synthetic polymers*, such as polyglycolic acid (PGA), polylactic acid (PLA) and poly (-lactic-co-glycolic acid) (PLGA). These classes of biomaterials have been tested in regard to their biocompatibility with primary human urothelial and bladder muscle cells.[17] Naturally derived materials and acellular tissue matrices have the potential advantage of biological recognition, while synthetic polymers can be reproducibly manufactured on a large scale with controlled properties of strength, degradation rate and microstructure.

Acellular Tissue Matrices

Acellular tissue matrices are collagen-rich matrices that are prepared by removing the cellular components from tissues. The matrices slowly degrade after implantation, and they are replaced and remodeled by ECM proteins synthesized and secreted by transplanted or ingrowing cells. Acellular tissue matrices have been shown to support cell ingrowth and regeneration of the urethra with no evidence of immunogenic rejection.[10,18] Since the structures of integral proteins (e.g. collagen, elastin) are well preserved, the mechanical properties of acellular matrices are not significantly different from those of native genitourinary tissues, such as bladder submucosa.[19] Additionally, these scaffolds retain other ECM features, such as growth factors, GAGs and glycoproteins, which are important for normal tissue regeneration.[20] More recently, these matrices have been seeded with wide cells from a variety of sources, such as foreskin epidermis, oral mucosa and voided urine.[21-24]

Nevertheless, collagen-based matrices also have some *inherent disadvantages*. First, although these constructs undergo a rigorous decellularization process, any retained cellular elements can stimulate an immunologic response that can lead to inflammation, fibrosis and ultimately stricture formation. Second, within a tubular construct for urethral replacement, the density of the collagen matrix that may be optimal for urothelial cell attachment and growth on the mucosal side may result in impaired muscle cell penetration on the serosal side. Additionally, there is inherent variability present in each group of matrices.[24]

Synthetic Polymers

Polyesters of naturally occurring α-hydroxy acids, including PGA, PLA and PLGA, are widely used in regenerative medicine. These polymers have gained Food and Drug Administration approval for human use in a variety of applications such as sutures.[25] The degradation products of PGA, PLA and PLGA are nontoxic, natural metabolites that are eventually eliminated from the body in the form of carbon dioxide and water.[25] Since these polymers are thermoplastics, they can be easily formed into 3D scaffolds with a desired microstructure, gross shape and specific dimensions using various techniques. To achieve the goal of having a scaffold with high porosity and a high ratio of surface area to volume, they are processed into configurations of fiber meshes and porous sponges.

The main drawback of synthetic polymers is the lack of biological recognition. As an attempt to incorporate cell recognition domains into these materials, copolymers with amino acids have been synthesized.[26-28] Other biodegradable synthetic polymers, including poly (anhydrides) and poly (ortho-esters), can also be used to fabricate scaffolds for genitourinary regenerative medicine with controlled properties.[29]

Comparison of Biological and Synthetic Materials

Studies of several biomaterials, both natural (i.e. bladder submucosa, SIS, collagen and alginate) and polymeric (i.e. PGA, PLA, PLGA and silicone), found that most did not induce significant cytotoxic effects, and cells grown on these materials exhibited normal metabolic function and cell growth *in vitro*.[17,30] In other work, Feng and colleagues compared the biomechanical properties of bladder submucosa, SIS, acellular corpus spongiosum matrix (ACSM) and PGA to rabbit urethra.[12] All the substances tested had similar Young's modulus and stress at break values compared to native tissue, with ACSM performing the best.

SYNTHETIC BIOMATERIALS IN URETHRAL RECONSTRUCTION

Various strategies have been proposed for the regeneration of urethral tissue with synthetic biomaterials. For example, woven meshes of PGA have been used to reconstruct urethras in canines. In one study, 3–4 cm of the ventral half of the urethral circumference and its adjacent corpus spongiosum were excised, and the mesh was sutured to the created defect.[31] After 2 weeks, the animals were able to void through the augmented urethra. At 2 months postreconstruction, the urothelium was completely regenerated. In addition, the mesh was completely absorbed after 3 months. No complications occurred, but the excised corpus spongiosum did not regenerate.[31]

Polyglycolic acid has also been used as a cell transplantation vehicle to engineer tubular urothelium *in vivo*. Cultured urothelial cells were seeded onto tubular PGA scaffolds and implanted into athymic mice. At 20 and 30 days polymer degradation was evident and the urothelium had formed, as evidenced by immunostaining for an urothelium-associated cytokeratin.[32] In another canine study, PGA mesh tubes coated with polyhydroxybutyric acid were used to reconstruct the urethra.[33] Eight to twelve months after reconstruction, there was complete regeneration of urothelium and adjacent connective tissue. All of the polymers disappeared within 1 year, and there were no anastomotic strictures or inflammatory reactions observed in any of the animals.[33]

Finally, while synthetic materials lack several components of natural ECM that serve as signals and anchors for overlying cells, some of these, including collagen type I and collagen type IV, can be reliably adsorbed onto some manufactured scaffolds.[34] Recent work has demonstrated that successful urethral repairs can be performed with cell-seeded PGA/PLGA scaffolds in the pediatric population.[35]

NATURAL BIOMATERIALS IN URETHRAL RECONSTRUCTION

Unseeded Matrices

Homologous free grafts of acellular urethral matrix have demonstrated excellent incorporation in a rabbit model.[36] While all tissue components were seen in the graft after 3 months, the smooth muscle was less developed and less well-oriented than native tissue. Bladder-derived acellular collagen matrix has also been extensively studied for urethral reconstruction. When applied as a ventral onlay, also in a rabbit model, results at 6 months showed a complete urothelial layer, normal appearing muscle fibers and no evidence of fibrosis.[10] Following this, Atala and colleagues used human-derived bladder acellular collagen matrix to repair urethral defects in males aged 4–20 years with a history of failed hypospadias reconstruction.[37] This was done by ventral onlay of segments ranging in size from 5 cm to 15 cm. At 3-year follow-up, three of the four patients had a successful outcome in regard to cosmetic appearance and function. The patient receiving the longest graft (15 cm) developed a subglandular fistula.[37]

Similar results have also been observed in patients with urethral stricture disease.[38] Twenty eight adults with anterior urethral strictures of multiple etiologies underwent urethral reconstruction using collagen-based inert matrix derived from human cadaveric bladder. The procedure was performed in the same manner as the previous study, with the neourethras ranging from 1.5 cm to 16 cm. At 4 months, normal-appearing urethral tissues were noted in 24 patients (85%), which included all patients with strictly bulbar strictures. The remainder of patients demonstrated minimal strictures, including 75% (three out of four) of those who originally had penobulbar strictures and 33.3% (one out of three) who had penile stricture only.

Matrix materials for urethroplasty have not been limited to genitourinary sources, as seen in the case of SIS. This material has been tested in both animals and humans. In rabbits, SIS has been successfully utilized as an onlay patch graft for urethroplasty, demonstrating better characteristics when compared to full-thickness preputial skin.[39] Comparable results have been obtained by utilizing SIS as the collagen scaffold in humans. One study involving 50 male patients treated with SIS in an onlay fashion for anterior strictures demonstrated a total success rate of 80% (40 out of 50 patients). Higher failure rates were seen in penile strictures (44.4%) versus penobulbar (16.1%) or bulbar (10%) strictures (length of defect ranged from 4 cm to 14 cm).[40] In other work, Palminteri and colleagues looked at 20 adult men with anterior strictures and performed urethroplasty, using a dorsal inlay technique in the vast majority.[11] They achieved 85% success, noting failures in penile and penobulbar stricture repairs (mean successful and unsuccessful stricture lengths were 2.6 cm and 5.7 cm, respectively).

Adequate spongiosum may be crucial to the regenerative capacity of the graft in that it may function as a robust blood reservoir for regenerating tissue, and its scarcity in the pendulous urethra, along with any concurrent ischemic fibrosis, may make that portion of the urethra poorly amenable to acellular graft repair.[11,40] Other studies have proposed an alternate explanation. El-Kassaby and colleagues randomized 30 adult patients with penile, bulbar or penobulbar strictures (length 2–18 cm) to substitution urethroplasty using either buccal mucosa or bladder acellular-matrix.[41] After 25 months follow-up period, they found that unsatisfactory outcomes tended to occur in patients with a history of more than one prior surgical intervention, irrespective of stricture location. In addition, all patients who received a buccal mucosa graft had a successful result, as opposed to only 33% of those receiving the acellular grafts. This is not surprising, since collagen scaffolds require healthy tissue in order to initiate and perpetuate the regenerative process.[41] These studies confirmed that the importance of a healthy, well-vascularized urethral bed for acellular collagen grafting cannot be overemphasized.

Seeded Matrices

It has been shown that while unseeded acellular matrix can be useful for onlay reconstruction, it is not sufficient for tubularized urethral repairs.[42] In a rabbit model, comparing replacement of the penile urethra with tubularized matrices with or without seeding of autologous bladder smooth muscle cells, all unseeded matrices developed strictures whereas none were seen in seeded cases. Gross examination of the cell-seeded urethral implants revealed normal-appearing tissue without any evidence of fibrosis. Histologically, these implanted matrices contained normal urethral tissue by 1 month, which consisted of a transitional cell layer surrounded by muscle cell fiber bundles, and the organization of the cells increased over time. Similar results have been seen, when the seeding is done with autologous foreskin epidermal cells or with oral keratinocytes.[21-23]

De-epidermized dermis seeded with *ex vivo* expanded oral keratinocytes has also been used as a graft material. After initial demonstration of the seeding process, Bhargava and colleagues implemented this technique for substitution urethroplasty in five male patients with strictures secondary to lichen sclerosis.[16,43] Although initial graft take was seen in all patients, two required either full or partial graft excision and the remainder required some form of urethral instrumentation (either dilatation or direct visual internal urethrotomy) for stricture recurrence and submeatal stenosis.

Based on the previously mentioned animal studies, cell-seeded matrices implanted as urethral replacement grafts are able to lengthen the distance over which normal tissue regeneration can occur, without initiating fibrosis. Studies in regenerative medicine have shown that very large defects (> 30 cm) can be successfully treated using cell-seeded scaffolds.[44] However, the maximum distance for normal regeneration over an unseeded scaffold, from any edge, is about 0.5 cm. This further explains the described experimental and clinical results noted with urethral repair. Unseeded matrices are able to replace urethral segments, when used in an onlay fashion, because of the short distances required for tissue in growth. However, if a longer or tubularized urethral repair is needed, the matrices need to be seeded with autologous cells in order to avoid the risk of stricture formation and poor tissue development.

FUTURE DIRECTIONS

Alternative Cell Sources for Scaffold Seeding

While fascinating research is being reported using the body as a bioreactor to grow a urethral substitute, or performing urethral transplantation with cadaveric tissue, the practicality of these approaches is severely limited.[45] The future lies in an "off-the-shelf" option for substitution urethroplasty. Several sources of cells for matrix seeding have been described in this chapter, but the process of harvesting these cells remains invasive and time-consuming. Zhang and colleagues recently demonstrated that voided urine specimens from patients contain urine-progenitor cells.[46] These cells express stem cell markers, including c-Kit, SSEA4 and CD44 and show genomic stability after serial cultures. Furthermore, they can be expanded to levels necessary for tissue engineering in a time-frame comparable to that of biopsy-derived cells (approximately 7 weeks), and the cost to obtain them is 100 times less than that of a biopsy.[46] Continued research has confirmed that these urine-progenitor cells are, in fact, stem cells (urine-derived stem cells or USCs), as they have self-renewal capability and can be stimulated to differentiate into multiple cell types.[47] In a recent study, USCs were stimulated to differentiate into urothelial cells and smooth muscle cells, and subsequently cultured in a layered fashion onto a 3D porous SIS scaffold.[24] The urothelial cells formed several layers on top of the smooth muscle cells, mimicking the histology of a normal urethra. These SIS scaffolds were then implanted into athymic nude mice without any adverse events (i.e. inflammation, extrusion). After 1 month, the urothelial and smooth muscle cells still stained for their respective markers. These studies suggest that USCs are a novel and viable source of cells for urethral tissue engineering.

Cell-seeded Synthetic Materials

Recently, a novel study has combined several aforementioned components including synthetic matrices, autologous cellular seeding and tubularized repair. Five males aged 10–14 years with urethral strictures **(Fig. 14.1)** secondary to pelvic trauma (n = 3) or failed posterior urethral repair (n = 2) were selected to undergo *ex vivo* urethral synthesis.[35] Epithelial and smooth muscle cells were obtained via bladder biopsies from these patients, and the cells were cultured and expanded *in vitro*. Next, tubularized PGA mesh **(Fig. 14.2)** was individually sized to the measured urethral defect in each patient, and it was then seeded with the autologous cells. Surgically, the stricture was completely excised and replaced with the tubularized urethral segment. Serial biopsies **(Figs 14.3A to E)** showed normal architecture, and up to 72 months later, excellent results were noted

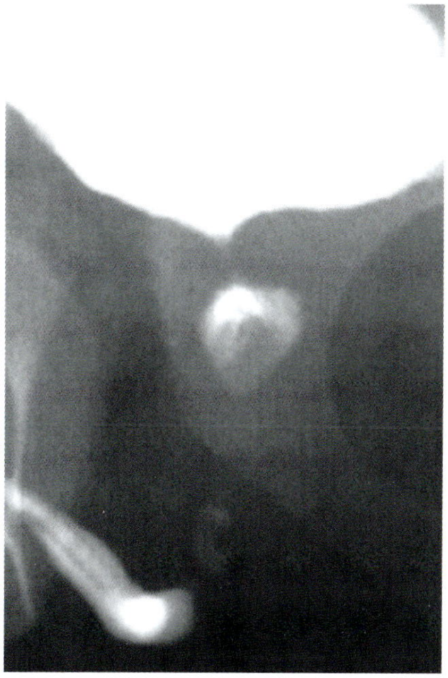

Fig. 14.1: Preoperative simultaneous retrograde urethrogram and micturating cystourethrogram of a 14-year-old patient

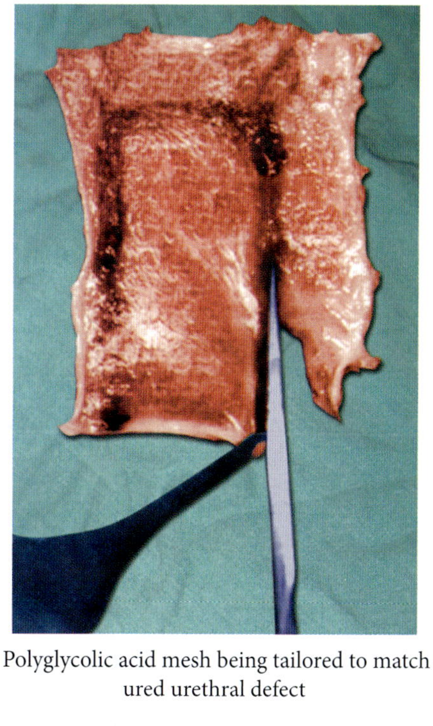

Fig. 14.2: Polyglycolic acid mesh being tailored to match the measured urethral defect

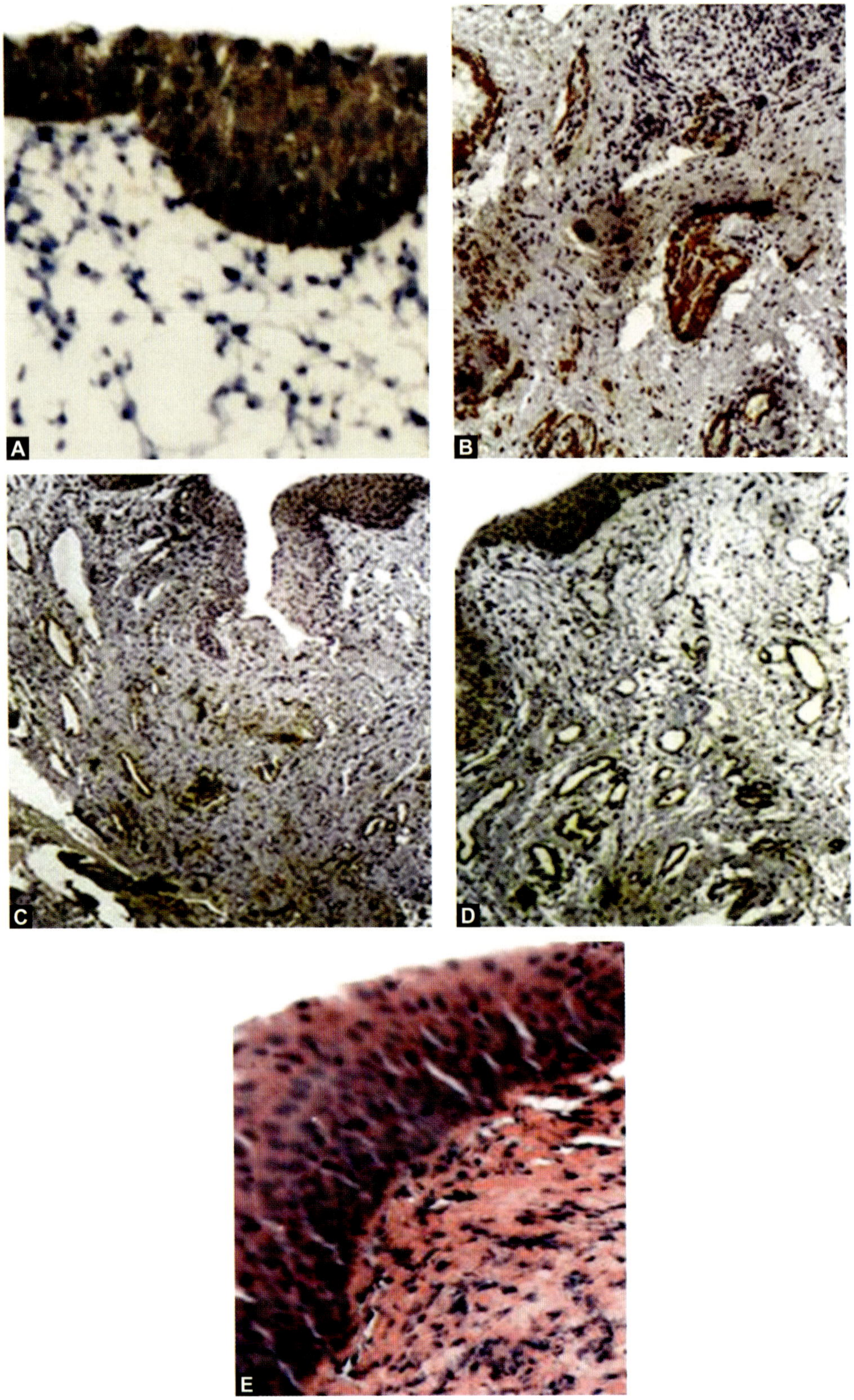

Figs 14.3A to E: Serial biopsies of engineered urethra for (A) AE1/AE3; (B) Actin; (C) Myosin; (D) Desmin; and (E) Hematoxylin and eosin

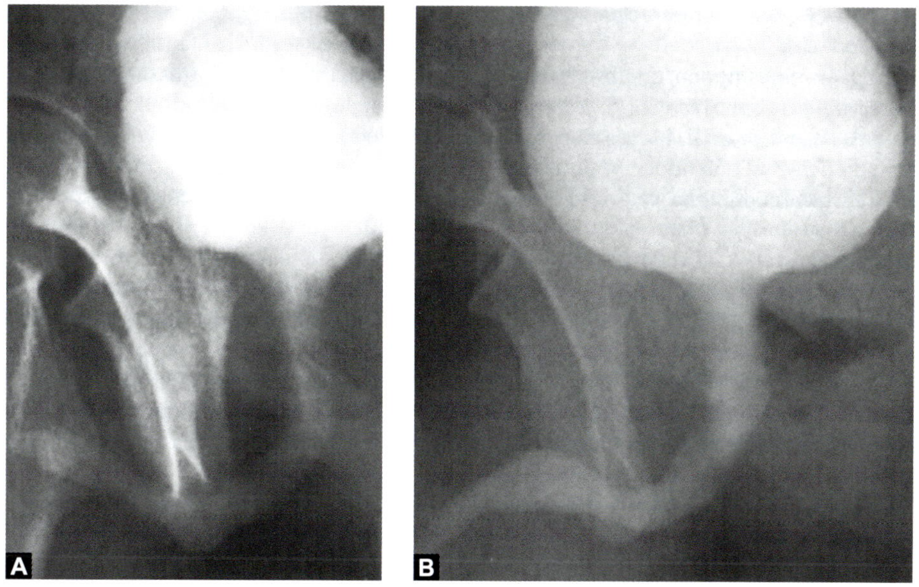

Figs 14.4A and B: (A) Postoperative voiding cystourethrogram (VCUG) at 2 months; (B) VCUG at 72 months (6 years postoperative follow-up)

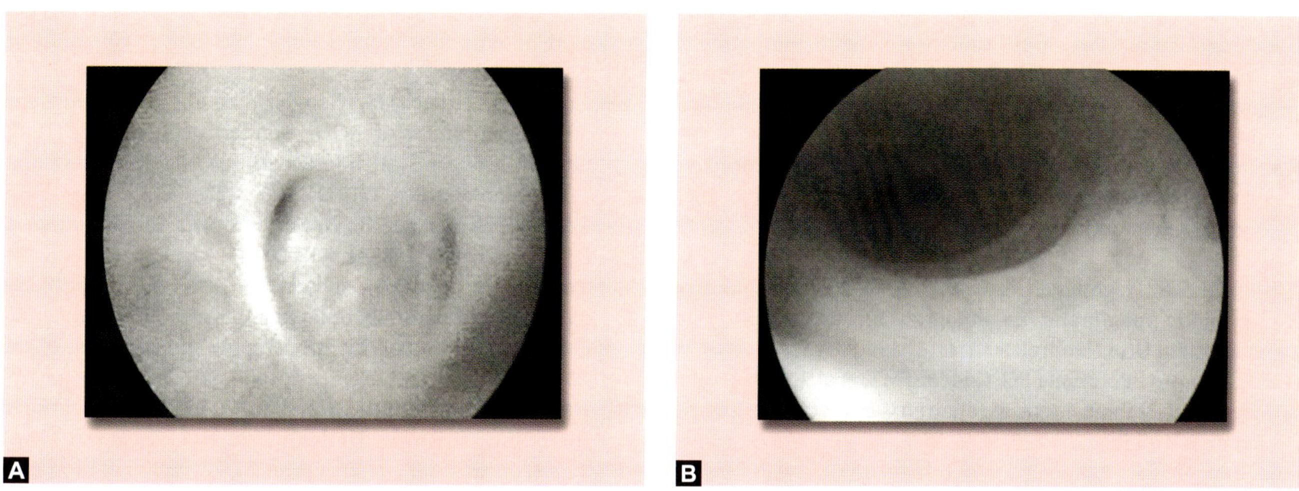

Figs 14.5A and B: (A) Preoperative cystoscopic view showing complete obliterative stricture; (B) Endoscopic view of the area, where tubularized cell seeded synthetic material (tubularized polyglycolic acid mesh seeded with autologous cells) was used to replace the strictured segment of the urethra

on voiding cystourethrogram **(Figs 14.4A and B)**, uroflowmetry and cystoscopic view **(Figs 14.5A and B)**. One patient experienced a small stricture at the proximal anastomosis site 4 weeks postoperatively, and this was most likely secondary to premature catheter removal. This was successfully treated with transurethral incision of the stricture with no subsequent complications.

REFERENCES

1. Santucci R, Eisenberg L. Urethrotomy has a much lower success rate than previously reported. J Urol. 2010;183(5):1859-62.
2. Terlecki RP, Steele MC, Valadez C, et al. Grafts are unnecessary for proximal bulbar reconstruction. J Urol. 2010;184(6):2395-9.

15

CHAPTER

From the Patients' Perspective

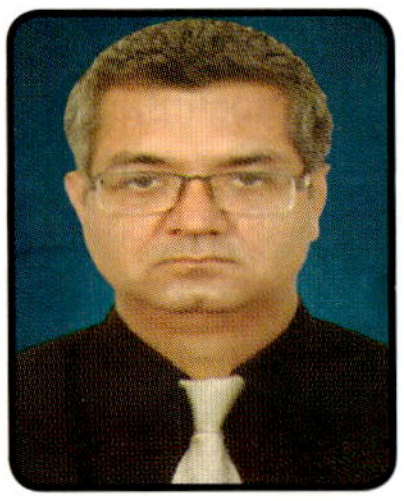

Rajesh Gulia

Rajesh Gulia

Abstract

Lot of books have been written from the angle of surgeons and urologists. But for a patient the big name of various urethroplasty procedures don't matter, not does it impresses him or even matter to him. He only knows that he has a urethral stricture and he wants to get "cured" not just "managed." So we as urethral surgeons should always put ourselves in the patient's shoes and then decide our approach. This chapter also explains the way and importance of patient counseling. It also explains how we as urologists can counsel the patient in a simple layman language. It also tells us what all is going on in the patients' mind, and to what all questions he expects answers. A must read, for not only gaining self-confidence but also soliciting patient confidence.

Keywords

www.stricturecure.com, Preoperative X-rays, Caliber of urethral lumen, Restricture, Native urethra, Narrowing, Endoscopic cut, Complex immunological problem, External genitalia, Loaded rectum.

We may talk of surgeries with big names like "Dorsal Free Graft Urethroplasty by Ventral Sagittal Urethrotomy Approach" or Webster's Augmented Urethroplasty with buccal mucosal graft (BMG), placed dorsal onlay graft (DOG), etc. But for the patient all this does not impress him or even matter to him. He knows he suffers from a urethral stricture and he wants to get cured not just managed.

I will always remember my Guru Prof HS Bhat sir's words. When you have more than one option in managing any medical problem, think as if your own relative is sitting in front of you. Then advice accordingly—you will never go wrong. Still if there is a confusion, imagine what would you like to get done on yourself, God forbid, had you been suffering from the same ailment. There are so many books written from the doctors, surgeons, teachers, perspective. I just thought to exchange roles and think as a patient, and what he expects from us as urethral surgeons regarding his problem of stricture urethra.

PATIENT

"First and foremost, the least I expect is an honest advice, with no false promises. Tell me the exact situation I am in, what are the options and their outcome. Further, if I was your relative sitting here, how would you have tackled my problem? Then is there any platform where I can see the X-rays of patients who have a similar problem as mine and what they have undergone and their outcome. That would be a big help."

DOCTOR

I think you need to visit a site, stricturecure.com. That site has no frills. Login as a patient or as a visitor. See where your type of stricture fits in. See their preoperative X-rays—I am sure you would say—this looks like mine. Then see the outcome of what surgery they have undergone, in the form of postoperative X-rays called retrograde urethrogram (RGU) and/or micturating cystourethrogram (MCU). You will see a remarkable difference in the caliber of the urethral lumen. This site is under construction. There may be lot of pitfalls. But we intend to work on it. All the patient's X-rays, including follow-up ones will be uploaded date wise.

www.stricturecure.com is especially dedicated to the patients of stricture urethra. Once it is fully constructed it will be a unique one with the following attributes:

- Patients will be able to see their own data, X-rays, follow-up investigations, etc. after they log in with a unique ID.
- A person suffering from stricture urethra will be able to identify himself with all such patients who have the same type of stricture as himself and see their surgical outcome (anonymity being maintained).

- Any patient/doctor can post/upload the RGU and MCU images and get expert opinion as to the type of management/surgery required. The experts panel is world famous urethral reconstructive surgeons.

This is my small effort toward Copenhagen, Nopenhagen, Hopenhagen. Our processing is technology driven. We have lowered the use of paper and X-ray films by over 75% thus reducing our carbon footprints.

WHAT AND HOW TO COUNSEL

Restricture

We all know the results of urethroplasty. Let's say a patient has undergone a ventral application of oral BMG for a 40 mm bulbar urethral stricture. Down the line he may develop bladder outlet obstructive symptoms. On investigations like RGU/MCU, he was now found to have strictures at either or both ends of the buccal graft where it is anastomosed to the native urethra. Now we all know this happens and the management is endoscopic cut one or two times. These are mucosal rings that generally settle down with one or two sittings of OIU. But from the patient's angle—he is disturbed and rightly so. Now we must go back and think—did we counsel this patient properly.

This is what I say to all my patients. You have a stricture of the urethra. Urethra is a very delicate organ of average length 20 cm. This is like a collapsible rubber pipe that opens up and gets filled while passing urine, at other times it remains collapsed. The 40 mm of your delicate pipe has gone bad. It has shriveled and no longer has the elasticity to expand. We cannot replace that segment, but we can attach a patch of delicate tissue which matches your urethral tissue to keep that segment open so that your urine passes freely. Though the patch portion of your urethra remains open, the two ends where they are attached to the native urethra, require regular monitoring, servicing and repair as and when any problem arises, as is the case with any machine. Only God can make a flawless machine that requires no regular servicing/repair.

Possible Problems

- There is narrowing at one or the two ends in which the repair is simple. A simple endoscopic cut should suffice.
- Initially we had put a patch on one of the walls of the shriveled portion which was at 12 o'clock, this worked and lasted for say "x" months. Now the other wall also requires a patch and we now require to put a patch at 6 o'clock.

Patient

Could you have not put both the patches last time itself, when I had taken off from work? It would have saved me both time and money.

Doctor

At that time your other wall looked good and did not warrant a patch. And you will see it has worked for these "x" months. You cannot repair anything anticipating it will not work. Now it seems is the time it requires a patch.

For patients suffering from balanitis xerotica obliterans (BXO), or stricture urethra because of lichen sclerosis, they need to be told—you have a very complex immunological problem. This is slowly progressive. And gradually affects all the tissues in and around your external genitalia area. So we will be putting a patch that is not known to be affected by this. Though this patch will remain unaffected, the areas where it joins the native urethra will be the weak points. If the patient comes back with a stricture at the proximal end of the graft, he needs to be told—look! initially you had a 40 mm long stricture. That is taken care of. Now what is left is only 2–3 mm of the problem for which a minimally invasive endoscopic procedure is required.

Sexual Function

Doctor

If you have preserved sexual function prior to your present problem, in all likelihood it will remain unaffected. There may be some temporary hitch but ultimately it all settles down. During the initial 2–3 weeks as long as the catheter is there, you have to avoid any sort of sexual stimuli, lest it puts a stress on the patch we have put and the sutures holding it. This may have a bearing on the result and outcome of our surgery. Even after the catheter has been removed, one is advised sexual abstinence/rest for a further period of 3 weeks.

Other Precautions

Avoid constipation as a loaded rectum predisposes to urinary tract infection. Take adequate catheter care. Fresh air and balanced diet will help in better wound healing. He should be educated about bladder spasms. These are sudden severe shooting pains, arising from the urinary bladder area and radiating along the penis, lasting for a couple of seconds. This may or may not be accompanied by leakage of urine by the sides of the catheter.

Index

Page numbers followed by *f* refer to figure